Major Problems in Obstetrics and Gynecology

A series of monographs designed to explore in depth specific problems in these related disciplines, and to offer reviews of the most complete and up-to-date information available on topics in the study of human reproduction and of the female reproductive system.

Other monographs in this Series:

Already published:

Cohen: *Laparoscopy, Culdoscopy and Gynecography: Technique and Atlas*

Plentl and Friedman: *Lymphatic System of the Female Genitalia*

Burrow: *The Thyroid Gland in Pregnancy*

Janovski and Paramanandhan: *Ovarian Tumors*

Roland: *Response to Contraception*

Burghardt: *Early Histological Diagnosis of Cervical Cancer*

Vollman: *The Menstrual Cycle*

Neuwirth: *Hysteroscopy*

Friedrich: *Vulvar Disease*

To be published:

Goldstein: *Gestational Trophoblastic Disease*

Bieniarz: *Angiography and Placental Localization*

Knapp: *Radical Surgery of Pelvic Cancer*

Brown: *Ultrasonography in Obstetrics and Gynecology*

Charles: *Infections in Obstetrics and Gynecology*

Perlmutter: *Human Sexuality*

Cavanagh, Comas and Rao: *Septic Shock*

Weinberger: *Hypertension in Pregnancy*

COLPOSCOPY

SANTIAGO DEXEUS, JR., M.D., F.I.A.C.

Director of the Department of Obstetrics and Gynecology,
Instituto Dexeus, Barcelona

JOSÉ M. CARRERA, M.D.

Chief of the Obstetric Service,
Instituto Dexeus, Barcelona

FERNAND COUPEZ, M.D.

Chief of the Cyto-Colposcopy Service, Créteil Hospital, and
Associate Professor of the School of Medicine, Paris

Translated by KARL L. AUSTIN, M.D.

VOLUME 10 IN THE SERIES

MAJOR PROBLEMS IN OBSTETRICS AND GYNECOLOGY

EMANUEL A. FRIEDMAN, M.D.
Consulting Editor

1977   W. B. Saunders Company   Philadelphia • London • Toronto

W. B. Saunders Company: West Washington Square
                          Philadelphia, PA 19105

                          1 St. Anne's Road
                          Eastbourne, East Sussex BN21 3UN, England

                          1 Goldthorne Avenue
                          Toronto, Ontario M8Z 5T9, Canada

Title of the original Spanish language edition:
Tratado y Atlas de Colposcopia
© 1973 Salvat Editores, S. A., Barcelona, Spain
Illustration rights held by Salvat Editores, S.A.

Colposcopy   ISBN 0-7216-3050-2

Last digit is the print number: 9   8   7   6   5   4   3   2   1

To Dr. José M.ª Dexeus

Foreword

Since the introduction of colposcopy by Hinselmann in 1925, this valuable technique has been widely accepted for use in evaluating cervical disease primarily in European and Latin American centers. That such an important tool has not heretofore won more popular appeal among English-speaking gynecologists is probably based on the misconception that it is somehow competitive with or duplicative of cytologic methods for screening. This is not the case at all. Colposcopy, as amply shown in this volume, stands between cytology and histology as an intermedium between population screening and definitive tissue diagnosis.

It is complementary to cytologic investigation in providing a most useful office-type procedure for elucidating problems relating to recognizing specific disorders of the cervix among patients preselected by cytologic approaches, determining indications for biopsy, locating sites for and extent of biopsy, and stipulating types of biopsy techniques. It has been shown to be valuable in avoiding overtreatment and excessively traumatic or inherently hazardous diagnostic methods (such as cervical conization) for handling otherwise minor or trivial lesions, while at the same time not overlooking significant ones which might thereby have been left untreated or inadequately managed. This applies especially in pregnancy when even simple punch biopsy may be associated with considerable hemorrhage and with harm, albeit remote, to the gestation. If its introduction does nothing more than minimize use of diagnostic conization operations, it will have demonstrated its worth by diminishing attendant hospital costs and delays in effecting definitive cancer treatment and in reducing the risks which are coassociated, such as those of anesthesia, bleeding, infection, cervical stenosis, and sterility.

Moreover, colposcopy has proved to be an important means for following patients after definitive surgical or radiotherapeutic management of cervical neoplasm as well as patients with benign, but suspicious or potentially serious, lesions of the cervix or the vagina. Included among the latter variety are women with vaginal adenosis which may have resulted from intrauterine exposure to maternally ingested stilbestrol and may, therefore, be at risk of developing clear cell carcinoma of the vagina. The special value of colposcopy in following the course of patients who have had irradiation for cervical cancer is based on the fact that post-radiation cytology is admittedly very limited by virtue of the distorting effect such treatment has on cell morphology.

This is a book written by recognized world authorities in the field with preeminence gained by a vast experience. Here they share with us their expertise derived from 15,000 colposcopies done in Barcelona. The rich heritage of the traditional German concepts with which their operating principles are deeply imbued has been built upon and expanded as a consequence of the extensive Spanish emphasis on and use of colposcopy. It is a real tribute to them that they have been able to show a 98 per cent accuracy in diagnosis of cervical lesions when colposcopy is used in combination with cytology. This is a level of accuracy to which all should strive to reach, and it is apparently feasible to achieve by their combined approach as described herein.

A special feature of this monograph is the profusion of excellent color photographs of specific lesions which leave no doubt as to the detailed characteristics of each lesion under surveillance. These instructive illustrations will serve as a ready, invaluable guide and resource for identifying cervical disorders, helping the practitioner to recognize the several specific variants of lesions he is likely to encounter. In addition they will aid him in correlating the magnified visual colposcopic pattern of a given disorder with both its histopathology and its biologic potential.

Needless to say, colposcopy is not a panacea and should not be expected to yield irrefutable results under all conditions, especially when the lesion sought is not on the exocervix or the lower cervical canal (as with lesions that originate high in the canal or occur in postmenopausal women), or is masked by superimposed acute cervicitis which alters the vascularity and makes the tissue bleed easily. Nevertheless, it does provide an excellent method for evaluating surface epithelial patterns and the network of the subsurface terminal vascular bed, offering a means for identifying the type of epithelium as well as its histologic characteristics. Patterns of surface atypicality can be coupled with definable disturbances of stromal vasculature to effect meaningful diagnoses.

This book ably affords the reader a working knowledge and operational skill in colposcopy which he can apply directly to his practice. Simultaneously, it integrates equally valuable complementary techniques relating to cytology and histology so that they can be optimally and appropriately utilized for diagnosis, management and follow-up. In this latter regard it puts colposcopy in its proper perspective among the important, utilitarian diagnostic tools available to the gynecologist today.

EMANUEL A. FRIEDMAN, M.D., MED.SC.D.

Preface

It was at the Créteil Hospital in Paris, more than ten years ago, that the history of this book began. The organization of postgraduate courses on the methods and results of colposcopy revealed a discrepancy between the concepts that we were developing and the classic approach found in the early literature. Arising out of these courses and the experience accumulated since that time, this book is essentially a distillate of our own thinking about the proper use of colposcopy and the intelligent evaluation of its results.

The first traditional doctrine that we should like to overthrow is the concept that colposcopy has as its only purpose the early detection of cervical carcinoma. In reality it is possible to discover, control, and help to treat a variety of benign cervical lesions as well, and in this way cervical cancer is effectively prevented in many instances.

It is our belief that colposcopic images are valuable only when they are considered within the context of cervical lesions. The early colposcopists and their modern followers describe images as if they could be separated from the lesions themselves, whereas we maintain that the lesions are what definitively characterize the images.

With this principle in mind, it will be clear that we reject the classic descriptions of colposcopic diagnosis, believing them to be incompatible with the fact of continuous dynamic change in the cervical mucosa. Attempts to differentiate a multitude of individual images, and to name each of them, have produced an esoteric kind of colposcopic language which in our opinion has been a major factor in causing gynecologists to abandon the use of this technique. Colposcopy, understood and utilized according to such rigid standards, resulted in a poor yield from a practical viewpoint, and required numerous biopsy procedures that confirmed a diagnosis of malignant disease on relatively few occasions.

Our terminology recalls that used by histologists simply because the lesions that we examine are the same. Colposcopy, like cytology, fills the gap between clinical and histologic examinations, and accordingly we have tried to establish the connection between colposcopic and cytologic findings whenever possible.

In addition to describing in detail each lesion seen by colposcopy, we have found it useful to explain its possible transformation and to review the method of management that is appropriate to each circumstance. The gynecologist interested in understanding colposcopy is more than likely a practitioner with a need to treat and not merely to diagnose. To include brief discussions of therapy, besides making this a practical book, will help to ensure that colposcopy takes its proper place within the diagnostic and therapeutic abilities of each reader.

Finally, the considerable confusion that has developed over the nomenclature of colposcopy has obliged us to include in each chapter a list of synonymous terms, in order to clarify matters for the reader who consults more than one work on the subject.

The statistical material assembled for this book has been compiled from the records of the Cancer Center of the Provincial Maternity Hospital of Barcelona, and we thank the hospital's medical director, Dr. Carceller, for the facilities which we have used in our daily work. The photographs were obtained by the authors in their clinical practices, and the excellent photoengraving work was performed by Tardiu, S.A. Dr. A. Fernandez-Cid has selected the majority of the histologic and cytologic views, and his help has been fundamental in establishing the histologic counterparts of some of the lesions seen at colposcopy.

Miss Carmen Baldrich, our cytotechnologist, has given many hours to the tedious task of data collection and statistical analysis. We also wish to express our most sincere gratitude to Mr. Eduardo Garcia for his personalized and efficient labor on behalf of this book; to Miss Esperanza Pous for help in reviewing the manuscript; and to Salvat Editores, S.A., for their confidence in us.

It would be unjust to finish these remarks without remembering the inspiration provided by Dr. J. Bret, who prompted the first efforts that led to the development of our present ideas about cervical pathology.

SANTIAGO DEXEUS, JR.
JOSÉ M. CARRERA
FERNAND COUPEZ

Contents

Chapter One

HISTORY, INSTRUMENTS, AND EXPLORATORY METHODS

HISTORY

In 1925, Hans Hinselmann, director of the gynecologic clinic of the University of Hamburg, invented an optical device that permitted him to examine the surface of the uterine cervix under great magnification. Prior observations of superficial epithelial atypia by Von Franqué, Shauenstein, Pronai, Rosthorn-Schottländer, and Rubin provided the stimulus that led to Hinselmann's invention, and an equally important part was played by technicians at Leitz and Zeiss, and at Moeller and Kern, in resolving the complex problems in physics that the idea presented.

With the aid of his new exploratory method, named colposcopy, Hinselmann described and systematized a number of cervical lesions that had been previously unknown. The great merit of his achievement is not simply the diagnostic instrument itself but the clearer understanding of cervical pathology that has resulted from its use. Performance of repeat biopsies and the correlation of histologic slides with colposcopic views permitted Hinselmann to develop a concept of the origin of cervical carcinoma that is still fundamental in the early diagnosis of this disorder (along with Papanicolaou's cytologic examination). It must be admitted that Hinselmann's preoccupation with this particular application of colposcopy led him to ignore its potential benefit in the study of many other lesions of the cervical mucosa as well.

Colposcopy was soon being widely practiced in Germany, where extensive series of examinations were reported and tabulated by Mestwerdt (1939), Haupt (1941), Treite (1942), Ganse (1949), and Limburg (1952). This occurred in spite of the fact that Schiller introduced his Lugol's staining test in 1927, which at first competed with colposcopy and retarded its early adoption. Through the work of Anderes (1936) and Wespi (1938), colposcopy was popularized in Switzerland, where such well-known practitioners as Glatthaar and de Watteville also described their experience in later years.

The procedure was introduced into Italy by Cattaneo's translation of Hinselmann's *Introduction to Colposcopy* in 1940, and into Austria by Antoine (1949), who tried to improve upon the technique by devising colpomicroscopy. Palmer made the virtues of colposcopy well known in France in 1950, and its position was strengthened when Funck-Brentano and de Watteville accorded it a preeminent position in their discussion of early diagnosis of cervical cancer in 1952. Since that time, important treatises have been written by Bret and Coupez (1960) in France and by Masciotta (1954) and Mossetti and Russo (1962) in Italy, and there have been notable atlases produced in Germany by Mestwerdt (1953), Ganse (1953), and Cramer (1956). Although significant papers appeared in England, notably the discussion by Youssef (1957), use of the method is still not widespread in that country. Adoption of colposcopy on a general basis in Australia was aided by the reports of Coppleson (1959), Browne (1960), Garret (1961), and Cope (1961).

Colposcopy was described relatively early in Spain—by Martínez de la Riva in 1944, Alba in 1947, and Varela in 1957—but its widespread use did not begin until the 1960's, following the reports of González-Merlo, Rodríguez-Soriano, and Mateu-Aragonés and Dexeus. All in all, the technique actually attained popularity more quickly in Latin America, where particularly important papers included those of Jurgens (1933), Jakob (1939), Goulart de Andrade (1940), Cruz (1941), Rieper (1941), Gori and Bayona (1943), and Rocha (1946).

In the United States, however, colposcopy encountered firm resistance, at least in part because it was considered to be a technique that competed with cytology. Scheffey (1955) was one of the first American authors to present his experience with the method; others were Lang and Rakoff (1956), Schmitt (1957), Trace (1959), Olson and Nichols (1960), Graham (1963), and Dampeer (1962). Coppleson and Reid suggested that, in addition to the great popularity of cytology and the lack of enthusiasm with which colposcopy was received by leading gynecologists, to explain the limited use of colposcopy in the United States one must point to the small number of publications in English and the restricted anatomic and pathologic training of the American gynecologist, to whom the complex nomenclature of the traditional colposcopists has been difficult to assimilate.

A common error among the pioneers of colposcopy, who described their methods in the years prior to World War II, lay in their wish to establish a histologic kind of nomenclature for colposcopic images. From Hinselmann on down, numerous and lengthy classifications of atypical epithelium have been created, but they seem to have resulted only in considerable terminologic confusion. Just as illustrative examples, we may cite Hinselmann's own scheme of simple and complex epithelial atypia, each of which was divided into two subgroups and a multitude of smaller divisions; Glatthaar's four-part classification into abnormal epithelium, active epithelium, atypical epithelium, and superficial carcinoma; Wespi's division of cervical appearances into simple epithelial atypia, active epithelium, complex noncancerous atypical epithelium, and aggravated cancerous atypical epithelium; and finally Mestwerdt's attempt at simplification that resulted in a classification of abnormal epithelium, hyperactive epithelium, atypical epithelium, and microcancer.

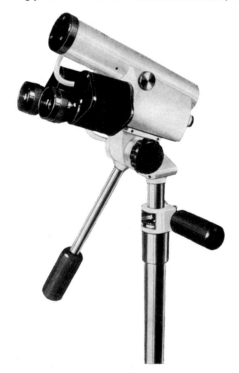

Figure 1. Leisegang colposcope, model I, with a magnification of 13.5 and a working distance of 24 cm. It is provided with a green filter and a mechanism for rapid focusing. The lighting is continuously adjustable over its entire range.

INSTRUMENTS

Colposcope

The colposcope is essentially a magnifying glass with a powerful light

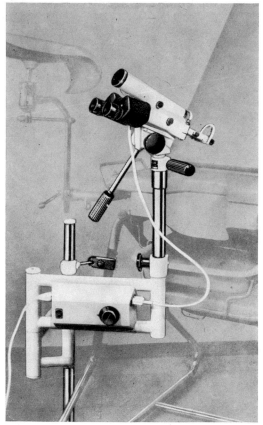

Figure 2. Leisegang colposcope, model Ia, similar to model I but with an articulated stand adaptable to any examination table.

trian (Reichert), one Swiss (Kern), and one French (B.B.T.), each maker offering several types. Leisegang, of Berlin, builds a range of colposcopes from the simple and economical Type IV, with a magnification of ×10, to the Type U IIIb, which incorporates stereophotographic equipment, magnification of up to ×50, and an intensive 50-watt light source. Entirely adequate for general practice are the Types I, Ia, and IIIb (Figs. 1 to 3), the last being the one we normally use. Two useful models from the Carl Zeiss firm are designated Types 1 and 6 (Figs. 4 and 5). The latter has an electric motor, operated by a foot pedal, that permits continuous variation of the magnification up to ×40 as well as focusing.

Auxiliary Instruments

In addition to the equipment required for cytologic sampling or biopsy, the colposcopic examination involves a set of atraumatic specula, dress-

source. Its fundamental parts are (1) an optical system that offers magnifications between 10 and 16 times; (2) an axial or parallax illumination system that can be brightened or dimmed at will; and (3) a mounting device that permits easy movement of the apparatus so that an adequate region of cervical mucosa can be examined. The focal length of the colposcope is 20 to 25 cm., and the width of the visual field should not be less than about 25 mm. For easier observation of the vascular system, the apparatus usually incorporates a green filter. A camera should be easy to attach, and with the help of an electronic flash, excellent pictures are not difficult to obtain. "Colpocinematography" would certainly be possible, but would not be helpful.

There are colposcopes available from four German manufacturers (Zeiss, Leitz, Moeller, and Leisegang), one Aus-

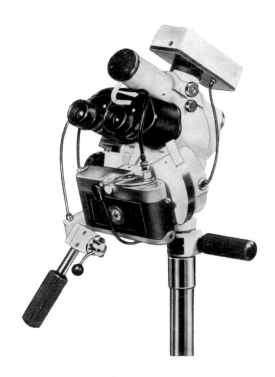

Figure 3. Leisegang colposcope, model IIIb. This type incorporates a device for stereophotography with a synchronized electronic flash, operating at a constant shutter speed of 1/800 second. The normal ×13.5 magnification can be increased to ×50 with the use of an auxiliary device.

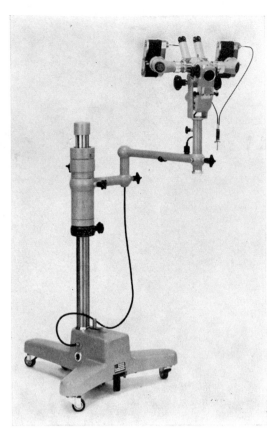

Figure 4. Zeiss type 1 colposcope, with a system for stereophotography and five different magnifications (×6, 10, 16, 25, and 40). The working distance can be adjusted between 50 mm. and 1 meter.

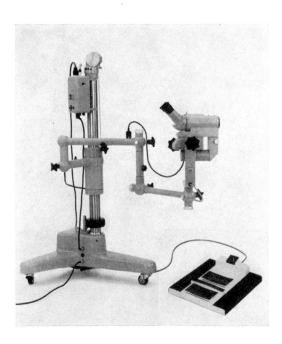

ing forceps with attached cotton swabs, Lugol's solution, 3 per cent acetic acid solution, and 1 per cent silver nitrate solution (Figs. 6 and 7).

METHODS

When colposcopy is performed without previous preparation of the cervical mucosa (so-called "direct colposcopy"), the presence of cervical mucus presents considerable difficulties. Hinselmann himself devised what he called "amplified colposcopy," in which a series of chemical reagents are used to dissolve the mucus for better visualization.

The speculum should be placed without previous vaginal exploration and should lie half open in the vagina. It should not be completely opened until the cervix has been visualized in order not to damage the unseen cervix. If the vagina is wide, a complementary lateral retractor may be necessary, and we have used Bret's retractor for this purpose. The speculum that is employed should have a dull-coated inner surface to prevent reflections of the colposcope light that will interfere with the examination.

The first procedure should be a naked eye examination of the cervix to evaluate its shape and size, the existence of any lacerations, and the presence of erythroplasia. At this time too, a cytologic specimen may be obtained, with care taken to avoid bleeding. We have not found it routinely necessary to take triple samples (vagina, ectocervix, and endocervix). It may also be useful to obtain a sample of the vaginal discharge to look for trichomonas, monilia, hemophilus, or other organisms, especially if the characteristics of the discharge are those that suggest an infection.

Direct colposcopic examination can then be done only after one has cleaned the mucus that usually coats the surface of the cervix. Diagnosis of a lesion by col-

Figure 5. Zeiss type 6 colposcope, similar to type 1 but equipped with electric motors for varying magnification and for focusing.

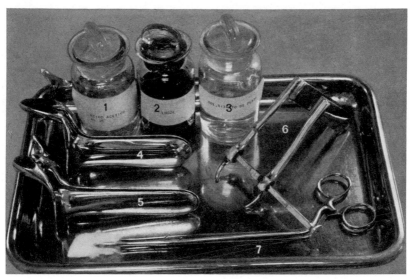

Figure 6. Instrument tray for colposcopy. Contents include (1) acetic acid solution, (2) Lugol's iodine solution, (3) silver nitrate solution, (4) and (5) specula of different sizes, (6) lateral vaginal retractor, and (7) forceps with cotton swabs.

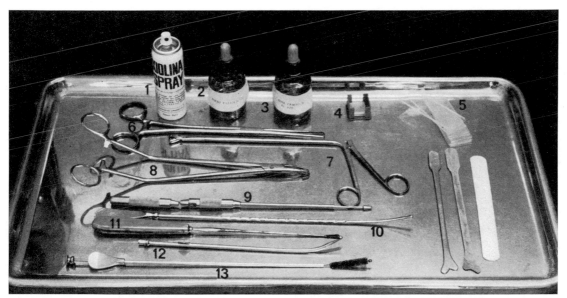

Figure 7. Additional instruments and materials for complementary examinations. (1) Cytologic fixative spray; (2) physiologic saline; (3) 10 per cent potassium hydroxide; (4) slide covers; (5) glass slides; (6) single-toothed cervical tenaculum (Fozzi); (7) and (8) punch biopsy forceps; (9) Gusberg forceps for endocervical biopsy; (10) uterine sound; (11) uterine biopsy curette; (12) tubular curette for endometrial biopsy; (13) endometrial cytology sampling brush. At the right are shown different types of spatulas, wood and metal, for cervical scraping and sampling of vaginal discharge.

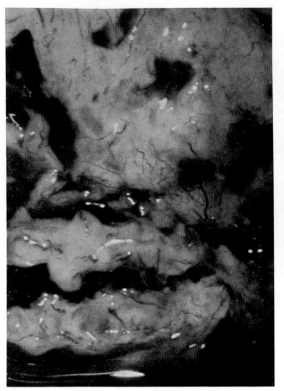 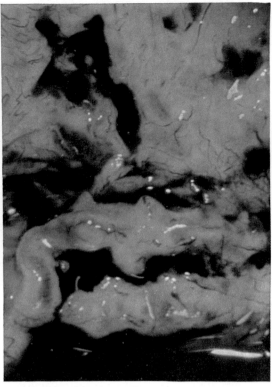

Figure 8. Use of a green filter. *A,* Colposcopic image without the filter, after application of mucolytic acetic acid. The image is clear, but the blood vessels are poorly seen. *B,* Better identification of the vasculature with the green filter interposed. Some of these vessels are frankly pathologic.

poscopy at this time can be taken as meaningful (Fig. 8).

Flooding the cervix with an aqueous solution of 3 per cent acetic acid is followed in 15 to 20 seconds by disappearance of the cervical mucus and a corresponding improvement in the clarity of the colposcopic image to the point where many lesions are revealed by this reagent (Figs. 9 and 10). Differences in cellular density, thickness and keratinization of the mucosa, breaks in the epithelium, and even the columnar papillae may be clearly seen after acetic acid has been applied. However, the vascular bed becomes less evident, perhaps due to arteriolar spasm (Ganse).

Various techniques have been proposed to obtain better visualization of the cervical blood vessels. Hinselmann recommended a fluorescent lamp, but this has had little or no acceptance. Kruger used ethyl chloride to differentiate typical vessels (which contract upon applica-

tion of that chemical) from the atypical ones of carcinoma (which do not). Majewski painted the cervix with a 1:1000 solution of epinephrine or norepinephrine and claimed that in 30 seconds the vascular network, especially the capillaries, became more evident. Mauler favored this method as well. We work with a colposcope that is equipped with a fluorescent lamp, and we have used both of the other techniques just mentioned. We believe, with Mateu-Aragonés, that a green filter over the lens provides the best visualization of the vascular bed of the cervix.

Madej has proposed substitution of 5 per cent lactic acid for the acetic acid, but there seems to be no advantage to this, except that it may make it easier to recognize instances of re-epithelialization.

After 2 minutes the effect of the acetic acid disappears, and reapplication becomes necessary. Also, if there is any

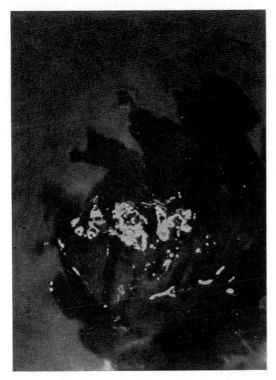

Figure 9. Without the use of acetic acid, the colposcopic picture lacks detail.

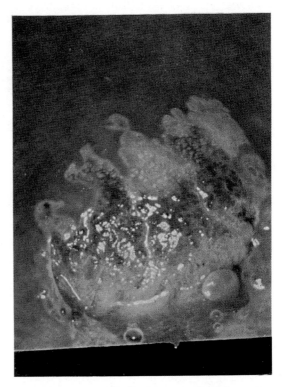

Figure 10. Added clarity and differentiation of the image after application of acetic acid.

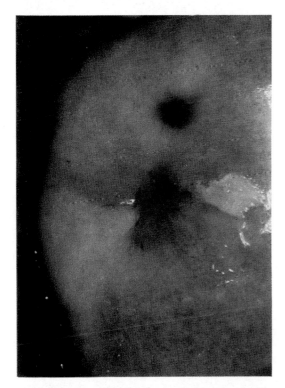

Figure 11. The borders of this dysplastic lesion are not sharp and clear, even after acetic acid solution has been applied.

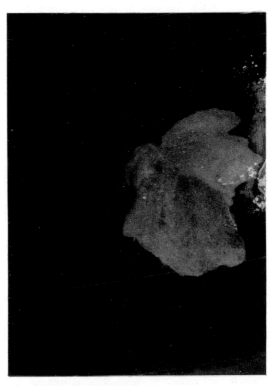

Figure 12. The usefulness of Schiller's test (application of Lugol's iodine solution) in delineating the borders of a cervical lesion is evident in this view.

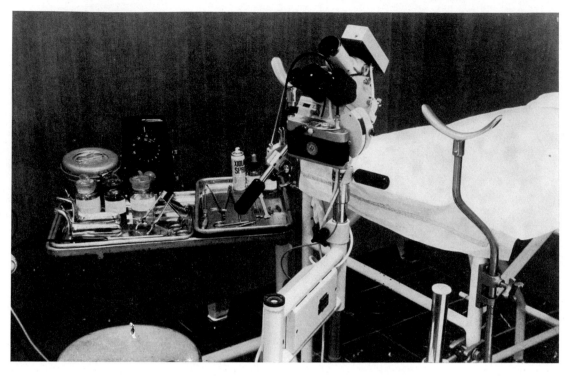

Figure 13. Placement of the colposcope and instrument trays for maximal efficiency in performing colposcopic examinations.

doubt regarding the integrity of the epithelium, application of a 1 per cent silver nitrate solution is useful at this time. This reagent will produce a whitish color in the denuded subdermis, offering clear visualization of the edges of the epithelium and permitting differentiation between an erosion and a red congested zone. An aqueous solution of metacresylsulfonmethane acid (50 per cent Negatol) may be used for the same purpose. We do not use this product as a colposcopic reagent or for hemostasis unless hemorrhage should follow biopsies. Neither agent should be used before the cervix has been examined, because their application will be followed by coagulation or scarification of the epithelium.

Lo Wan-Hua has proposed an in vivo staining method to be applied after the acetic acid solution. It consists of hematoxylin solution for 1 to 2 minutes and then 0.5 per cent hydrochloric acid for 1 minute. A positive test, implying malignancy, consists of a deep blue stain of any part of the cervix. A light blue color is read as negative. Lo Wan-Hua claims a 94 per cent accuracy in early diagnosis of cervical cancer.

Schiller's test (use of Lugol's solution) is not essential if the examiner has obtained what he believes to be sufficient information from the procedures outlined so far. However, it is a useful adjunct in the differentiation of some atypical images which look alike superficially, such as ground structure found with vaginitis. Application of Lugol's solution also makes it possible to define the exact limits of a lesion and to study its degree of maturation as well as the extent of regularity of the epithelium (Figs. 11 and 12). In principle it would be useful if every colposcopist used this test, for it does reveal lesions that might not be evident to a less experienced observer. However, Gonzalez-Merlo has emphasized the lack of specificity of Schiller's test, and we agree that an experienced colposcopist will derive little benefit from it.

The fundamental principle of Schiller's test is that only mature tissues, containing stores of glycogen, take up iodine; carcinomatous epithelium is iodine-negative. However, in addition to malignant or atypical epithelium, iodine will also not stain young epithelium (as in a normal re-epithelialization zone), columnar epithelium (ectopy), and involuted epithelium (senile atrophic mucosa), all of which lack glycogen but are normal tissues and not malignant. In spite of its limitations, the use of Lugol's solution has some notable defenders, such as Nyberg and Wyss.

Finally, selective exocervical biopsy is done, using a biopsy forceps that permits the volume of tissue obtained to include both epithelium and the subjacent stroma. The best forceps for this purpose are those of Gaylor, Faure, Schubert, and Tischler, and the articulated types of Karl Storz, Dovay, Luer, and others (Fig. 14).

Colposcopic patterns have traditionally been grouped in two classes, typical and atypical (Table 1). Still used by many practitioners (González-Merlo, Calvo de Mora, and others), this classification attempts the definitive separation of totally benign findings from those which imply the existence of histologic disorders more or less related to cancer. Although we recognize the simplicity and clarity of such a scheme, we should like to propose that it has two important drawbacks.

The first of these is terminologic. It is important and significant to distinguish "images" from "lesions." A colposcopic image, the basis for the examiner's evaluation, is but one element of a lesion or disorder, others being the histologic picture and the result of the cytologic examination. Thus it is impossible to put images and lesions on the same plane. The classic grouping of colposcopic findings confuses the two by including under one "atypical" heading some that are only images (mosaic structure, ground structure, etc.) and others that are true lesions (such as typical re-epithelialization).

The second objection is to the rigid alternatives raised by the usual classification. We have found it difficult or impossible to assign to either category some dystrophic processes such as deciduosis and endometriosis, and also polyps and papillomas. Some authors have included endocervical polyp, for example, among the atypical images (González-Merlo),

Table 1. Traditional Classification of Colposcopic Findings

TYPICAL	ATYPICAL
Original mucosa	Leukoplakia
Ectopy	Ground structure
Typical re-epithelialization	
	Mosaic
Atrophic mucosa	Erosion
Vaginitis	Vascular irregularities
Benign excrescence	Atypical re-epithelialization
	Carcinomatous proliferation

while others group it with the typical appearances and consider it benign (Mateu-Aragonés). Consequently, tabulation of the typical and atypical colposcopic pictures classified by different authors pro-

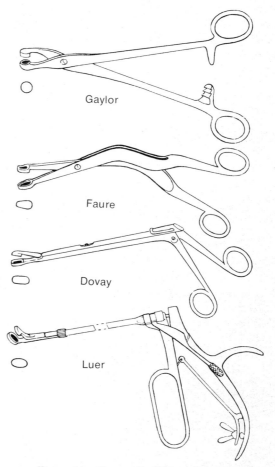

Figure 14. Exocervical biopsy forceps.

Table 2. Frequency of Occurrence of
Typical Colposcopic Images

Figuero et al. (1971)	80.34%
González-Merlo (1966)	81.20%
Guerrero et al. (1957)	82.00%
Zamarriego et al. (1966)	87.40%
Youssef (1957)	87.80%
Mateu-Aragonés (1971)	91.37%
Hernández-Alcántara et al. (1971)	92.10%
Calvo de Mora et al. (1971)	92.80%
Our Series (1971)	83.14%

duces a wide range of results (Tables 2
and 3).

To avoid these difficulties, we have
devised a new classification using four
groupings: inflammatory pathology, mechanical and restorative pathology, abnormal reparative processes, and destructive processes. Mestwerdt has proposed a
division into physiologic, inflammatory,
and malignant states. For purposes of
prognosis, we have also used a classification of benign, doubtful, and malignant.
At present, we distinguish five groups of
lesions: inflammation, dystrophy, ectopy
and its normal repair, dysplasia, and neoplasia. We continue to use the classic
"typical" and "atypical" classification for
statistical purposes, for comparison with
other series; the first three of our pathologic groups belong within the "typical"
class, and the last two are "atypical."

At the first World Congress of Colposcopy and Cervical and Uterine Pathology
at Mar del Plata (November, 1972) it was
proposed that colposcopic findings be
classified in three groups: (a) normal or

Table 3. Incidence of Atypical
Colposcopic Images

Calvo de Mora (1971)	6.67%
Hernández-Alcántara et al. (1971)	7.8%
Mateu-Aragonés (1971)	7.96%
Guerrero et al. (1957)	8.0%
Mestwerdt (1958)	8.0%
Figuero et al. (1971)	8.1%
Stafl et al. (1967)	8.3%
Rodríguez Soriano (1958)	9.2%
Dietel and Focken (1955)	10.0%
Kern (1964)	10.56%
Cramer (1958)	11.2%
Zamarriego et al. (1969)	12.13%
Gil Vernet et al. (1969)	16.41%
González-Merlo (1966)	19.02%
Limburg (1958)	20.0%
Mossetti and Russo (1962)	31.0%
Our Series (1971)	15.61%

typical appearances (original mucosa,
ectopy, zone of re-epithelialization, and
atrophic mucosa), (b) pathologic images
not related to malignancy (vaginitis, polyps, endometriosis, condyloma, sequelae
of coagulation, etc.), and (c) pathologic
images compatible with malignancy (leukoplakia, ground structure, mosaic, erosion, zone of atypical transformation,
atypical vascularization, uncharacteristic
iodine-negative zone, carcinoma).

This provisional international classification suffers, in our judgment, from
several drawbacks: It classifies images
and lesions conjointly; it introduces the
expression "uncharacteristic iodine-
negative zone," which to us seems rather
unfortunate; and it neglects some colposcopic appearances peculiar to gestation.
Notwithstanding, it seems to us useful
as a point of departure leading to future
terminologic unification. Therefore we
have begun the statistical registration of
our observations in the three proposed
groups, but are making some slight variations in the terminology of the subgroups.

A. *Normal or typical appearances*

1. Original mucosa
2. Ectopy
3. Zone of atypical re-epithelialization
4. Atrophic mucosa

B. *Pathologic appearances not directly
related to malignancy*

1. Vaginitis and other inflammatory
   appearances
2. Polyps and papillomas
3. Endometriosis, deciduosis, coagulation sequelae (dystrophy)
4. Other dystrophies

C. *Pathologic appearances compatible
with malignancy*

1. Zone of atypical re-epithelialization
2. Zone of atypical transformation
3. Uncharacteristic leukokeratotic or
   vascular images
4. Carcinomatous exophytic or endophytic growth

Recording of the observations is
commonly done by means of symbols

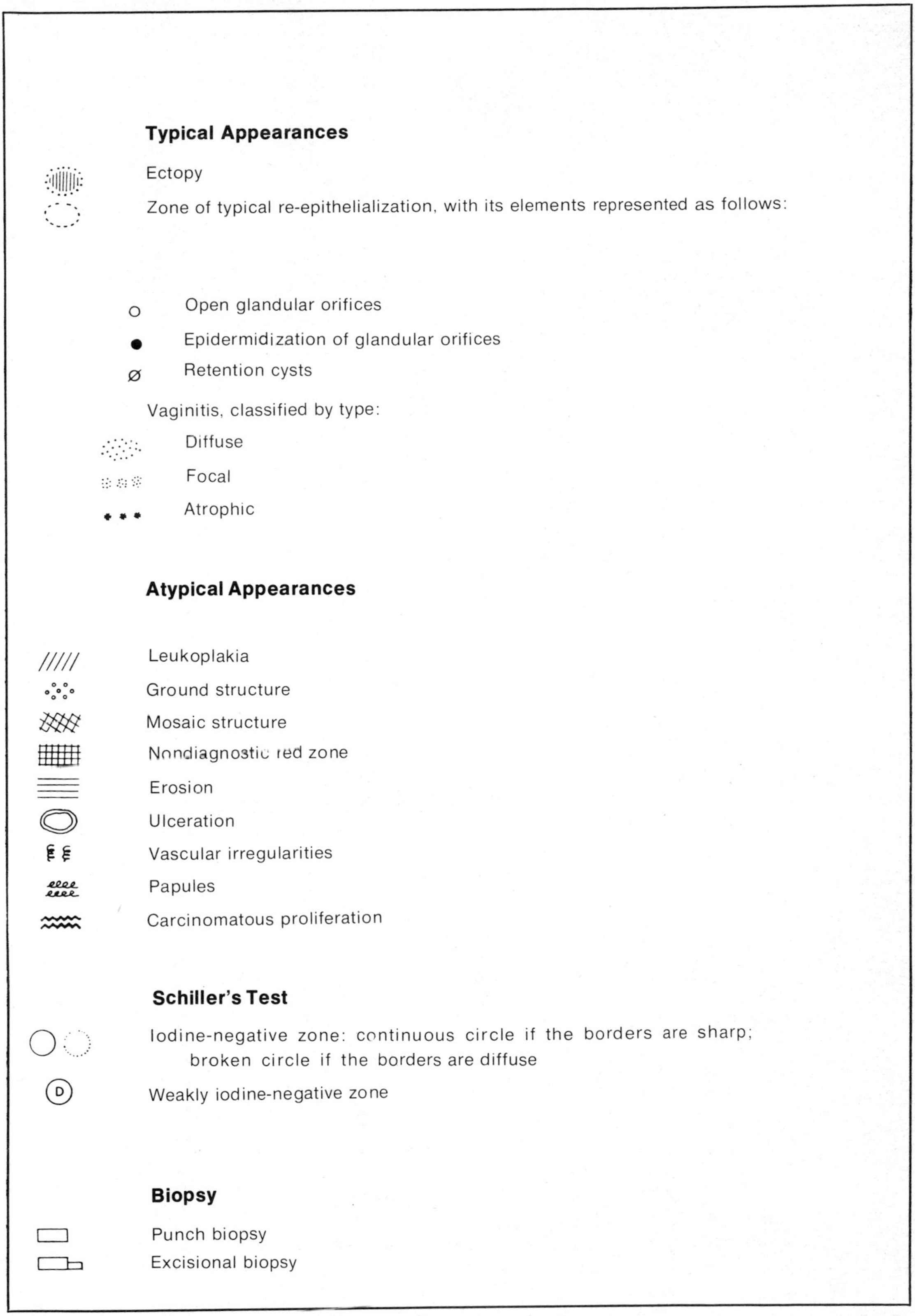

Typical Appearances

Ectopy

Zone of typical re-epithelialization, with its elements represented as follows:

o   Open glandular orifices

●   Epidermidization of glandular orifices

ø   Retention cysts

Vaginitis, classified by type:

Diffuse

Focal

Atrophic

Atypical Appearances

Leukoplakia

Ground structure

Mosaic structure

Nondiagnostic red zone

Erosion

Ulceration

Vascular irregularities

Papules

Carcinomatous proliferation

Schiller's Test

Iodine-negative zone: continuous circle if the borders are sharp; broken circle if the borders are diffuse

Weakly iodine-negative zone

Biopsy

Punch biopsy

Excisional biopsy

Figure 15.   Symbols of colposcopic findings as devised by the Zurich group and modified by us.

Table 4. Abbreviations Used in Colposcopy

Typical Appearances	Atypical Appearances

Original mucosa: O.M.
   papillary elevation: p.e.
Ectopy: E.
Vaginitis: V.
   red punctate vaginitis: r.p.v.
   white punctate vaginitis: w.p.v.
   focal vaginitis: f.v.
Atrophic mucosa: A.M.
   petechial vaginitis: p.v.
Typical re-epithelialization zone: T.R.Z.
   regular re-epithelialization: T.R.Z.r
   irregular re-epithelialization: T.R.Z.i.
   wax drops: w.d.
   white rings: w.r.
   glandular cysts: g.c.
	Leukoplakia: L.
	Ground structure: G.
	Mosaic: M.
	True erosion: T.E.
	Ulceration: U.
	Vascular irregularities: V.I.
	Atypical re-epithelialization zone: A.R.Z.
	Stable atypical scar: S.A.S.
	Atypical transformation zone: A.T.Z.
	Carcinomatous proliferation: Ca.

devised some years ago by the Zurich group and partially modified by Palmer (Fig. 15), although a set of simple abbreviations would be just as useful when the examiner and the gynecologist in charge of the patient are not the same person. Hammond has proposed the use of a radial diagram to note the exact location of the lesion.

The final report of the colposcopist should include both a description of the colposcopic image, using the symbols of Figure 15 or an understandable set of initials, and a provisional diagnosis taking into account the peculiarities of the cervix being examined. Recommendations as to follow-up and treatment of symptoms should be added as well (Fig. 16).

REFERENCES

Ahumada, J. C.: Carcinoma in situ del cuello uterino: Cancer en la patología femenina. Bibl. Canc. Arg. Colec., *1*:15, 1960.

Alba Menendez, C.: ¿ Cual es el valor de la colposcopia? An. Casa de Salud Valdecilla, *10*:133, 1947.

Anderes, E., and Wespi, H. J.: Der heutige Stand der Früherfassung des Portiokarzinoms mittels der Kolposkopie. Geburtsh. u. Frauenheilk., *3*:248, 1941.

Antoine, T., and Grünberger, V.: Die Auflichtmikroskopie in der Gynäkologie. Klin. Med., *4*:575, 1949.

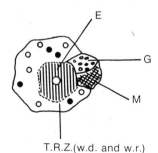

Schematic description of observations

E

G

M

T.R.Z.(w.d. and w.r.)

Diagnosis

    Coarse-grained median ectopy in the course of typical re-epithelialization (irregular) and atypical re-epithelialization (ground structure and mosaic over slight leukoplakia).

Recommendations

    Follow-up colposcopy and cytologic examination are advisable within three months. During the interval it would be well to improve tissue nutrition.

Figure 16. Colposcopy report, including description, diagnosis, and recommendations.

Antoine, T., and Grünberger, V.: Atlas der Kolpomikroskopie. Stuttgart, Georg Thieme Verlag, 1956.

Bolten, K. A., and Jacques, W. E.: Introduction to Colposcopy. New York, Grune and Stratton, 1960.

Brandl, K., and Kofler, E.: Die Krebsfrüherkennungsmethoden bei 230 Fällen mit Kollumkarzinom. Geburtsh. u. Frauenheilk., 19:415, 1959.

Bret, J.: Colpophotographie et stéréocolpophotographie. Rev. Franç. Gynéc. Obstét., 59:275, 1964.

Bret, J., and Coupez, F.: Colposcopie. Paris, Masson et Cie., 1960.

Bret, J., and Coupez, F.: Colposcopy of cervicitis and endocervicitis. Acta Cytol., 5:40, 1961.

Browne, J. C., and Wachtel, E.: Frühdiagnose und Behandlung des Cervixcarcinoms. Med. Press, 243:581, 1960.

Chalfant, R. L.: Use of the colposcope in gynecological practice. South. Med. J., 55:449, 1962.

Cope, I.: The place of colposcopy in cancer detection. Med. J. Australia, 2:164, 1961.

Coppleson, M.: The use of colposcopy in the early detection of carcinoma of the cervix. Med. J. Australia, 2:65, 1959.

Coppleson, M.: The value of colposcopy in the detection of preclinical carcinoma of the cervix. J. Obstet. Gynaec. Brit. Comm., 67:11, 1960.

Coppleson, M., and Reid, B. L.: Preclinical Carcinoma of the Cervix Uteri: Its Origin, Nature and Management. Oxford, Pergamon Press, 1967.

Cramer, H.: Die Kolposkopie in der Praxis. Stuttgart, Georg Thieme Verlag, 1956.

Cruz, H.: La colposcopía en el diagnóstico precoz del cáncer del cuello del útero. Bol. Soc. Chil. Obstet. Ginec., 6:237, 1941.

Dampeer, T. K., Jr.: Colposcopy. South. Med. J., 55:445, 1962.

de Andrade, C. G.: A colposcopia no diagnóstico do câncer do colo uterino. Thesis, A. Noite, Rio de Janeiro, 1940.

de Watteville, H., and Danon, L.: L'influence des hormones génitales sur la biologie du vagin. Gynéc. Obstét., 47:437, 1948.

de Watteville, H.: Cellules cancéreuses dans les sécrétions vaginales: Démonstration du test de Papanicolaou. Schweiz. Med. Wschr., 79:553, 1949.

Dexeus, S., Jr., Fontane, F. G., and Carrera, J. M.: Resultados obtenidos en nuestras 500 primeras colposcopias. Progr. Obstet. Ginec., 7:486, 1965.

di Paola, G., and Vasquez Ferro, E.: Comentario sobre 2000 colposcopias. Bol. Soc. Obstet. Ginec. Buenos Aires, 37:140, 1958.

Dietel, H., and Focken, A.: Das Schicksal des atypischen Epithels an der Portio. Geburtsh. u. Frauenheilk., 15:593, 1955.

Fegerl, H. E.: Use of colpophotogram. Am. J. Obstet. Gynec., 89:827, 1964.

Foote, F. W., and Li, K.: Smear diagnosis of in situ carcinoma of the cervix. Am. J. Obstet. Gynec., 56:335, 1948.

Funck-Brentano, P.: Le problème actuel de l'épithélioma intra-épithélial du col utérin. Gynéc. Obstét., 59:5, 1960.

Funck-Brentano, P., Moricard, R., Palmer, R., and de Brux, J.: L'épithélioma pavimenteux intra-épithélial du col utérin. Bull. Féd. Soc. Gynéc. Obstét., 4(Suppl. 1): 80, 1952.

Ganse, R.: Kolpofotogramme zur Einfuhrung in die Kolposkopie. Vol. I and II. Berlin, Akademie Verlag, 1953.

Ganse, R.: Einfuhrung in die Kolposkopie. Jena, Gustav Fischer, 1963.

Garret, W. J.: The efficiency of present cancer detection methods. Med. J. Australia, 2:166, 1961.

Glatthaar, E.: Kolposkopie. In Seitz-Amreich: Biologie und Pathologie des Weibes. Vienna, Urban und Schwarzenberg, 1955.

Gonzalez-Merlo, J.: Colposcopia de las lesiones benignas del cuello uterino. Toko-Ginec. Práct., 20:220, 1961.

Gori, R. M., and Bayona, E.: Contribución de la colposcopia a la profilaxis del cáncer del cuello uterino. An. Inst. Matern. Asist. Social, 5:151, 1943.

Graham, R. M., Schmitt, A., and Graham, J. B.: Screening for cervical malignancy in a cancer hospital. Am. J. Obstet. Gynec., 84:1013, 1962.

Haupt, W.: Zur Leistungsfähigkeit der Kolposkopie. Zbl. Gynäk., 65:669, 1941.

Hinselmann, H.: Der Nachweis der aktiven Ausgestaltung der Gefässe beim jungen Portiokarzinom als neues differentialdiagnostisches Hilfsmittel. Zbl. Gynäk., 64:1810, 1940.

Hinselmann, H.: Colposcopy. Wuppertal-Elberfeld, Verlag W. Girardet, 1955.

Jakob, A.: La profilaxis del cáncer de cuello: El periódo de latencia. Día Méd., 11:51, 1939.

Janisch, H., Klein, R., and Kremer, H.: Die Früherfassung des Gebärmutterhalskrebses: Ihre Organisation und Problematik. Geburtsh. u. Frauenheilk., 19:63, 1959.

Jürgens, O.: La colposcopia de Hinselmann. Rev. Med. Quir. Pat. Fem., 2:801, 1933.

Kern, G.: Colposcopic findings in carcinoma in situ. Am. J. Obstet. Gynec., 82:1409, 1961.

Kern, G.: Preinvasive Carcinoma of the Cervix. Berlin, Springer-Verlag, 1968.

Kraatz, H.: Farbfiltervorschaltung zur leichteren Erlernung der Kolposkopie. Zbl. Gynäk., 63: 2307, 1939.

Krüger, E. H.: Über die Topographie kolposkopischer Befunde und histologischer Epithelveränderungen an der Portio uteri. Zbl. Gynäk., 79:789, 1957.

Lagrutta, J., Laguens, R. P., and Quijano, F.: Cáncer de Cuello Uterino: Estados Primarios. Buenos Aires, Editorial Intermedica, 1966.

Lang, W. R.: Colposcopy and early diagnosis of carcinoma of cervix. CA: Bull. Cancer Prog., 6: 205, 1956.

Lang, W. R.: Benign cervical erosion in nonpregnant women of childbearing age: A colposcopic study. Am. J. Obstet. Gynec., 74:993, 1957.

Lang, W. R.: Role of colposcopy in cervical atypism and cancer. Proc. Third National Cancer Conference. Philadelphia, J. B. Lippincott Co., 1957.

Lang, W. R.: Colposcopy—neglected method of cervical evaluation. J.A.M.A., 166:893, 1958.

Lang, W. R., and Rakoff, A. E.: Colposcopy and cytology: Comparative values in the diagnosis of cervical atypism and malignancy. Obstet. Gynec., 8:312, 1956.

Limburg, H.: Die Fruhdiagnose des Uteruskarzinoms, Histologie, Kolposkopie, Cytologie, Biochemische Methoden. 3rd ed. Stuttgart, Georg Thieme Verlag, 1956.

Lo Wan-Hua: Rapid and simple in vivo staining method for diagnosis of carcinoma of cervix and its use in combination with colposcopy. Zhonghua Fu-Chainke Zazhi, 11:408, 1965.

Madej, J.: Die Anwendung der Milchsäurelösung

als Kontrastmittel in der erweiterten Kolposkopie. Geburtsh. u. Frauenheilk., *22*:1427, 1962.

Majewski, A.: Die Noradrenalinprobe als neues Hilfsmittel der Kolposkopie. Geburtsh. u. Frauenheilk., *20*:983, 1960.

Martinez de la Riva, A.: La colposcopia en la profilaxis del carcinoma del cervix. Rev. Españ. Obstet. Ginec., *1*:16, 1944.

Masciotta, A.: La Colposcopia nella Lotta Contro Il Cancro e nella Diagnosi Ginecologica. Bologna, Licinio Cappelli, 1954.

Mateu-Aragonés, J. M.: Las imágenes colposcópias atípicas: Su correlación histologica. Acta Gynaec. Obstet. Hisp. Lusit., *10*:69, 1961.

Mateu-Aragonés, J. M.: Importancia del cuadro vascular en la exploración colposcópia; Clasificación de las imágenes vasculares. Acta Gynaec. Obstet. Hisp. Lusit., *13*:231, 1964.

Mateu-Aragonés, J. M.: Metódica exploratoria: La correcta preparación del cuello. Rev. Esp. Obstet. Ginec., *26*:103, 1967.

Mauler, H.: Über den Wert der Noradrenalinprobe als Zusatzuntersuchung der Kolposkopie zur besseren Darstellung atypischer Gefässe. Zbl. Gynäk., *87*:1256, 1965.

Mayer, M., Lieveauz, A., and Camenen, Z.: Colposcopie. Edition Sandoz, 1962.

Menken, F.: Photokolposkopie und Photodouglaskopie. Wuppertal-Elberfeld, Verlag W. Girardet, 1955.

Mestwerdt, G.: Atlas der Kolposkopie. Jena, Gustav Fischer, 1953.

Mossetti, C., and Russo, A.: Definizione dei rapporti fra reperto macroscopico e colposcopico nella patologia della portio uterina ai fini di un razionale indirizzo per la diagnosi precoce del cancro. Attualitá Ostet. Ginec., *4*:1283, 1958.

Mossetti, C., and Russo, A.: La Colposcopia nella Diagnostica Ginecologica. Torino, Ediz. Minerva Medica, 1963.

Navratil, E.: The value of simultaneous use of cytology and colposcopy in the diagnosis of early carcinoma of the cervix of the uterus. *In* Meigs, J. V., and Sturgis, S. H. (eds.): Progress in Gynecology. Vol. III. New York, Grune and Stratton, 1957.

Navratil, E.: Colposcopy. *In* Gray, L. A. (ed.): Dysplasia, Carcinoma In Situ and Micro-invasive Carcinoma of the Cervix Uteri. Springfield, Ill., Charles C Thomas, 1964.

Nyberg, R., Törnberg, B., and Westin, B.: Colposcopy and Schiller's iodine test as an aid in the diagnosis of malignant and premalignant lesions of the squamous epithelium of the cervix uteri. Acta Obstet. Gynec. Scand., *39*:540, 1960.

Olson, A. W., and Nichols, E. E.: Colposcopic examination in a combined approach for early diagnosis and prevention of carcinoma of the cervix. Obstet. Gynec., *15*:372, 1960.

Olson, A. W., and Nichols, E. E.: Leukoplakia of the cervix—the mosaic and papillary pattern. Am. J. Obstet. Gynec., *82*:895, 1961.

Palmer, R.: Sur la colposcopie et les biopsies dans le diagnostic des cancers du col uterin. Acta Gynaec. Obstet. Hisp. Lusit., 8:315, 1959.

Palmer, R., and Wenner-Mangen, H.: Quelques considérations pratiques sur l'interprétation et les résultats de la colposcopie, C. R. Soc. Franç. Gynéc., *24*:23, 1954.

Plasse, G., Martin-Laval, J., and Dajoux, R.: Colposcopie et colpophotographie dans la pratique gynécologique. Bull. Féd. Soc. Gynéc. Obstét., *19*:255, 1967.

Przybora, L. A., and Plutowa, A.: Histological topography of carcinoma in situ of the cervix uteri. Cancer, *12*:263, 1959.

Rieper, J. P.: Câncer incipiente do colo uterino descoberto pelo colposcopio. Anais Brasil. Ginec., *11*:143, 1941.

Rocha, A. H.: A colposcopia no diagnostico precoce do cancer do colo. Obstet. Ginec. Lat. Amer., *4*: 728, 1946.

Rodríguez-Soriano, J. A., and Márquez, M.: La colposcopia como medio de exploración en ginecología. Anal. Med. (Sec. Cirug.), *47*:366, 1961.

Rodríguez-Soriano, J. A., Serradel Terreres, E., and Márquez, M.: La colposcopia en el diagnóstico precoz del cáncer cervical uterino. Toko-Ginec. Práct., *17*:584, 1958.

Rubin, I. C.: The pathological diagnosis of incipient carcinoma of the uterus. Am. J. Obstet. Dis. Wom. Child., *62*:668, 1910.

Ruge, C., and Veit, J.: Der Krebs der Gebärmutter. Stuttgart, Ferdinand Enke, 1881.

Scheffey, L. C., Bolten, K. A., and Lang, W. R.: Colposcopy: Aid in diagnosis of cervical cancer. Obstet. Gynec., 5:294, 1955.

Scheffey, L. C., Lang, W. R., and Tatarian, G.: An experimental program with colposcopy. Am. J. Obstet. Gynec., *70*:876, 1955.

Schiller, W.: Jodpinselung und Abschabung des Portioepithels. Zbl. Gynäk., *53*:1056, 1929.

Schmitt, A.: The value of colposcopy in the diagnosis of cancer of the cervix. Proc. Third National Cancer Conf., Philadelphia, J. B. Lippincott Co., 1957.

Schmitt, A.: Colposcopy detection of atypical and cancerous lesions of the cervix. Obstet. Gynec., *13*:665, 1959.

Señor, J. C.: Valor de la colposcopia en el diagnóstico del cáncer ectocervical. Anal. Med. (Sec. Cirug.), *47*:372, 1961.

Trace, R. J., Brew, B. A., Rollins, J. H., and McCall, M. L.: Preliminary report of colposcopy in gynecology and obstetrics. Surg. Forum, *10*:736, 1959.

Treite, P.: Über kolposkopische Farbenphotographie. Zbl. Gynäk., *65*:22, 1941.

Varela Uña, M.: La colposcopia en el diagnóstico precoz del cáncer del cuello del utero. Toko-Ginec. Práct., *16*:501, 1957.

von Franqué, O.: Die Frühdiagnose der Genitalkrebse der Frauen. Med. Klin., *27*:491, 1931.

von Franqué, O.: Carcinoma uteri und Schwangerschaft. Monatschr. Krebsbekämpf., *2*:129, 1934.

Wespi, H. J.: Erfahrungen mit der systematischen Kolposkopie an der Zürcher Frauenklinik. Zbl. Gynäk., *62*:1762, 1938.

Wespi, H. J.: Kolpophotographie. Gynaec., *131*:65, 1951.

Wyss, H.-J.: Zusammenhang zwischen kolposkopischen und histologischem Befund in der Schillerschen Abschabung. Arch. Gynäk., *194*: 365, 1961.

Youssef, A. F.: Colposcopy: The results of its routine employment in 1,000 gynaecological patients. J. Obstet. Gynaec. Brit. Emp., *64*:801, 1957.

Zimmer, S.: Früherfassung und Früherkennung des Kollumkarzinoms in der Allgemeinärztlichen Praxis. Leipzig, Georg Thieme Verlag, 1962.

Chapter Two

NORMAL CERVIX

DEFINITION

Included in "normal cervix" are two kinds of epithelium: (a) the squamous epithelium of the exocervix, colposcopically identified as *original mucosa;* and (b) the columnar epithelium which coats the inner portion of the cervical canal, known also as *papillary* or *endocervical mucosa.* The extent of visibility of the latter depends upon the degree of cervical opening. The two kinds of epithelia meet at the squamo-columnar junction, at the external os.

When we refer to papillary endocervical mucosa we definitely do not include any columnar epithelium which invades the exocervix. Such a finding is pathologic and is known to colposcopists as ectopy. We reserve the term for the endocervical mucosa located above the anatomic external os of the cervix. In the strictly normal cervix the anatomic external os corresponds exactly with the histologic external os (Figs. 17 and 18).

SYNONYMS

Normal Cervix. Ideal cervix. Standard cervix. Perfectly healthy cervix.
Original Mucosa. First colposcopic image of Hinselmann. Normal original mucosa. Normal mucosa.
Papillary Mucosa. Cervical mucosa. Endocervical mucosa.
Squamo-columnar Junction. Inter-epithelial limit. Transition zone. Squamo-columnar ring.

We retain the classic term "normal cervix" because it has been so very widely used. But there is no doubt that, due to the infrequency with which it is found, it would theoretically be better to speak of the "ideal" or "standard" cervix (Barcellos and Nahoum).

On the contrary, we believe it would be less accurate to use the expression "perfectly healthy cervix" coined by Dohnal and Kotal, because it implies that the cervix with epithelial borders different from the normal one is pathological or diseased, which is not the case.

The mucosa that covers the normal exocervix was first called "original mucosa" by Hinselmann. We believe that this term should be retained without the qualification of "circular" which was attached to it in the earliest texts. The expression "first colposcopic image," used by Hinselmann, has since been employed by others (Ahumada), but it is evident that besides leading to confusion, it lacks any descriptive power.

There are no major objections to the word "normal," but the traditional term does not imply a judgment regarding the frequency of appearance that might be conveyed by the word "normal."

The most graphic expression for the endocervix is "endocervical papillary mucosa," which simultaneously expresses its morphologic appearance and its origin. The expression "cervical mucosa" is clearly imprecise, and "endocervical mucosa" lacks colposcopic significance.

Lastly, there is no objection to the indiscriminate use of several different terms to describe the site where the squamo-columnar epithelia meet. The expression that we prefer is "transitional zone."

15

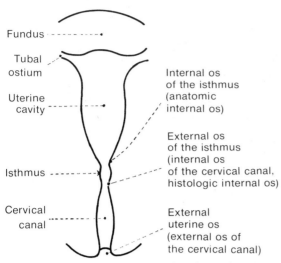

Fundus

Tubal
ostium

Uterine
cavity

Internal os
of the isthmus
(anatomic
internal os)

External os
of the isthmus
(internal os
of the cervical canal,
histologic internal os)

Isthmus

Cervical
canal

External
uterine os
(external os of
the cervical canal)

Figure 17. Topographical relationship between the uterine corpus, isthmus and cervix.

Table 5. Frequency of Occurrence of Original Mucosa in Colposcopy

Berger and Wenner-Mangen (1952)	1.7%
González-Merlo (1966)	4.1%
Arenas et al. (1961)	7.3%
Figuero et al. (1971)	8.3%
Fernández Laso et al. (1960)	10.0%
Youssef (1957)	12.2%
Mateu-Aragonés (1969)	14.8%
Guerrero et al. (1957)	15.0%
Our Series (1972)	11.0%

dard cervix in relation to the hormonal condition of the female, reached the surprising conclusion that instead of being a reflection of endocrine equilibrium, a "standard cervix" indicated hormonal insufficiency. Contrary to what is believed, women who have small areas of ectopy conceive readily because their endocrine regulation is excellent.

FREQUENCY

It is strange that what we describe as "normal cervix" is a rare finding, seen in only 11 per cent of our colposcopic observations. Several authors cite similar figures (Youssef 12.2 per cent, Fernández Laso et al. 10 per cent), but in the literature it is possible to find both extraordinarily low percentages and notably higher ones (see Table 5). In our experience, only in the virgin or the young nullipara is it possible to observe original mucosa exclusively on the exocervix in a large percentage of cases (32 per cent).

Dohnal and Kotal, while investigating the incidence of the normal or stan-

COLPOSCOPIC APPEARANCES

Original Mucosa. The original mucosa has a uniform pink color and its surface is smooth and moist. Without prior preparation, the subepithelial vascularization is barely visible, except in special hormonal circumstances (pregnancy for example), in which it becomes more evident.

As a normal element of the original mucosa, Hinselmann described the so-called superficial papillary elevation. This morphologic detail is present in a

Anatomic external cervical os
↓

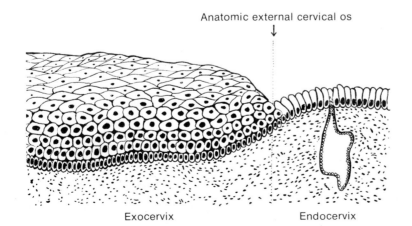

Figure 18. Sketch of a normal cervix. Observe the exact correspondence between the anatomic external os and the histologic external os.

Exocervix   Endocervix

considerable number of patients (14 per cent of our colposcopies) and takes one of two forms: vascular (present in 29 per cent of cases during pregnancy) and avascular (commonly seen in menopause). It has the appearance of a series of whitish points, somewhat larger than those seen with white punctate vaginitis (p. 34) and always situated along the cervical orifice (Fig. 21). Generally, it is not extensive. The classification refers to the presence or absence of a small central capillary. Generally, this form of elevation arises in response to irritation. Superficial papillary elevation corresponds to the histologic findings of circumscribed and nonkeratinized thickenings of the squamous epithelium, limited by minute conjunctival papillae, which extend close to the superficial epithelial layers (Mestwerdt).

After flooding with acetic acid, the usual pink color of the original mucosa pales a bit, even though it remains rigorously homogeneous (Fig. 20). The mucus that generally covers the cervix is dissolved and details are better seen. Hence, after a few minutes it is possible to see the terminal capillaries which cover the exocervix in a manner suggesting a head of delicate hair.

The terminal capillary vessels seen through the colposcope may have either of two appearance aspects (Koller). (1) The forked or hairpin type, in which ascending and descending branches are observed, is not easily seen when the capillary loop is perpendicular to the surface, but it is clearly demonstrable when the capillary is parallel to the surface, as it is in about 20 per cent of cases. (2) The plexus or network type is more common in the cervix of a pregnant woman. The terminal capillaries are distributed irregularly, producing vascular pseudoanastomoses, which give them a reticular or net-like appearance (Fig. 19). This is referred to as "hyperemic original mucosa."

With Schiller's staining, the cervix takes on an intense, homogeneous chestnut color. Coloration is less remarkable at the level of the vaginal vault. At the interepithelial junction, the color disappears because the columnar epithelium does not fix iodine (Fig. 22).

Physiologic Variations. The original mucosa displays some colposcopic variation according to the age of the patient. In the newborn, besides its frequent coexistence with "congenital ectopy," the original mucosa is particularly congested, resembling that of the pregnant subject. Schiller's test reveals great fixation of iodine, probably due to hyperplasia of the intermediate layer at this stage of development.

In the girl before the age of puberty, colposcopy reveals a very thin and hypotrophic original mucosa, which is similar to the atrophic epithelium of advanced menopause. Just as in that case, the vascular net is more apparent than usual. Schiller's test is practically negative.

At puberty the original mucosa recovers its thickness, is filled with glycogen, and acquires an intense pink color. The mucosa is more moist and congested. In some cases, a somewhat superficial and circumoral maceration is observed, caused by the frequent ectopies of hormonal origin that appear at this time in life.

In the process of sexual maturation, and in the absence of obstetric trauma,

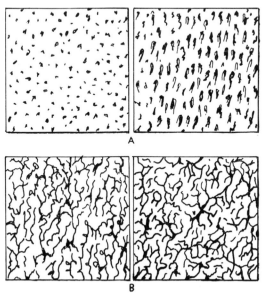

Figure 19. The terminal capillaries of the exocervix, according to Koller. *A,* Forked capillary vessels. *B,* Vessels in the form of a network or plexus. The latter are frequently seen in the congestive or hyperemic original mucosa of pregnancy.

the original mucosa undergoes small variations during the ovarian cycle. Hence, around the time of ovulation it is possible to observe a wider opening of the anatomic external os (Perloff) and an increase in the mucus. This is accompanied by a slight epithelial congestion, which is accentuated during the premenstrual phase when the mucosa takes on a much deeper violet color than usual. Also at this time, the blood vessels become more evident.

During pregnancy, the original mucosa appears more hyperemic, with an increased number of vessels that are more clearly visible and in a plexiform arrangement (Fig. 23). Its surface is less smooth than usual, and it is not rare to see epithelial or stromal deciduosis (see p. 239).

At the menopause, the progressive atrophy of the vaginal cervical mucosa has a clear colposcopic correlation. The original mucosa is much paler, smooth, without elevations, and dull rather than shiny. The subepithelial vascular network is much more visible than usual, and bleeding can be provoked much more readily (see p. 57).

Finally, during senility, the vaginal epithelium reaches an extreme degree of thinness, and as it also is very poor in glycogen, it gives the colposcopic appearance of "senile vaginitis" (p. 59).

Endocervical Papillary Mucosa. In many patients, especially those who have had no children, the endocervical papillary mucosa is only faintly visible, except in those cases where a special colposcopic technique is used to expose the endocervical canal. However, in the majority of multiparas, and even when the epithelial border maintains its relation with the anatomic external os, it is possible to observe a small strip of normal endocervical mucosa, which we call papillary mucosa. Even without prior preparation, this papillary mucosa is promptly recognized because of its irregular surface and its intense brilliant red color, even brighter than the exocervix itself. The mucus layer which usually covers it is responsible for this brilliance and the numerous reflections that usually appear on colpophotography (Fig. 26).

The presence and abundance of mucus that comes from the cervical canal varies according to the time in the cycle and the local hormonal circumstances. Colposcopically, it can be proved that this cervical mucus does not mix in any way with the menstrual blood (Mestwerdt) and that the production of the two substances has a distinct rhythm and intensity (Fig. 24). On the contrary, hemorrhagic lesions of the endocervix give rise to a bloody effusion that does mix with the cervical mucus.

Flooding with acetic acid makes it possible to visualize the papillae proper of the endocervical mucosa (Fig. 27), among which glandular depressions can be detected. The colposcopic characteristics of these grape-like papillae are similar to those of ectopy, which will be described later (p. 85), even though they are smaller and are grouped in folds separated by breaks (evaginations and recesses).

After applying Lugol's solution, the papillary mucosa appears unchanged, being iodine-negative (Fig. 28).

Squamo-columnar Junction. The boundary between the endocervical columnar epithelium and the squamous epithelium of the exocervix follows an undulating line. The possibility of observing this boundary in its entirety depends on the shape of the os, which in turn is influenced by several factors, most notably parturition (Fig. 25).

The os is round and regular in the nullipara, making observation of the endocervix difficult. Visualizing the endocervix is practically impossible if, besides being a nullipara, the patient is premenopausal. In this case the boundary between the two kinds of epithelium is poorly defined.

By contrast, in the multipara the cervical os is not circular but elongated transversely. This affords visibility of the endocervical papillary mucosa and also most of the length of its junction with the original mucosa.

The epithelial border is sharply defined by colposcopy, and the transitional zone described by the histologists is usually not seen (p. 24). It may be visible as a small strip of plain circumoral epithelium, slightly paler than usual, which blends smoothly into the original mu-

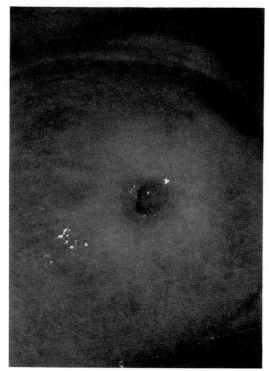

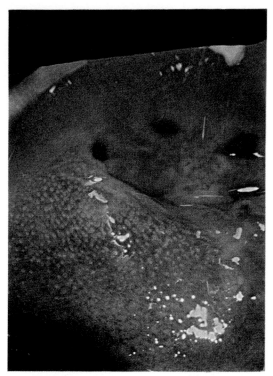

Figure 20. Original mucosa after application of acetic acid. Note the homogeneous pink color, in the undisturbed mucosa. The vascular network is barely visible.

Figure 21. Original mucosa with an apparent circumoral papillary elevation of Hinselmann, of a vascular type.

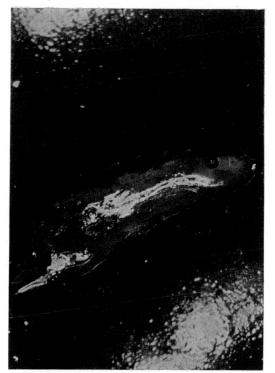

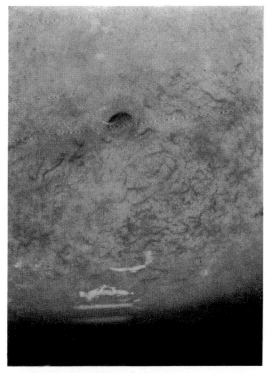

Figure 22. Original mucosa subjected to Schiller's staining (Lugol's solution) takes on a uniform maroon color.

Figure 23. Original mucosa in a pregnant cervix, showing plexiform disposition of the terminal vascularization and many pseudoanastomoses.

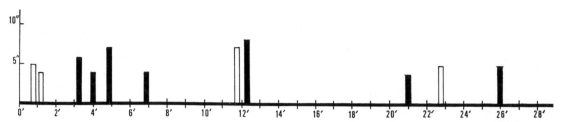

Figure 24. Representation of a 30-minute colposcopic observation of the emission of menstrual flow and cervical mucus, after Mestwerdt. The ejection of the menstrual flow (black columns) does not mix with the cervical mucus (white columns), each being produced at different times.

cosa. More frequently seen in practice is a more or less extensive zone of metaplastic re-epithelialization (Fig. 29).

Even in the absence of true invasion of the exocervix by columnar epithelium (ectopy), the junction between the two types of epithelium may be displaced caudally. This may be caused either by the existence of an eversion of the endocervical mucosa or by cervical lacerations after delivery. In these instances, the original mucosa near the cervical os is more congested than ordinarily, and the transitional zone is not uniform, but rather presents a saw-toothed irregular border.

If there has been displacement of the epithelial junction, the colposcopist may visualize a more extensive area, including not only the squamo-columnar junction throughout its length, but also an important segment of the endocervical canal (Johnson et al.). Opening the speculum may exaggerate this state of affairs, leading the untrained colposcopist to a false diagnosis of ectopy when there is simply an exteriorization of the transitional zone. The opposite phenomenon, upward displacement of the interepithelial border, is less frequent (Fig. 30). However, it is easily observed after circumoral coagulation and in the menopause.

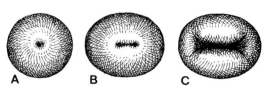

A   B   C

Figure 25. Shapes of the external os. *A,* Virginal; *B,* primiparous; *C,* multiparous.

HISTOLOGIC CORRELATIONS

Original Mucosa. Even though the description of the cervicovaginal mucosa is extremely complex, the most practical way to study it in the adult woman is to divide it into three layers: basal, intermediate and superficial (Fig. 31).

BASAL LAYER. Two zones are differentiated. (1) The deep basal or germinative zone formed by one layer of columnar cells in a palisade, resting perpendicularly upon a basal plate which separates them from the stroma. These cells are relatively small and they have a large nucleus which stains intensely and occupies the major portion of the cell. Mitotic figures may be observed.

(2) The external basal zone or deep horny layer, formed by various layers of oval-shaped cells, joined together by intercellular bridges and oriented in an irregular manner (Fig. 32). The nuclei of these cells are also large and vesicular, but the cytoplasmic volume equals or surpasses the nuclear. The layer takes ordinary tissue stains well (from which arises the term "dark zone," by which it is also known). In this layer it is still possible to observe mitoses which are not seen more superficially under physiologic conditions.

INTERMEDIATE LAYER OR SUPERFICIAL HORNY LAYER. This is formed by numerous rows of flat, fusiform cells, which are also linked together by intercellular bridges. The cytoplasm is clear and very often occupied by vacuoles. The nucleus remains clear and vesicular, but less so than in the underlying layer. There is relatively more cytoplasm than nucleus in the cells of this layer, from which has arisen the name "clear zone."

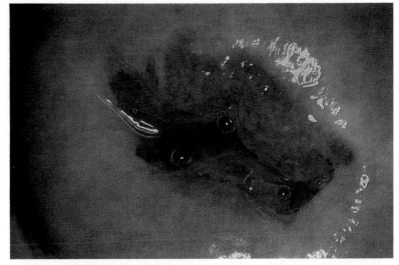

Figure 26. Endocervical papillary mucosa seen without preparation. Its boundary with the squamous epithelium of the exocervix is not clear.

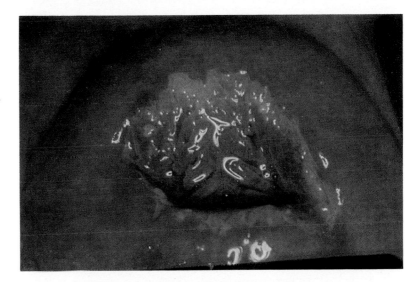

Figure 27. Endocervical mucosa after application of acetic acid. It is clearly distinguished from the exocervical original mucosa by its color and by its irregular papillary surface.

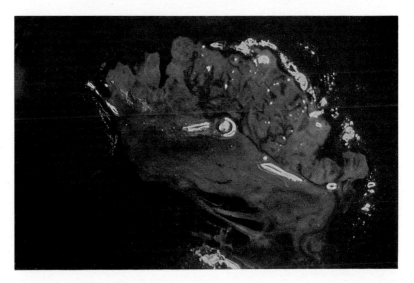

Figure 28. Papillary endocervical mucosa after Schiller's staining. Its total iodine negativity is demonstrated, and it contrasts with the positive reaction of the exocervical mucosa around it.

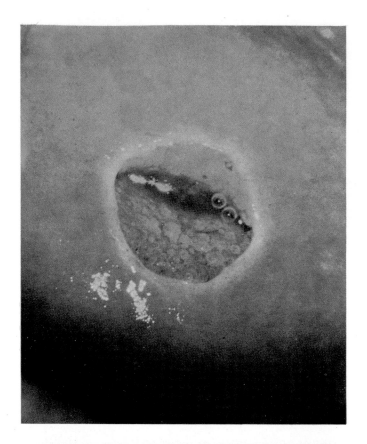

Figure 29. Transition zone with colposcopic distinctness. Around the endocervical papillary mucosa a small band of exocervical original mucosa is seen, albeit much paler than usual.

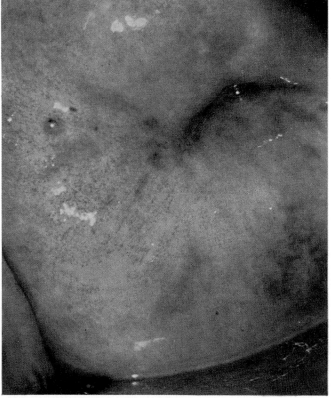

Figure 30. Upward displacement of the transition zone (entopy), as a consequence of the coagulation of an ectopy. The endocervical papillary mucosa cannot be seen.

SUPERFICIAL LAYER. This layer can be distinguished from the intermediate layer because its cells are much flatter and have marked karyopyknosis. Even though it possesses less glycogen, the cytoplasm contains variable quantities of keratin, which is responsible for its acidophilic quality.

Immediately beneath this three-layered epithelium is the so-called basement membrane, which, even though difficult to visualize with the normal staining techniques, may still be made evident by special methods which stain the reticulum and the mucopolysaccharides of the ground substance of the connective tissue.

Papillary Mucosa. The endocervical epithelium which constitutes the architectural base of the papillary mucosa, visible with the colposcope, is formed by a solitary layer of tall columnar cells which covers the surface of the endocervical canal and its glandular formations (Fig. 33). There is no submucosa; hence these cells lie directly above the fibrous stroma of the cervix.

Each cellular element has a height of 20 to 35 microns and a width of 5 to 10 microns. The nucleus is generally found in the lower third of the cell, even though when active secretion occurs (as in ovulation and pregnancy) they ascend significantly. The nucleus has an oval shape, with a characteristic apical concavity.

The cytoplasm is regularly occupied by fine mucous vacuoles which tend to join into one large vacuole. This occupies the supranuclear portion of the cell and is responsible for the apical concavity of the nucleus. It stains intensely with the periodic acid–Schiff stain and takes on a pale color with hematoxylin and eosin.

Some cells are ciliated, but this has no pathological significance.

The papillary mucosa presents some fissures of variable depth and direction, which constitute the openings of the endocervical glands. These creases and fissures are covered by a columnar epithelial lining, identical to the one that covers the free surface of the endocervix. However, it is not unusual to find squamous epithelial elements in the depths of the

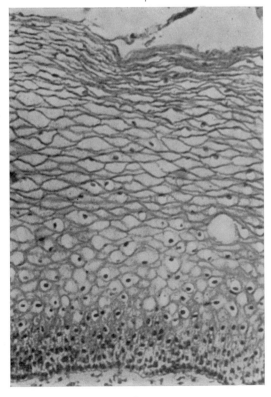

A

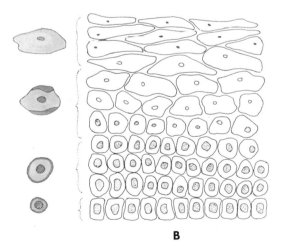

B

Figure 31. Histology of the exocervical original mucosa. *A*, Histologic preparation, in which the three characteristic cellular layers are seen. *B*, Schematic drawing of the histologic structure and of the appearance of each cell type once desquamated. From top to bottom: superficial, intermediate, parabasal, and basal cells.

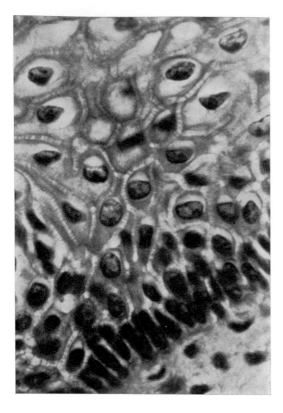

Figure 32. Histologic preparation that shows the entire thickness of the basal layer and part of the superficial stratum spinosum (intermediate layer). Intercellular bridges are seen.

fissures, a condition which has been attributed to metaplastic transformation (Fluhmann).

Generally these depressions are remote from the external cervical os and are rarely found in the visible area of papillary mucosa. In the proximity of the transitional squamo-columnar zone, it is possible to observe small groups of cuboidal cells, with large nuclei and scarce cytoplasm, between the columnar cells and the basement membrane. We refer to them as "reserve cells" (p. 109).

Squamo-columnar Junction. According to studies by Fluhmann which today are accepted without reservation, there are two histologic types of squamo-columnar borders. In almost all girls and young nulliparas, a simple line separates the plain stratified epithelium from the columnar. The junction is abrupt, and histologically it is possible to see that the layer of columnar cells abuts without any break directly against the germinal layer

of the squamous epithelium. This type of border is always apparent due to the distinctly different appearance of the epithelium on both sides (Fig. 34*A*).

In the majority of adult women (73 per cent of pregnant adults, 88 per cent of all gravidas, and 83 per cent of postmenopausal women) the junction between the two types of epithelium is not sudden because of the existence of a transitional zone of variable thickness (Figs. 34*B* and 35). Fluhmann has determined that this represents epithelium in different stages of development (p. 109), and that its width varies between 1 and 10 mm.

This immature metaplastic epithelium which occupies the transitional zone is much flatter, denser and darker than the normal squamous epithelium. It merges in an imperceptible manner with the more or less mature, although still hypotrophic, metaplastic epithelium (of de Brux), which forms the common circumoral "re-epithelialization zone," and which has intermediate histologic characteristics between the transitional zone and that of the original mucosa. The transitional zone actually constitutes the area in which advancement of the re-epithelialization is occurring. Its epithelium has not yet achieved secretory activity and is easily traumatized. This explains why it may not be found in some histologic preparations. Its stroma frequently shows a leukocytic infiltration, which should not be attributed to an ordinary inflammatory process, but rather to the turmoil of this zone, where processes of destruction and regeneration occur concomitantly.

In a given cervix, both types of squamo-columnar junction may coexist.

The strict concordance between the anatomic external os and the squamo-columnar junction, which conceptually is what is considered normal, is an exceptional finding in practice. Schneppenheim et al. say they have never found it.

CYTOLOGIC CORRELATIONS

The cytologic smear, corresponding to the original mucosa observed in an adult woman, consists mostly of super-

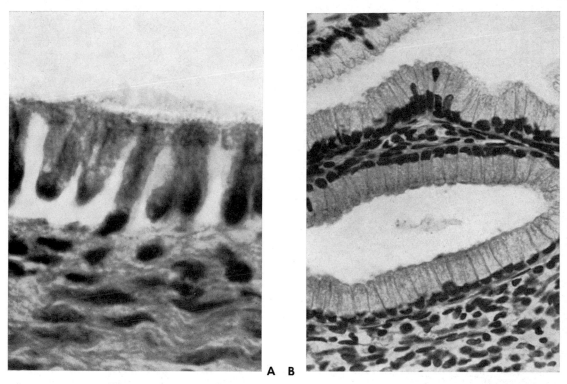

Figure 33. Histology of the endocervical papillary mucosa. *A,* Row of columnar cells in a palisade arrangement covering the endocervical canal. *B,* Glandular formation covered by columnar cells, identical to those that line the surface of the endocervix.

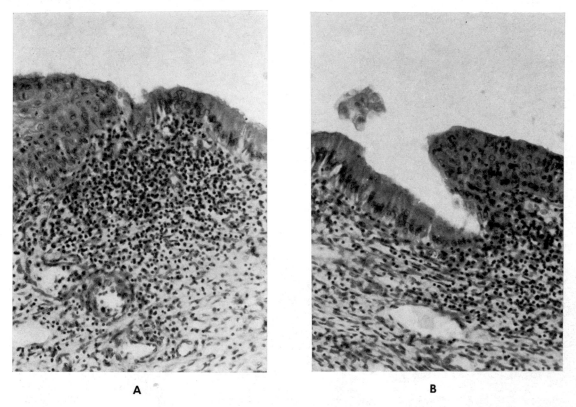

Figure 34. Histology of the squamo-columnar junction. *A,* Linear form: abrupt change from squamous epithelium to endocervical. *B,* The junction is between normal columnar epithelium and immature squamous-type metaplastic epithelium.

ficial eosinophilic or cyanophilic cells, which desquamate either individually or in more or less dense clusters.

Along with the superficial cells, a certain number of intermediate cells are found. Their numbers, as well as the characteristics of the superficial desquamation, will depend on the time of the cycle in which the sample is obtained and the age of the woman (Fig. 36).

The majority of cytologic smears fall within Papanicolaou's Class I (Table 6). The small percentage of doubtful or neoplastic smears generally come from menopausal patients, whose interepithelial junction has been displaced up into the endocervical canal, making it impossible to see dysplastic or malignant processes in this critical area by colposcopy.

Desquamated cylindrical cells of the endocervical papillary mucosa will only rarely appear (Fig. 36). If the anatomic external os really corresponds with the histologic, and there is no overt endocervical pathology, this finding is present in only 5 per cent of cases.

Table 6. Cervical Cytology in Association with Original Mucosa

Papanicolaou Class	
Class I	71 %
Class II	27 %
Class III	1.6%
Class IV or V	0.3%

REFERENCES

Ahumada, J. C.: El Cáncer Ginecológico. Libreria "El Ateneo" Editorial, Buenos Aires, 1954.

Barcellos, J. M., and Nahoum, J. C.: Cuello uterino: Notas de nomenclatura: Concepto de cuello normal y de tercera mucosa. Acta Ginec., 16:315, 1965.

de Brux, J.: Histopathologie Gynécologique. Paris, Masson et Cie., 1971.

Dohnal, V., and Kotál, L.: Über die ideal platten-

epithelbedeckte Portio vaginalis uteri und ihre Beziehung zu Fortpflanzungs-Funktionen. Geburtsh. u. Frauenheilk., 27:485, 1967.

Fluhmann, C. F.: The Cervix Uteri and Its Diseases. Philadelphia, W. B. Saunders Co., 1961.

Hamperl, H., and Kaufmann, C.: The cervix uteri at different ages. Obstet. Gynec., 14:621, 1959.

Johnson, L. D., Easterday, C. L., Gore, H., and Hertig, A. T.: The histogenesis of carcinoma in situ of the uterine cervix: A preliminary report of the origin of carcinoma in situ in subcylindrical cell anaplasia. Cancer, 17:213, 1964.

Koller, O.: The Vascular Patterns of the Uterine Cervix. Oslo, Universitetsforlaget, 1963.

Kos, J.: Gefässanordnung in der Portio vaginalis cervicis uteri unter normalem gesunden Plattenepithel. Zbl. Gynäk., 82:1849, 1960.

Mateu-Aragonés, J. M.: Lesiones atípicas del epitelio cervical. Estudio clínico e histológico. Acta Gynaec. Obstet. Hisp. Lusit., 18:1, 1969.

Mateu-Aragonés, J. M.: La exploración colposcópica en la práctica ginecológica: Lesiones benignas. Orbe Ginec. Obstet., Mar.-Apr. 1971, p. 19.

Mestwerdt, G.: Die Funktion der Zervix in der Geburtsmotorik. Zbl. Gynäk., 76:1377, 1954.

Mikoláš, Vl., Štafl, A., and Linhartová, A.: Das terminale Gefässbild der Portio vaginalis uteri bei Schwangeren. Zbl. Gynäk., 84:524, 1962.

Mossetti, C., and Russo, A.: La Colposcopia nella Diagnostica Ginecologica. Torino, Ediz. Minerva Medica, 1963.

Ober, K. G., Schneppenheim, P., Hamperl, H., and Kaufmann, C.: Die Epithelgrenzen im Beriche des Isthmus uteri. Arch. Gynäk., 190:346, 1958.

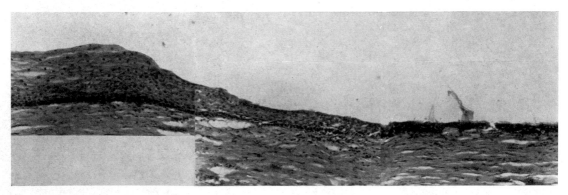

Figure 35. Transitional form of the squamo-columnar junction. Between the normal columnar epithelium (right) and the mature squamous epithelium (left), there exists a strip of immature squamous epithelium of metaplastic origin.

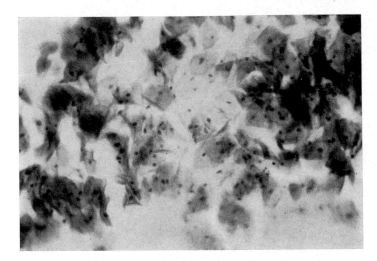

Figure 36. Cytology of the normal cervix. *A*, Totally normal cytologic smear (Papanicolaou's Class I), which corresponds to the post-ovulatory phase of a sexually active woman. *B*, Endocervical columnar cells, observed in two distinct projections in the same smear. This finding in a woman who has a strictly normal cervix is infrequent (less than 5 per cent of all cases).

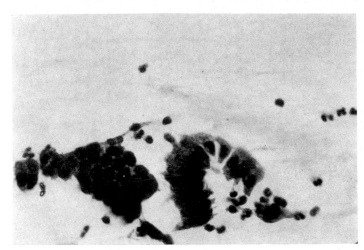

Rosenthal, A. H., and Hellman, L. M.: The epithelial changes in the fetal cervix, including the role of the "reserve cell." Am. J. Obstet. Gynec., *64*:260, 1952.

Sjövall, A.: Untersuchungen über die schleimhaut der cervix uteri. Acta Obstet. Gynec. Scand., *18*(Suppl. 4):13, 1938.

Wollner, A.: A preliminary study of the cyclic histologic changes of the human cervical mucosa in the intermenstrual period. Am. J. Obstet. Gynec., *32*:365, 1936.

Zinser, H. K., and Rosenbauer, K. A.: Untersuchungen über die Angioarchitektonik der normalen und pathologisch veränderten Cervix uteri. Arch. Gynäk., *194*:73, 1960.

Chapter Three

INFLAMMATORY CERVIX

DEFINITION

In the category of inflammatory cervix we group the consequences of mechanical or traumatic irritation, chemical insults, bacterial infections, and other offenses. However, in practice, only the study of infections and infestations is of interest, because the other inflammatory conditions have nonspecific colposcopic signs.

We can distinguish primary inflammation of the cervix from secondary inflammation. The first term is reserved for the inflammatory reaction (generally of microbial origin) of the squamous epithelium of the exocervix, in the absence of previous anatomical lesions preparing the way for the infection. Under secondary inflammation we include all inflammatory processes originating from mucosal changes which diminish resistance and create a favorable setting for contamination.

SYNONYMS

Inflammatory Cervix. Cervicitis. Inflammatory erosion. Cervical infection. Vaginitis. Colpitis. Cervicovaginitis.

The term cervicitis, widely used clinically and theoretically correct, should not be used to describe a colposcopic image because it tends to confuse. Standard textbooks include in "cervicitis" lesions as different as ectopy and its complex typical and atypical reparative

processes, traumatic ectropion, and in general any cervical erythroplasia. The term should be reserved for purely clinical inflammatory disease of the cervix, visible to the naked eye and involving a specific type of leukorrhea.

The term "inflammatory erosion" may refer to two distinct concepts. If it refers to inflammatory "true erosion," to be described later in this chapter, the term is colposcopically correct. It should not be used for the classical idea of cervical erosion, which includes all reddish cervices, supposedly de-epithelialized and inflammatory.

"Cervical infection" refers exclusively to contamination of the uterine cervix by microbes. It has no colposcopic significance.

Vaginitis and colpitis are synonymous, signifying "inflammation of the vagina" without referring to etiology, extent or severity. Both terms have been profusely used in colposcopy, referring to certain visible lesions at the exocervical level.

ORIGIN

The elements capable of producing or favoring an inflammatory reaction of the cervicovaginal mucosa are many. They may be classified as follows.

Mechanical. These include contraceptive devices, pessaries, and in general any type of foreign body in the cervix or vagina. Each of these, if left permanently or over a long period, is capable of producing necrosis or local lesions due to mechanical compression, variations in blood flow or stagnation of secretions. Hence, maceration of the exocervix is not unusual, and it prepares the tissues for future bacterial colonization. In this group also may be listed uterine prolapse, cervical elongation, cystocele, and any other disorder that predisposes to infection.

Traumatic. Obstetrical tears can enlarge a small cervical os into a wide crevice, which secretes alkaline mucus in abundance and which is highly macerating to the squamous epithelium. In a widely opened cervix, without the normal protection of the mucus plug and scarred from trauma, the possibility of an endocervicitis is enhanced. This infection will be accompanied secondarily by an exocervicitis (Fig. 37).

Chemical. Irritating substances introduced into the vagina for contraception or hygienic purposes, or alterations of the pH of the vagina, can create a favorable environment for bacterial infection.

The normal vaginal pH is around 4, and if it rises above 5, conditions become optimal for bacterial growth (Fig. 39). This can be due to the presence of soap or to hypersecretion of the alkaline endocervical mucus.

Excessive acidification (pH below 3.5) of the vaginal contents can cause

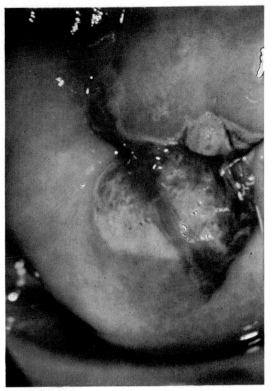

Figure 37. Lacerated cervix with a permanently infected ectopy. The anatomical conditions were responsible for the cervical infection and the difficulty in its eradication.

local discomfort as well. We believe in the possibility of "vaginitis without vaginitis" due to an evident lowering of the vaginal pH, and this in turn due to

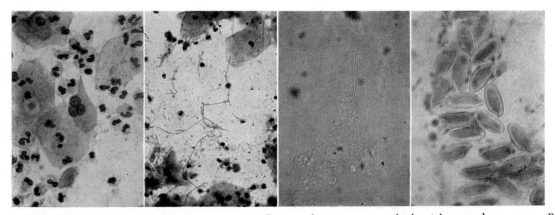

Figure 38. Causes of infectious vaginitis. *A,* Papanicolaou smear in which trichomonads are seen. *B,* Papanicolaou smear showing Leptothrix. *C,* Candida albicans in a fresh sample. *D,* Oxyuris eggs.

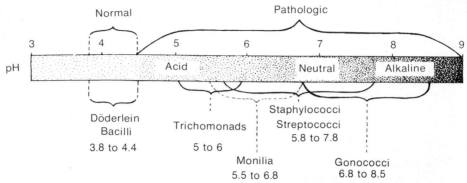

Figure 39. Variations in vaginal pH favor different bacterial infections.

massive transformation of glycogen to lactic acid in the vaginal epithelial cells. This would represent an exaggeration of the normal self-cleansing process of the vagina caused by a true or relative hyperestrogenism, or to a global hyperhormonal state (as in the premenopause or pregnancy). The phrase "without vaginitis" refers to the absence of bacteria, and to the minimal inflammatory signs which are found. By colposcopy the only observations are a hyperemic and congestive mucosa, in contrast to the numerous complaints of the patient.

This aseptic acidification should not be confused with the fall in pH which tends to follow a vaginal infection by

trichomonads or fungus. In this case acidification is the result and not the cause of the infection. As has been demonstrated by Lang, these microorganisms are capable of directly attacking the glycogen and transforming it into acid metabolites.

Infections. Undoubtedly, this is the most significant group (Fig. 38). The responsible organisms may arrive from outside (as in venereal diseases), from the corpus uteri (as occurs with septic abortions), or from the blood and lymphatics (though this possibility is minimal).

In our experience (Fig. 40) the most frequent microorganisms found in the inflammatory cervix are:

1. Nonspecific flora, made up of cocci, bacilli, and others; these are especially frequent in so-called "secondary inflammations."

2. Fungi, particularly Monilia and Leptothrix.

3. *Trichomonas vaginalis,* alone or associated with one of the preceding groups. Such an association constitutes the most frequently observed cause of primary inflammation.

4. *Haemophilus vaginalis.* The importance of this organism increases as we improve our diagnostic methods.

5. Herpes simplex virus, especially type II.

6. Organisms which cause venereal disease are the exception, although at present there is a resurgence in the incidence of these diseases.

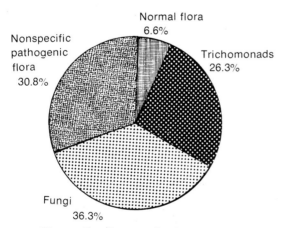

Figure 40. Causes of infectious leukorrhea. As can be seen the principal organisms are Trichomonas and Monilia.

FREQUENCY

Inflammation is an extraordinarily frequent colposcopic finding, appearing in approximately 30 per cent of cases. However, in two-thirds of these the inflammation is secondary, due to common organisms infecting pre-existing lesions. As the lesions are what attract the colposcopist's attention, the superimposed inflammation is not usually made part of the statistical record. In the majority of cases, cervical ectopy is accompanied by inflammatory signs.

Other cases of inflammation are primary. Their frequency is diversely estimated (Table 7). While some authors such as Mateu-Aragonés report low figures (in the 2 per cent range), many others indicate a much higher incidence (Guerrero et al., 26.6 per cent; Arenas et al., 26.4 per cent). In our experience, the approximate incidence is 10 per cent. Almost all of these primary lesions are represented by cervicovaginitis (9.32 per cent of all colposcopic observations), and only a few (less than 0.6 per cent) by inflammatory erosions and ulcerations (Table 8).

COLPOSCOPIC APPEARANCES

Primary Inflammation. This condition was more frequent when venereal disease was not as well controlled as it is today. Nevertheless, it is possible to confirm a primary inflammatory lesion in almost 10 per cent of all patients who attend a gynecologic service. The lesion may be one of three types: vaginitis (very frequently), erosion (rarely), and ulceration (exceptionally).

VAGINITIS. Besides the atrophic petechial vaginitis, which is described later (p. 60), we distinguish three fundamental types of infectious vaginitis: diffuse or red punctate, vaginitis of the lymphoid follicles or white punctate, and focal vaginitis. To these we add the mixed form, having characteristics of all three types, and the so-called rare forms (vesicular, hypertrophic, papillar, emphysematous).

Red Punctate Vaginitis. This type of vaginitis has a characteristic pattern. Over a pale pink background some red dots are seen, which extend diffusely over the cervix and the rest of the vaginal mucosa (Figs. 41 and 42). When such vaginitis persists for a long time, the "strawberry spots" are accompanied by hyperemia and an increased subepithelial vascularization. One type of colposcopic image is the one we call "geographical vaginitis." While in one area the red spots persist, in others they are in regression or may disappear entirely. The picture resembles a map, from which its name is derived (Fig. 43). On occasions the grouping is linear, which becomes especially evident if there are small perivascular hemorrhages as a consequence of the exploration.

The cervix which harbors this type of cervicovaginitis is bathed with abundant secretions. When trichomonads are the responsible agents, the discharge is frothy, yellow and bubbly (Fig. 44), while it is white and in lumps if the infection is fungal (Fig. 50).

On occasion the so-called "double crested capillaries" described by other colposcopists (Koller, Bergsjö and Kolstad) are seen. The capillary loop, which constitutes the central element of each red punctate lesion, divides as it reaches the surface, forming a double loop (Figs. 45 and 46). However, in many cases this type of capillary is not visible (60 per cent of our patients). Sometimes, before the capillary loop reaches the surface, it runs for a short distance parallel to the

Table 7. Frequency of Vaginitis

Mateu-Aragonés (1971)	2.1%
Guzmán Llovet et al. (1967)	4.1%
Berger and Wenner-Mangen (1952)	5.7%
Figuero et al. (1971)	13.3%
González Merlo (1966)	15.6%
Nagel et al. (1970)	20.0%
Arenas et al. (1961)	26.4%
Guerrero et al. (1957)	26.6%
Our Series (1972)	9.3%

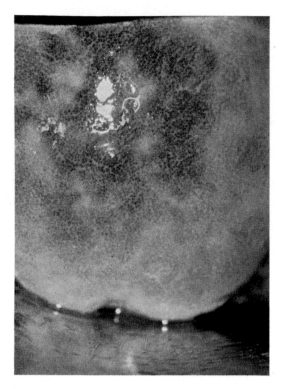

Figure 41. Red punctate vaginitis. With the application of acetic acid the red dots diffuse along the major part of the exocervix.

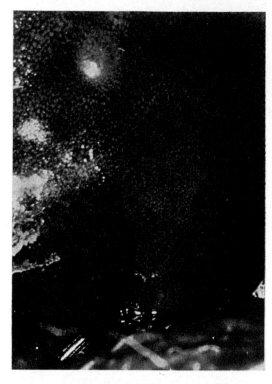

Figure 42. After Schiller's test all the exocervical mucosa takes up iodine except the red dots of the vaginitis.

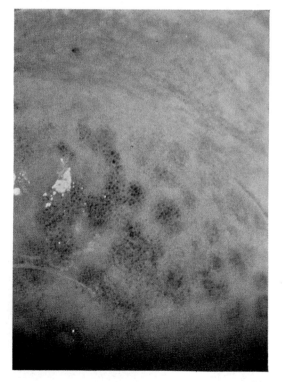

Figure 43. Geographic vaginitis. Areas with red punctate vaginitis alternate with practically unaffected areas.

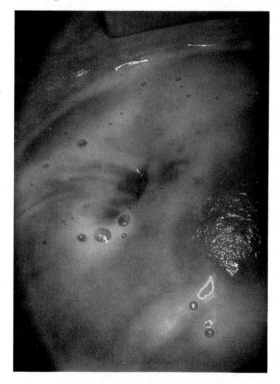

Figure 44. Leukorrhea in a case of red punctate vaginitis due to Trichomonas. Its bubbly appearance is very characteristic.

surface. Then the image of a double crested capillary is even more apparent. To improve the image, a green filter or a lens giving a magnification of ×40 or 50 may be used, even though much light is lost with the latter.

This type of vaginitis must be distinguished from the atypical lesion called ground structure (p. 140). The latter is also made up of reddish spots, but the image differs from that of vaginitis in three fundamental ways. The red spots are much coarser and lack the double-looped capillary; the lesion is isolated and well defined; and the whole region is iodine-negative (Fig. 205, p. 141).

Doubt may persist, even after the application of Lugol's solution, when the cervicovaginitis affects a zone of "initial typical re-epithelialization" (p. 111). The fact that the spots are found over a whitish iodine-negative area makes the differential diagnosis more difficult.

This variety of vaginitis cannot be attributed to any particular microorganism, even though the most frequently implicated agent is Trichomonas (49.1 per cent of cases). Other cases involve fungi (25.1 per cent), nonspecific flora (22.9 per cent), or a mixture of fungi and trichomonads (2.7 per cent) (Table 9).

The double-crested capillary image is very frequent when Trichomonas is the causative microorganism (Carrera and Dexeus). On the contrary, it is not seen in cases of mycotic infestation or nonspecific vaginitis. This colposcopic differentiation permits the establishment of an etiologic correlation which is accurate in 80 per cent of cases. In a lesser number of patients (around 20 per cent), the colposcopist should limit himself to making a presumptive diagnosis (red punctate vaginitis without double capillary loops or other elements that permit guessing its cause).

The regularity of the vaginitis, both in distribution and in the sizes of the red spots, points to a trichomonal infection.

White Punctate Vaginitis. In this variety the dots are white or yellowish-white, again situated on a more or less

Table 8. Colposcopic Aspects of Cervical Inflammation

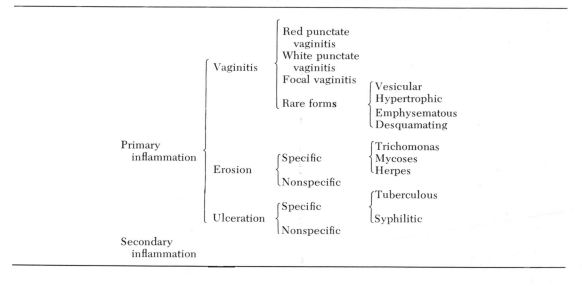

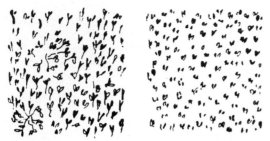

Figure 45. Sketch of the double crested capillaries observed in cases of red punctate vaginitis caused by Trichomonas (after Koller).

hyperemic mucosa. In the center of each white dot there is a single capillary loop, without bifurcation. These white dots are slightly elevated and are distributed with notable regularity over the major portion of the cervical portio and the vagina (Figs. 47 and 48).

This cervicovaginitis should not be mistaken for the "wax droplets" or the "white rings" of the typical irregular re-epithelialization zone. Nor should it be confused with "superficial papillary elevation," whose etiology is irritative. These lesions are not widespread, but are usually localized around the cervical os; also they are accompanied by other findings that facilitate the diagnosis. On the other hand, the white spots seen in those disorders are much coarser than those of cervicovaginitis. Schiller's test differentiates the papillary elevation, which takes up iodine and hence becomes invisible, from the vaginitis, which does not take up Lugol's solution, so that the lesion becomes evident over an iodine-positive background (Fig. 49). Both images may coexist.

This variety of cervicovaginitis is caused almost exclusively by fungi (94 per cent of cases) and to a lesser extent by Trichomonas (4.2 per cent) and nonspecific flora (1.7 per cent) (Table 9). However, the colposcope does not always show these well defined images when the bacteriologic examination of the vaginal discharge reveals mycosis. We estimate that in 25 per cent of infestations of this type, the colposcopic examination does not show anything more than a congested epithelium, or one proceeding toward

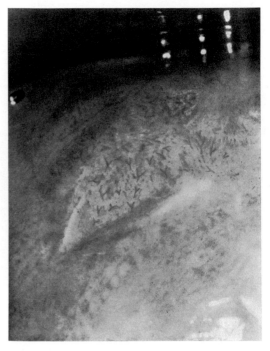

Figure 46. Colpophotography in which red punctate vaginitis is seen with double capillary loops.

maceration. It is surprising that this occurs very often in recurrent mycosis. Undoubtedly, the milieu is of great importance.

When the etiologic agent is a fungus (generally *Candida albicans*), pseudo-membranous plaques are formed by desquamated epithelium, fibrin, necrotic tissue, inflammatory cells, bacteria, and budding yeasts. On occasion, when these separate to create the lesions seen at colposcopy, superficial bleeding may occur. In place of the separated plaque, an opaque zone will be seen for some time, with a somewhat irregular surface (sometimes having a mosaic-like appearance), whose colposcopic image may be useful in defining the etiology of the process, when the vaginitis is nonspecific. Persistence over many years of such a mycotic infestation can cause a monilial granuloma which affects the submucous layer and even the muscular layer, but whose colposcopic characteristics are poorly defined.

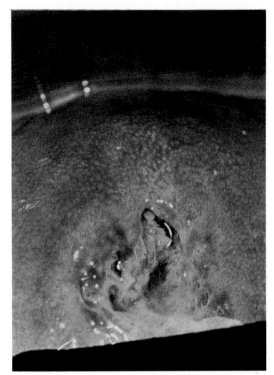

Figure 47. White punctate vaginitis after application of acetic acid, showing the white, diffuse, homogeneous dots.

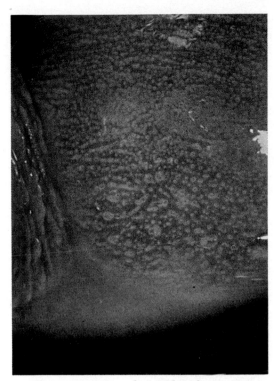

Figure 48. White dots of less homogeneous appearance, creating an image that vaguely resembles a mosaic.

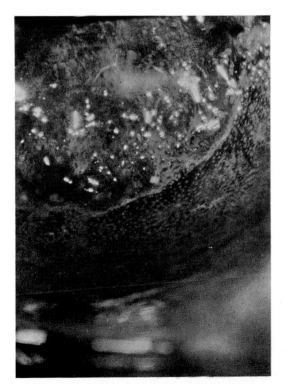

Figure 49. White punctate vaginitis after application of Lugol's solution.

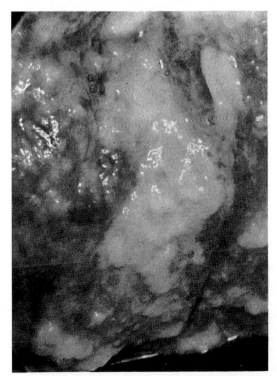

Figure 50. Mycotic leukorrhea with pseudomembranous plaques.

There are two ways in which red and white punctate cervicovaginitis can be confused. (1) The density of the red dots may be such that they appear to be grouped, and consequently the white undamaged mucosa appears by contrast as a dotted area, overlying the apparent reddish background. We are convinced that many diagnoses of white punctate vaginitis due to Trichomonas infection have arisen from colposcopic errors of this nature. (2) In some red punctate vaginitis, there is a small "cotton-like halo" around the terminal portion of the capillary loop, which can give the colposcopist some concern. However, the observation of the capillary can resolve this, because it is precisely in these cases when, at least in some areas, it travels a path parallel to the surface, it will reveal the presence of a double capillary loop.

Focal Vaginitis. In these cases the colposcopist observes some spots or stains (which are also visible to the naked eye) and which speck the cervicovaginal mucosa. Some authors (Magendie and Leger, Bredland) have likened this appearance of the cervix to a leopard skin, and it has also been compared with the surface of a strawberry (Figs. 52 and 53).

Each spot or inflammatory islet is formed by a group of red points, similar to those of diffuse vaginitis but set above a notably more hyperemic mucosa. The spaces of the mucosa that are found between these spots are practically undamaged, even though they are seen to have increased vascularity. This is visible only in the first stages of the inflammation. Later it is difficult to see, because the congestion of the stroma effaces the vascular paths.

Mestwerdt insisted that the blood vessels were interrupted at the borders of the cones or spots without passing through them, but in fact such an interpretation is very seldom correct.

Each hyperemic "core," full of "red punctations," is elevated above the exocervix. This is especially apparent in those islets that are situated far from the os, near the cervical borders, when they are silhouetted as small humps. Then the fact that they exude a serous liquid is also evident, and this secretion is seen in the form of small drops which remain adherent to each core.

Focal vaginitis almost always has a trichomonal origin (98.4 per cent of cases). Focal vaginitis can progress to granular vaginitis (Fig. 54) and even to certain forms of cervical inflammatory papilloma (Figs. 55 and 56).

"Mixed vaginitis" is the term used to describe the presence of more than one type of lesion. It may originate as the result of multiple infections (Trichomonas, fungus, etc.) or, as frequently occurs, represent different stages of evolution of a single inflammatory process on the same cervix. For example, it is not infrequent to observe a red punctate and a white punctate vaginitis in fungal infections (Fig. 57) and coexisting focal vaginitis and red punctate vaginitis in trichomonal infections (Fig. 58).

Figure 51. Cytologic smear with trichomonads (May-Grünwald stain) at high magnification.

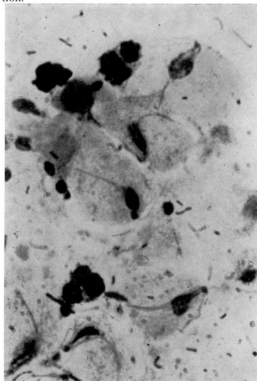

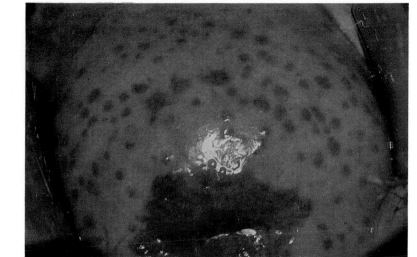

Figure 52. Focal vaginitis after application of acetic acid.

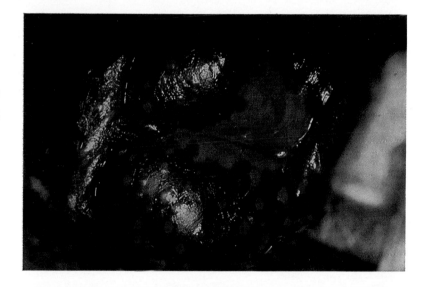

Figure 53. Observation of focal vaginitis after Schiller's test. The iodine negativity of each focus vividly contrasts with the rest of the undamaged mucosa.

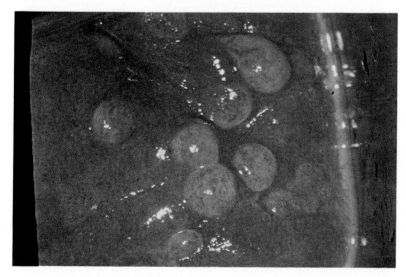

Figure 54. Focal vaginitis with a hypertrophic or granular conversion. Each focus has slowly become elevated.

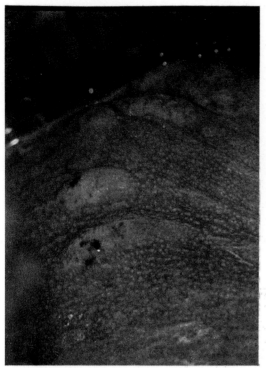

Figure 55. Areas of an old focal vaginitis in the process of transformation into inflammatory papillomatous elements (condyloma acuminata).

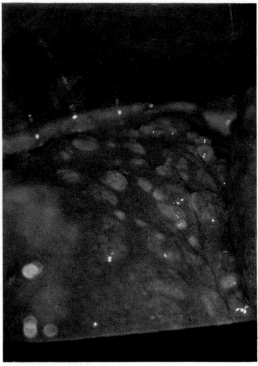

Figure 56. Diffuse papillomatosis, secondary to an old focal vaginitis.

Rare Forms of Vaginitis. Some varieties of vaginitis, even though well defined colposcopically, are only exceptionally seen.

Vesicular Vaginitis. Small vesicles are seen, filled with a serous fluid (Fig. 60). Sharply defined and clearly limited, they are perfectly disposed in groups, which are preferentially found on the periphery of ectopy or a recently re-epithelialized zone. Hyperemic mucosa with inflammatory lesions of another type may be jointly seen. On occasion, the coexistence of inflammatory cores and vesicles suggests a common origin.

Extraordinarily infrequent is the observation of herpes simplex vesicles, due to the fact that they burst quickly, and what is usually found are the resulting erosions. The moist surface of the vagina and the trauma of coitus explain the rapid ruptures. In only one case have we been able to disclose this virus disease in its acute phase, confirming the existence of multiple vesicles arrayed in a rosette form, and circled by a distinct erythematous zone. We have never seen the excrescent, granulomatous type of lesion described by Josey et al.

Even though cytologic smears permit a general etiologic orientation (Stern, Naib, Varga and Browell), identification of the virus by culture is difficult, due to the rapid evolution of the disease (Stern, González-Merlo et al.). Usually, the patients are malnourished individuals who practice cunnilingus. The disease appears as a result of a febrile illness, hormonal disturbances, or a general toxic state.

Hypertrophic or Granular Vaginitis. The vagina and to a lesser extent the cervix are seen with reddish bleeding papules, slightly larger than the spots of

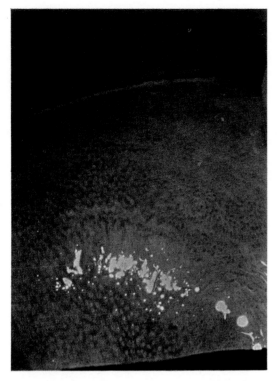

Figure 57. Mixed vaginitis of mycotic origin, with coexistence of red and white punctations.

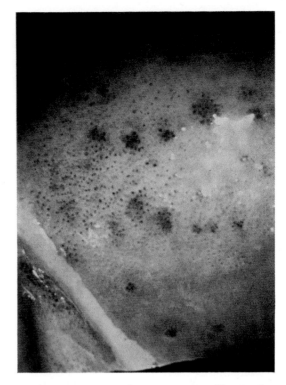

Figure 58. Mixed vaginitis caused by Trichomonas. Besides a characteristic punctate vaginitis, red punctations are interspersed.

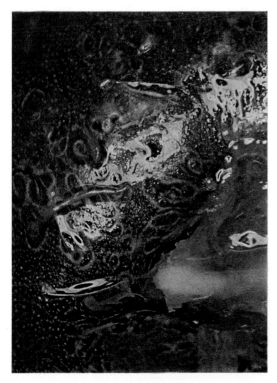

Figure 59. Mixed vaginitis after Schiller's test, with a striking mosaic-like appearance.

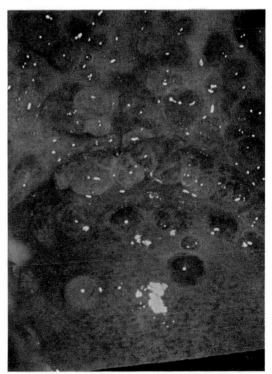

Figure 60. Vesicular vaginitis. Vesicles are disposed in groups or bunches which clearly stand out over a hyperemic exocervical mucosa.

focal vaginitis and with greater elevation. We are convinced that this type of vaginitis is almost always secondary to the focal variety and appears subsequent to repeated infections, generally trichomonal (Fig. 61).

Papillary Vaginitis. This is an acute form of vaginitis, barely visible without preparation but very evident after the application of acetic acid (Fig. 62). Some small whitish papillae are seen, disposed in a "gloved finger" array which becomes extraordinarily prominent above the more or less undamaged exocervical epithelium. Each papilla has a clearly visible microvascular axis. This lesion is almost always limited to the cervix. It lacks a specific etiology. Even though it is possible to confuse it with white punctate vaginitis, it differs by its greater elevation of the fingering, its scanty blood supply, and its topographical limitation.

Emphysematous or Cystic Vaginitis. Over the cervicovaginal epithelium some small cysts are seen of approximately the size of a lentil, and of a yellow or whitish color, unless small intracystic hemorrhages have occurred. Generally the content of these cysts is gaseous. Their rupture at the time the speculum is introduced produces a characteristic crepitation (Whalen, Wilbanks).

The intercystic vaginal mucosa does not usually present other inflammatory lesions, except for marked edema. On the rare occasions in which we have seen this variety of vaginitis, it appeared in pregnant women in which metabolic or toxic factors prevailed over the purely infectious (Shenker, Gardner). One of our patients had typhoid fever in pregnancy. However, there are reported cases in the literature of this type of vaginitis in nonpregnant patients (Mleziva).

Another rare disorder and even more poorly characterized colposcopically is desquamating vaginitis. This well defined entity (characterized by burning or itching, with a notable percentage of basal cells on cytologic smears, despite a normal ovarian function) was first described in 1965 by Gray and Barnes. In our three identified cases, it was most peculiar to see a thin cervicovaginal mucosa (which recalls the atrophic mucosa of the senile female), affected by an acute inflammation with congestion and hyperemia. The epithelium was so brittle that simply placing the speculum caused it to come away in extensive areas, leaving a visible bleeding stroma.

The etiology of this vaginitis is still to be determined. Gray and Barnes suggested a possible viral infection which causes an alteration of the superficial cells.

TRUE EROSION. This term implies the total or partial disappearance of the squamous epithelium in a more or less extensive portion of the cervix. The stroma is visible but not altered. The qualification "true" is used to make it clear that pseudoerosions are not included. This latter clinical expression corresponds in the majority of cases to what we call "ectopy."

There are four varieties of erosions: inflammatory (the ones we will now study), traumatic, dystrophic, and neoplastic.

Inflammatory true erosion is seen

Table 9.   Bacteriologic Correlation of Colposcopic Appearances of Vaginitis

	FUNGUS	TRICHOMONAS	FUNGUS AND TRICHOMONAS	NONSPECIFIC FLORA (COCCI, BACILLI, HAEMOPHILUS)
Red punctate	25 %	49 %	2.7%	22.9%
Focal	1.5%	98.4%	0	0
White punctate	94 %	4.2%	0	1.7%
Mixed	22.7%	12.5%	59 %	5.6%
Rare forms	0	28.5%	14.2%	57.2%

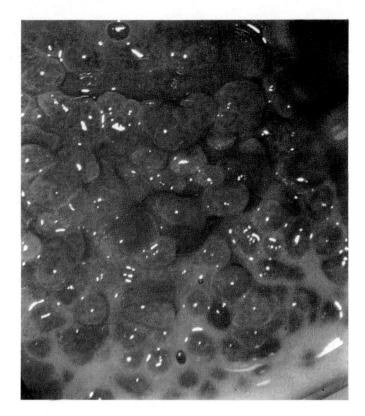

Figure 61. Granular (hypertrophic) vaginitis on the cervix of a pregnant woman. Observe the presence of a typical trichomonal leukorrhea.

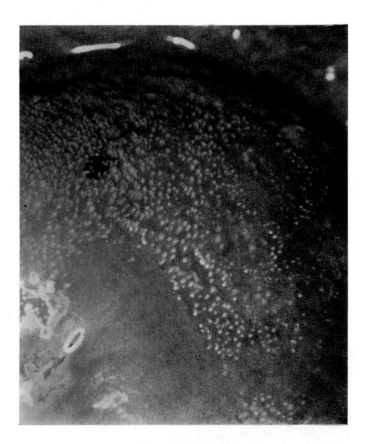

Figure 62. Papillary vaginitis, characterized by whitish fingerlike projections over a limited area of the exocervix. Each one has a vascular axis, not visible in this colpophotograph.

colposcopically as a red zone, without definite analyzable characteristics, which bleeds upon contact. Its surface is smooth, and generally there is no appreciable increase in its vascularity. The acetic acid test and, better yet, the silver nitrate test certify the absence of epithelium as well as verifying the observation of the denuded stroma, with many vessels of uniformly small caliber (Fig. 63). Some of these vessels form part of the papillae that constitute the lesions of a previous vaginitis.

On occasion, the erosions are numerous, minute, and close together, in which case we speak of "inflammatory microerosions" (Fig. 64).

Trichomonas vaginalis is usually the microorganism responsible for inflammatory erosion.

After a significant increase in the epithelial vascularization, inflammatory erosion gives way to an intraepithelial edema, inflammatory infiltration of the stroma, and papillitis, which can lead to superficial necrosis and loss of epithelium in large areas. During pregnancy, it is possible to observe these trichomonal lesions with greater frequency, creating patterns having dysplastic characteristics which may confuse the colposcopist (Savin, Carrera and Dexeus).

With less frequency, herpes simplex virus may cause this type of erosion. When this occurs, it is due to tiny erosions which are grouped or tend to coalesce and form a single one, covered by fibrin. Lesions in various stages may be seen, from one which preserves its vesicular epithelial cover, to another which has already initiated its re-epithelialization (Josey, Nigogosyan, Nowakovsky and others).

Inflammatory erosion may be prematurely concealed by an atypical re-epithelialization process (p. 146), without there being a possibility, in most cases, of demonstrating a first stage of cure by regrowth of normal columnar epithelium. We have seen this especially in young, nulliparous women who are very active sexually.

Differential diagnosis is not always easy, and the following details may be helpful. Inflammatory erosion is generally accompanied by other similar images: vaginitis, mucosal hyperemia, etc. It is not near the cervical os (which would lead to a suspicion of malignancy), no residue of flat epithelium is found around the periphery (which would suggest trauma), and the residual mucosa is not necessarily atrophic, nor does it present an intense petechial vaginitis (which would certify its dystrophic origin).

In the presence of a presumptive inflammatory erosion, a course of antimicrobial therapy is necessary, and if the appearance of the lesion does not improve, a biopsy should be done. Remember Limburg's data: 9 cancers in 24 erosions.

Exploring with a probe and verifying the presence of a normal and elastic chorion will help to rule out neoplastic origin. The destructive cancerous erosion is known to have a fragile and woody consistency (p. 220).

ULCERATION. This is a rare lesion, and due to its infrequency it is usually difficult to diagnose. Many times the colposcopist thinks it to be a malignant process, not because he observes well characterized atypias, but rather because he cannot be sure what he is seeing. The stroma is not only denuded, but also participates actively in the inflammatory process.

From a colposcopic viewpoint, ulceration refers to sharply limited lesions with elevated borders and a varied background in response to the particular etiologic agent (Fig. 65). In general the lesions are set on a healthy mucosa, far from the cervical os and lacking the vascular irregularities which would lead one to consider the adaptive vascular hypertrophy of malignant processes. If this is not the case, histopathologic study is warranted.

An etiologic diagnosis may be attempted, taking into consideration the following factors:

Tuberculous ulceration is usually not single but multiple, constituting a series of ulcers like links in a chain. Its edges are rolled and purplish. Its center is gray but sturdy and does not bleed easily due to the fact that, contrary to what occurs in neoplastic ulceration, vascular development is slight. It is characteristic for the base of the ulcer to be elevated like a mushroom and encircled by a uniform edge. Mestwerdt showed that the probe slides off this lesion, indicating its lack of fragility. Confusing tuberculous with neoplastic ulcers is still common (Dexeus, Robecchi).

The syphilitic ulcer or chancre is shaped like an oval funnel. The edges are thickened, and the base is pink with plaques which ooze with a serous or bloody discharge. Its color is whitish and it may be coated with necrotic-appearing tissue which may be separated with difficulty by using a cotton swab. In the periphery of this complex, the mucosa is edematous, and induration becomes evident.

Schiller's test demonstrates weak iodine fixation in an inflammatory ring. The bottom of the ulcer fixes iodine only slightly, as if it were made up of young reparative tissue (Caplier). Blood vessels are not seen.

Along with syphilitic ulcerations, on occasions one sees leukoplakic zones of a gray-white color, level, neither nacreous nor sharply limited, but surrounded by a very vascular area (Mestwerdt).

Nonspecific inflammatory ulceration is usually secondary to previous erosion. Almost always, it is made up of level, oval-shaped ulcerations, which are encircled by a reddish areola and a reactive periulcerative edema. Its surface may be covered with scales.

Secondary Inflammation. In at least 20 per cent of all colposcopic examinations, inflammatory signs are seen superimposed upon anatomic or pathologic alterations. All cervical lesions offer a fertile ground for bacterial colonization by altering tissues. Inflammation adds to the observed characteristics of the original lesions. Swelling, vascular hypertrophy, suppuration, and necrosis can alter the original appearance of the cervix, causing diagnostic difficulties (Fig. 66).

Some examples will illustrate this. If a simple diffuse vaginitis is localized over an area of initial re-epithelialization, the lesion will look much like ground structure (p. 111), even after the acetic acid test. The infectious destruction of a plaque of ectopy leaves an ulceration surrounded by an elevated rim, whose nature is not colposcopically identifiable. A typical re-epithelialization zone in a maceration (p. 122) with glandular infection may resemble an atypical transformation zone. Deciduosis (pp. 239 and 245) occurring over the glandular sequelae of re-epithelialization resembles an atypical transformation zone, if infection coexists.

In the attempt to define the benign or malignant nature of a lesion it may be useful to study the vascular network by means of the green filter or using special methods such as the reaction to hydrogen peroxide (Carretero).

Especially during pregnancy, an inflammatory complication may even induce a false diagnosis of malignancy (Nesbitt, Coupez). When decidual transformation is superimposed on an exuberant ectopy of pregnancy (p. 245), along with a considerable inflammatory component, the resulting images may be really impressive, giving the colposcopist the false idea of an excrescent epithelioma. Prudence is essential, and we encourage a thorough search for intact glandular elements and preserved papillae of ectopy. A course of anti-inflammatory treatment will probably clear up any doubts. If these persist after therapy, biopsy is indicated.

HISTOLOGIC CORRELATIONS

There are histologic patterns common to all types of vaginitis, but there are also some very specific ones. In the majority of cases with vaginitis, histologic examination reveals an epithelium with a thin covering, much traumatized by the inflammatory process. The stroma is very edematous and is occupied by a neutrophilic or round cell infiltration, according to the stage of evolution of the infection.

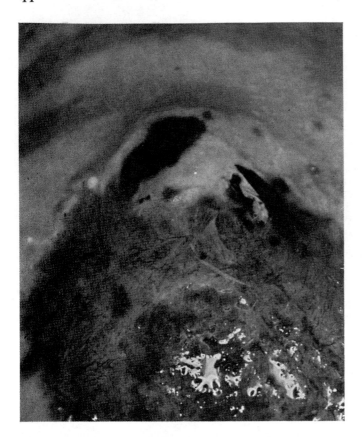

Figure 63. Inflammatory erosion. Besides the evident lack of epithelium, the congestive and hyperemic appearance of an inflammatory reaction is quite striking.

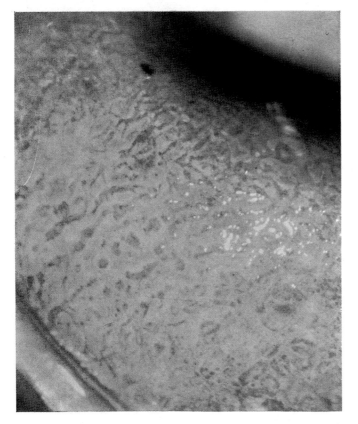

Figure 64. Pseudomosaic inflammatory microerosions. Anti-inflammatory treatment caused disappearance of this lesion is less than two weeks.

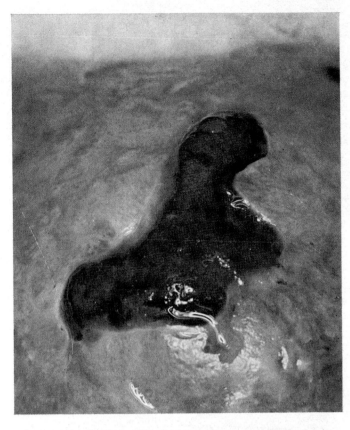

Figure 65. Nonspecific ulceration with well defined edges. The stroma is affected by an inflammatory process, while the undamaged mucosa has a normal appearance.

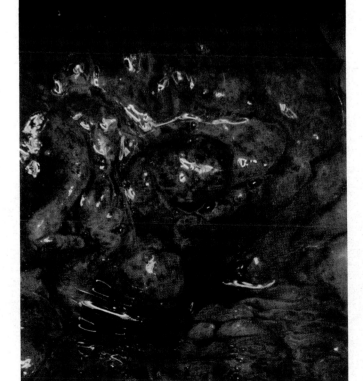

Figure 66. Secondarily infected ectopy. The granular appearance may lead the inexperienced to suspect a malignant lesion.

If there are glandular openings on histologic preparation, they will be filled by a purulent exudate and the periglandular stroma will appear infiltrated. The blood vessels are quite dilated and their endothelium is swollen and encircled by an inflammatory membrane. Because there are fewer layers in the epithelial cover, the vessels are much closer to the surface than usual. Edema and infiltration of the stroma also contribute to this picture (Fig. 67).

Histologic differentiation between the different types of vaginitis is established by observing the vascular openings. Fernandez-Cid has demonstrated that in the case of the red punctate vaginitis with double crested capillaries, there is a "double capillary unit" which is visible on transverse section (Fig. 68). In the nonspecific red punctate vaginitis, and also in the white punctate vaginitis, on the contrary, there is only one "simple capillary unit" (Fig. 69).

Even though Mestwerdt described a special type of vaginitis of the lymphoid follicles (similar to our white-punctate form), sometimes taking the form of real microabscesses, it is not specific for any particular vaginitis, and we have seen it in almost all varieties (Fiocchi) (Fig. 70).

Where erosions and ulcerations are concerned, by describing their colposcopic characteristics we have delineated their most distinguished pathologic features as well. Fundamental differences exist between these lesions: an intact epithelium in the former, and an inflammatory injured mucosa in the latter.

Erosion caused by the herpes simplex virus is preceded by a stage of multilocular vesicles, beginning with degeneration of the cells which swell and lose their intercellular bridges. Their mem-

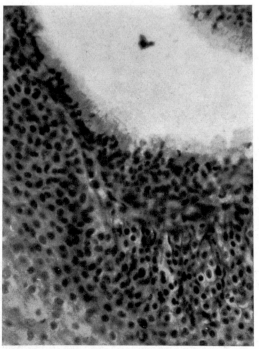

Figure 67. Histology of nonspecific vaginitis. There is a notable round cell infiltration of the stroma.

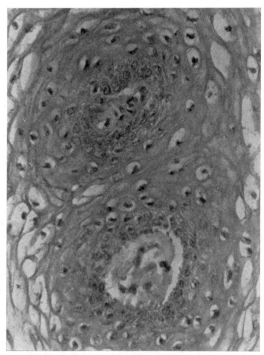

Figure 68. Histologic section in which a "double capillary unit" is observed, the pathologic equivalent of red punctate vaginitis with a double capillary loop. This is a pathognomonic sign of trichomonal vaginitis.

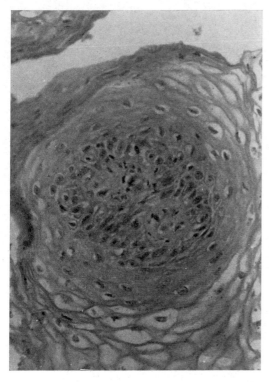

Figure 69. Histologic section of a diffuse non-specific vaginitis. Besides the inflammatory infiltration of the stroma there is a "simple capillary unit."

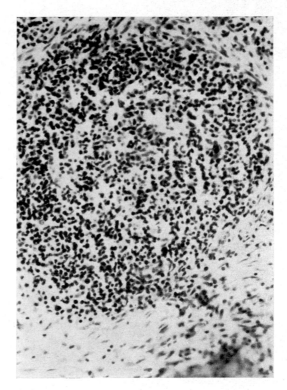

Figure 70. Histology of vaginitis exhibiting a typical lymphoid follicle.

branes are broken by the edema. Nuclear inclusions are characteristic of the process (Nowakovsky).

Tuberculous ulceration, in addition to its obligatory chronic inflammatory infiltration of the stroma, also shows total loss of the epithelium as well as some typical tubercles with epithelioid and giant cells. During advanced stages more or less extensive caseous degeneration is seen (Sered et al.).

leukocytes and histiocytes, vaginal cells with inflammatory characteristics (perinuclear halos, leukocytic inclusions, vacuolated cytoplasm) and bacteria in abundance, as those responsible for vaginitis (Fig. 71).

The existence of a large number of basilar cells suggests a vaginal mucosa severely damaged by an inflammatory process.

In 13.6 per cent of samples, the desquamated cells are practically normal;

CYTOLOGIC CORRELATIONS

In our experience, 85 per cent of the smears corresponding to colposcopically described lesions have evidence of inflammation which makes us classify the smear in Papanicolaou's Class II (Table 10). As such, we accept the presence of

Table 10. Cytologic Correlation of Vaginitis Seen Colposcopically

Class I	13.6%
Class II	85 %
Class II–III and III	1.3%
Class IV and V	0

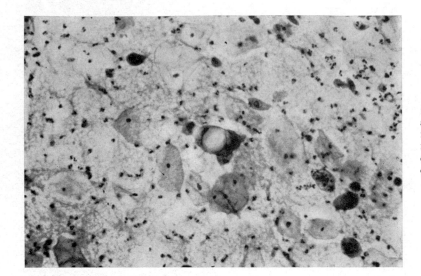

Figure 71. Nonspecific inflammatory smear. Alongside abundant inflammatory elements (leukocytes, histiocytes, mucus, detritus), some basilar cells and intensely vacuolated cells are seen.

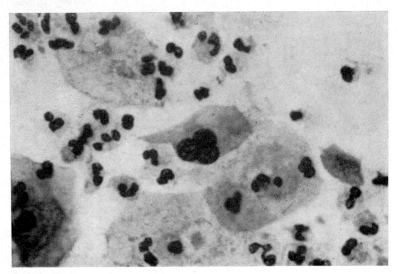

Figure 72. Inflammatory smear demonstrating trichomonads. Besides these microorganisms, cellular alterations are outstanding (multinucleation and perinuclear halos).

hence, even in the presence of considerable numbers of leukocytes and microorganisms, we classify these in Papanicolaou's Class I (Carrera and Dexeus). The majority of these represent vaginitis caused by nonspecific organisms (65 per cent) or by Monilia (30 per cent).

When the infection is very severe, the cytologic picture may be frankly suspicious (1.3 per cent of cases). This is seen frequently in trichomonal vaginitis (Van Niekerk, Panella, Lindenschmidt and Stoll, and others) (Figs. 51 and 72).

The cytologic alterations typical of herpes simplex virus also lead to confusion if they are not known. Actually, the nuclear vacuolization, the ground glass appearance of the nucleus, and the existence of basophilic and eosinophilic intranuclear inclusions, may lead one to include the sample in Class III of Papanicolaou (Figs. 73 and 74).

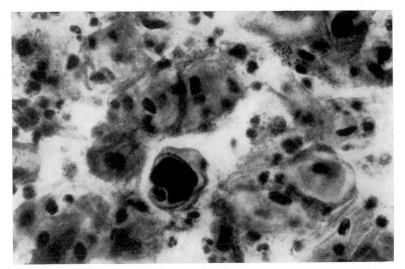

Figure 73. Vaginal viritis at low magnification.

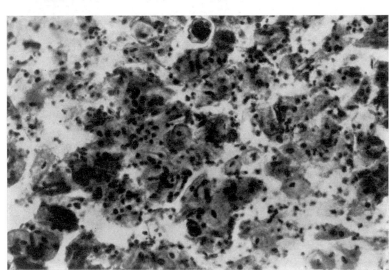

Figure 74. Vaginal viritis at high magnification, demonstrating notable nuclear alterations (inclusions).

CLINICAL COURSE

Inflammation of the cervicovaginal mucosa may follow one of three paths.

Cure After the Acute Phase. This is the rule with primary inflammation which has been duly diagnosed and correctly treated. In our experience 80 per cent are cured with the first therapeutic attempt.

The evolution of an acute vaginitis differs according to the etiology. In the case of trichomonal infection, the mucosa responds with a red punctate vaginitis, developing double capillary loops. If the inflammation tends to heal either spontaneously or with adequate therapy, the mucosa regains its normal appearance, after a brief stage of "geographic vaginitis," which should then be considered as a phase of recovery. Later colposcopic views do not show sequelae.

The acute phase of a mycotic vaginitis is also represented by red punctation, each having a single capillary element. In more advanced stages of the infestation, each red dot is circled by a small white area. This appearance then gives way to that of white-punctate vaginitis, which generally does not leave any sequelae when cured.

Chronic Persistence. If primary acute vaginitis finds the proper fertile ground for its development and the proper course of therapy is not followed, it gives rise to a chronic condition whose colposcopic appearance is a focal or spotty vaginitis. This may still respond to therapy, or may lead after several years to a hypertrophic granular vaginitis. In such cases the vaginal mucosa never recovers its normal colposcopic appearance, but instead looks dull and shows evident vascular irregularities (Fig. 75). The possibility that this epithelium is extraordinarily susceptible to cancer is the object of extensive discussion (Simeckova, Pereyra, Koss, Skacel, and others).

In a colposcopic study, Szell observed that the incidence of atypical patterns doubled in patients with trichomonal infection (49.3 per cent), while the incidence of subsequent neoplasia quintupled (0.33 per cent as compared to 0.06 per cent of the group free of trichomonal infection).

In a series of over 60,000 cytologic samples, Meisels observed that the incidence of both dysplastic and carcinomatous lesions increases if trichomonal infection exists (Table 11).

The possibility that herpetic vesicular cervicitis favors the appearance of carcinoma in situ has also been suggested (Naib, Rawls et al.).

Cervical inflammation, which is favored and maintained by trauma ("secondary inflammation") and has experienced multiple reparative attempts and is found to be affected by vascular and glandular sequelae of failed metaplastic processes, does not tend to disappear. Cure of the inflammatory process will not be possible until the damaged tissues are removed (Fig. 76).

Extension to Other Areas of the Genital Tract. At first the infection is limited to the exocervical mucosa, and colposcopically it is possible to confirm that the mucus in the cervical canal remains clear and transparent, not mixed with the infected vaginal contents. When infection persists and especially when there are favorable anatomic conditions (such as tears) endocervicitis will develop and, will be announced clinically by the emission of an abundant mucoid and sticky discharge (Fig. 78). Colposcopically, the papillar endocervical mucosa is much more congested and irregular than usual.

The hypersecretion of an inflamed mucosa should not be mistaken for physiologic cervical hypersecretion (hydrorrhea), which flows in the form of a cascade through the cervical os and which is clear and sterile (Fig. 77).

The possibility of this infection ascending to the corpus uteri is practically nonexistent in cervicovaginal inflammation other than the gonococcal variety.

Table 11. Correlation Between Vaginal Trichomonal Infection and Cytologic Diagnosis (Meisels, 1969)

	TRICHOMONAL INFECTION				
CYTOLOGIC DIAGNOSIS	*Present*		*Absent*	*Total*	*P*
Negative	6,528	(10.5%)	55,756	62,284	–
Dysplasia	256	(22.4%)	887	1,443	<0.001
Carcinoma in situ	75	(25.9%)	214	289	<0.001
Invasive carcinoma	25	(16.2%)	129	154	<0.05
Total	6,884	(10.8%)	56,984	63,870	–

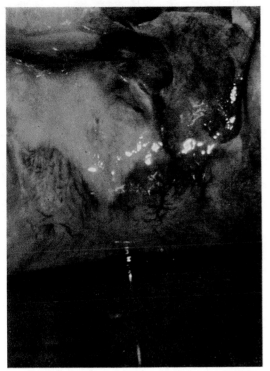

Figure 75. Vascular irregularities in a cervix that had been infected with a trichomonal vaginitis a few months earlier.

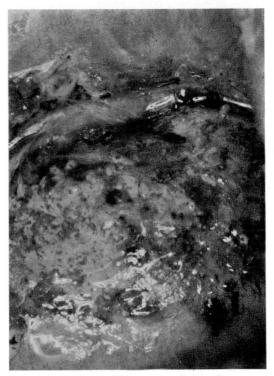

Figure 76. Stubborn secondary inflammation in a cervix with multiple glandular and vascular sequelae.

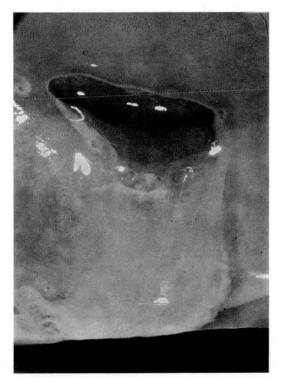

Figure 77. Clean cervical mucus, practically colorless.

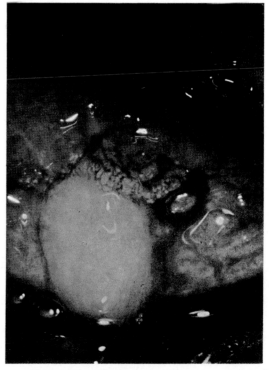

Figure 78. Thick, dirty and creamy cervical mucus is often of septic origin.

Table 12. Role of Anovulatory Agents
in Vaginitis

Incidence	
Expected frequency of vaginitis	9.32%
Frequency during anovulatory therapy	21.10%
Responsible microorganism	
Monilia	37%
Nonspecific flora	35%
Trichomonas	21%
Leptothrix	5%
Haemophilus	3%
Differences according to the agent used	
Classical anovulatory agents	32.7%
Sequential anovulatory agents	10.7%

Thanks to its menstrual desquamation the endometrium is spared serious effects of any infections that spread superficially. Parametritis and salpingitis due to lymphatic spread are also seldom seen during the acute phase of pancervicitis.

FOLLOW-UP

The more thorough the assessment, the more effective will be the treatment of a given case of inflammation of the cervicovaginal mucosa. Careful evaluation of the symptoms, identification of the organism causing the observed lesions, and the type and intensity of the lesions are of value. In practice, colposcopy permits the gynecologist to confirm the clinical impression of cervicitis, to obtain an exact description of the lesion, and to establish the etiologic agent with exactness.

On many occasions fresh samples and even stained smears are negative a few days after specific anti-inflammatory treatment is established, but colposcopy shows persistence of the lesion. In these cases to abandon treatment is an error because, clinically and bacteriologically, the infection will reappear.

The treatment to be used in the presence of a specific type of vaginal inflammation is beyond the scope of this book, but irrigations and baths, which at one time were the mode, are no longer used. They contribute to epithelial maceration and interfere with the vaginal self-cleansing. Topical medication should be administered in the form of suppositories or creams.

Once the acute stage of the infection has been overcome, and the vagina has been made sterile, local circumstances that favor infection should be sought with the colposcope. Generally these are typical but torpid re-epithelialization with multiple glandular sequelae; extensive ectopy; multiple lacerations; or polyposis. Management is then directed toward eliminating these elements, either by coagulation or surgery.

Finally, the possibility of a hormonal imbalance should be considered, for this would alter the vaginal biology and create favorable conditions for the propagation of an infection. We have observed on several occasions, as have other authors (Catterall), that the frequency of vaginitis diagnosed by colposcopy is increased threefold in patients taking anovulatory medication over long periods of time (Table 12). Suspension of that therapy for an indefinite period is an obligatory step toward effecting recovery of the injured vaginal mucosa.

REFERENCES

Adair, F. L., and Hesseltine, H. C.: Histopathology and treatment of vaginitis: I. Histopathology. II. Biochemical approach in treatment. Am. J. Obstet. Gynec., 32:1, 1936.

Ayre, J. E.: Role of the halo cell in cervical cancerigenesis: A virus manifestation in premalignancy? Obstet. Gynec., 15:481, 1960.

Bechtold, E., and Reicher, N. B.: The relationship of trichomonas infestations to false diagnosis of squamous carcinoma of the cervix. Cancer, 5:442, 1952.

Bergsjö, P., Koller, O., and Kolstad, P.: The vascular pattern of trichomonas vaginalis cervicitis. Acta Cytol., 7:292, 1963.

Bredland, R.: Die kolposkopische Diagnose der

gynäkologischen Trichomoniasis. Geburtsh. u. Frauenheilk., *25*:815, 1965.

Bret, J., and Coupez, F.: Colposcopie. Paris, Masson et Cie., 1960.

Bret, J., Durieux, R., and Guerci, P.: Dysplasie du col utérin et infection vaginale. Rev. Franç. Gynéc. Obstét., *60*:195, 1965.

Burnett, R. G., and Purdon, T. F.: Pyovesiculosis as a cause of chronic vulvovaginitis: Report of 3 cases. Obstet. Gynec., *26*:508, 1965.

Carrera, J. M., and Dexeus, S., Jr.: Diagnóstico colposcópico de las vaginitis infecciosas: Su correlación colpocitológica y bacteriológica. Acta Ginec., *22*:71, 1971.

Carrera, J. M., Palacín, A., and Dexeus, S., Jr.: Cambios morfologicos inducidos en el frotis vaginal por los anovulatorios orales. Acta Ginec., *19*:869, 1968.

Carretero Moreno, L.: Investigacion de hidroperoxidasas en el ectocervix: I. Estudio de reaccion de catalasas con el colposcopio. II. Estudio de la reaccion bencidina − H_2O_2 con el colposcopio. Acta Ginec., *15*:461, 467, 1964.

Catterall, R. D.: Candida albicans and the contraceptive pill. Lancet, *2*:830, 1966.

Catterall, R. D., and Nicol, C. S.: Is trichomonal infestation a venereal disease? Brit. Med. J., *1*: 1177, 1960.

Cianci, S., and Marotta, N.: Le displasie epiteliali della portio nella trichomoniasi vaginale. Clinica Ginec., *7*:331, 1965.

Davis, C. H.: Trichomonas vaginalis infections: A clinical and experimental study. J.A.M.A., *157*: 126, 1955.

Dexeus, S., Jr., and Fontane, F. J.: Tuberculosis cervical: A propósito de un error diagnóstico. Acta Ginec., *15*:99, 1964.

Dexeus, S., Jr., and Carrera, J. M.: Cambios inducidos en la bacteriologia vaginal por los anovulatorios. Progr. Obstet. Ginec., *14*:257, 1971.

Fiocchi, E.: Sulla presenza di noduli linfatici pseudofollicolari nella muccosa del collo uterino. Archivio "De Vecchi" L'Anatomia Patologica, *35*:683, 1961.

Fuchs, K., and Levy, E.: Vaginitis emphysematosa. Gynaec., *149*:361, 1960.

Gardner, H. L.: Desquamative inflammatory vaginitis: A newly defined entity. Am. J. Obstet. Gynec., *102*:1102, 1968.

Gardner, H. L., and Fernet, P.: Etiology of vaginitis emphysematosa: Report of ten cases and review of literature. Am. J. Obstet. Gynec., *88*:680, 1964.

González-Merlo, J.: Colposcopia de las lesiones benignas del cuello uterino. Toko-Ginec. Práct., *20*:220, 1961.

González-Merlo, J., and Biaza, F.: Estudio colposcópico del cervix uterino en 3306 casos. Acta Ginec., *14*:463, 1963.

González-Merlo, J., Montalvo, L., Vilar, E., and Botella, J.: Cinco años de experiencia en el diagnostico precoz del cancer cervical uterino. Prog. Obstet. Ginec., *7*:441, 1964.

Gray, L. A., and Barnes, M. L.: Vaginitis in women, diagnosis and treatment. Am. J. Obstet. Gynec., *92*:125, 1965.

Josey, W. E., Nahmias, A. J., and Naib, Z. M.: Viral and virus-like infections of the female genital tract. Clin. Obstet. Gynec., *12*:161, 1969.

Josey, W. E., Nahmias, A. J., Naib, Z. M., Utley, P. M., McKenzie, W. J., and Coleman, M. T.: Genital herpes simplex infection in the female. Am. J. Obstet. Gynec., *96*:493, 1966.

Kleger, B., Prier, J. E., Rosato, D. J., and McGinnis, A. E.: Herpes simplex infection of the female genital tract: I. Incidence of infection. Am. J. Obstet. Gynec., *102*:745, 1968.

Koller, O.: The Vascular Patterns of the Uterine Cervix. Oslo, Universitetsforlaget, 1963.

Kolstad, P.: The colposcopical picture of trichomonas vaginitis. Acta Obstet. Gynec. Scand., *43*: 388, 1964.

Kos, J.: Gefässanordnung in der Portio vaginalis cervicis uteri unter normalem gesunden Plattenepithel. Zbl. Gynäk., *82*:1849, 1960.

Koss, L. G., and Wolinska, W. H.: Trichomonas vaginalis cervicitis and its relationship to cervical cancer: A histocytological study. Cancer, *12*: 1171, 1959.

Laffont, A., and Martin-Laval, S.: Quelques images colposcopiques particulières au cours de l'infection du col. Gynéc. Obstét., *66*:621, 1967.

Lang, W. R.: Colposcopy − neglected method of cervical evaluation. J.A.M.A., *166*:893, 1958.

Lang, W. R., and Ludmir, A.: A pathognomonic colposcopic sign of trichomonas vaginalis vaginitis. Acta Cytol., 5:390, 1961.

Limburg, H.: Comparison between cytology and colposcopy in the diagnosis of the early cervical carcinoma. Am. J. Obstet. Gynec., *75*:1298, 1958.

Limburg, H.: Die Frühdiagnose des Uteruskarzinoms, Histologie, Kolposkopie, Cytologie, Biochemische Methoden. 3rd ed. Stuttgart, Georg Thieme Verlag, 1956.

Lindenschmidt, W., and Stoll, P.: Occurrence of dyskaryotic cells in trichomonas infestation. Acta Cytol., *2*:11, 1958.

Magendie, J., and Leger, H.: La colpite a trichomonas: Son diagnostic colposcopique et son histologie. C. R. Soc. Franç. Gynéc., *32*:469, 1962.

Mateu Aragonés, J. M.: La exploración colposcópica en la práctica ginecológia: Lesiones benignas. Orbe Ginec. Obstet., 19, 1971.

Meisels, A.: Microbiology of the female reproductive tract as determined in the cytologic specimen: III. In the presence of cellular atypias. Acta Cytol., *13*:64, 1969.

Mestwerdt, G.: Atlas der Kolposkopie. Jena, Gustav Fischer, 1953.

Mestwerdt, G.: Enfermedades del hocico de tenca y del cuello uterino. *In* Schwalm and Döderlein (Eds.), Clínica Obstétrico-Ginecológica, Vol. 5, 1st Edit. Madrid, Editorial Alhambra, 1966.

Mleziva, J., and Štafl, A.: Vulvovaginitis emphysematosa. Zbl. Gynäk., *86*:1667, 1964.

Naib, Z. M.: Exfoliative cytology of viral cervicovaginitis. Acta Cytol., *10*:126, 1966.

Nesbitt, R. E. L., Jr.: Benign cervical changes in pregnancy. Clin. Obstet. Gynec., *6*:381, 1963.

Nigogosyan, G., and Mills, J. W.: Herpes simplex cervicitis. J.A.M.A., *191*:496, 1965.

Nogales, F., Beato, M., and Martinez, H.: Cervix-tuberkulose. Arch. Gynäk., *203*:423, 1966.

Nowakovsky, S., McGrew, E. A., Medak, H., Burlakow, P., and Nanos, S.: Manifestations of viral infections in exfoliated cells. Acta Cytol., *12*:227, 1968.

O.M.S. (W.H.O.): Recommendaciones finales del Seminario Interregional de Praga, 1970.

Panella, I., Di Leo, S., and Marotta, N.: La trichomoniasi vaginale quale causa di diagnosi citologiche "false positive" di epitelioma della portio. Clinica Ginec., 7:16, 1965.

Pereyra, A. J.: The relationship of sexual activity to cervical cancer: Cancer of the cervix in a prison population. Obstet. Gynec., *17*:154, 1961.

Peterson, W. F., Hansen, F. W., Stauch, J. E., and Ryder, C. D.: Trichomonal vaginitis: Epidemiology and Therapy. Am. J. Obstet. Gynec., 97: 472, 1967.

Pinkerton, J. H. M.: Chronic inflammatory lesions of the cervix. Clin. Obstet. Gynec., 6:365, 1963.

Porter, P. S., and Lyle, J. S.: Yeast vulvovaginitis due to oral contraceptives. Arch. Derm., 93:402, 1966.

Rawls, W. E., Gardner, H. L., and Kaufman, R. L.: Antibodies to genital herpesvirus in patients with carcinoma of the cervix. Am. J. Obstet. Gynec., *107*:710, 1970.

Robecchi, E.: Tubercolosi e pseudotubercolosi collo dell'utero. Minerva Ginec., *16*:761, 1964.

Savin, S., Popesku, K., Rusu, A., and Tsopa, E.: Correlations between dysplasia of the uterine cervix and vaginal trichomoniasis (colposcopic and histopathological investigation). Akush. Ginek., 38:35, 1962.

Sered, H., Falls, F. H., and Zumno, B. P.: Recent trends in the management of tuberculosis of the cervix. J. Internat. Coll. Surg., 20:409, 1953.

Shenker, L., and Blaustein, A.: Emphysematous vaginitis: A theory of its pathogenesis and report of a case. Obstet. Gynec., 22:295, 1963.

Simeckova, M., Lonser, E., Nichols, E. E., and Rubinstein, I. N.: Chronic trichomoniasis and cervical cancer. Obstet. Gynec., 20:410, 1962.

Simon, T. R., Koss, L. G., and Wolinska, W. H.: Trichomoniasis and its relation to cervical atypia. First Internat. Cytol. Congress, Chicago, 1956.

Skácel, K.: On the significance of trichomoniasis in precancerous states of the uterine cervix. Neoplasma, 4:297, 1957.

Skindzuka, A.: Growth and life cycle of Trichomonas vaginales and the mechanism of recurrence of Trichomonas vaginalis vaginitis. J. Jap. Obstet. Gynec. Soc., 2, 1955.

Stern, E., and Longo, L. D.: Identification of herpes simplex virus in a case showing cytological features of viral vaginitis. Acta Cytol., 7:295, 1963.

Széll, I., Traub, A., Ember, M., Palánkai, G., and Schmidt, I.: Die Rolle der Trichomoniasis in der Entstehung der Präblastomatosen der Portio uteri. Zbl. Gynäk., 89:312, 1967.

van Niekerk, W. A.: Atypical basal-cell nuclei in cervical smears caused by Trichomonas vaginalis. S. Afr. Med. J., 37:582, 1963.

Varga, A., and Browell, B.: Viral inclusion bodies in vaginal smears. Obstet. Gynec., *16*:441, 1960.

Watt, L.: Trichomoniasis. Bull. Inst. Technicians Venereol., 7:67, 1966.

Wespi, H. J.: La colposcopie dans le diagnostic des leucorrhées. C. R. Soc. Franç. Gynéc., *26*:49, 1956.

Whalen, J. P., and Ziter, F. M. H., Jr.: Emphysematous vaginitis. Obstet. Gynec., 29:9, 1967.

Wilbanks, G. D., and Carter, B.: Vaginitis emphysematosa: Report of 4 patients. Obstet. Gynec., 22:301, 1963.

Zajacová, E.: The effect of vaginal trichomonas infection on the genesis of atypical epithelium on the vaginal portion of the uterus: III. Trichomonas colpitis in the colposcopic and microscopic pictures. Bratislavské Lekárske Listy, *44*:480, 1964.

Chapter Four

DYSTROPHIC CERVIX

DEFINITION

We consider a cervical dystrophy to be any histologic alteration of the cervical mucosa, morphologic or functional, which has as its basis a trophic disorder caused by circumstances such as dystopia, asynchrony, or hormonal or nutritional disturbance. It refers, hence, to a heterogeneous group of cervical perturbations.

CLASSIFICATION

The dystrophic process may involve any of the elements that form the mucosa which covers the cervix: epithelium, glands, stroma, and vessels—hence the reason for an anatomic classification which uses as its basis the altered element (Table 13).

SYNONYMS

These lesions have rarely been grouped under the ample criteria we have defined. The term "cervical dystrophy" has scarcely been used by colposcopists, and only irregularly by pathologists. Some do not use it (Novak, Fluhmann), and others give it different meaning (de Brux, Gompel).

It is therefore impossible to list either histologic or colposcopic synonyms.

Classical treatises on colposcopy study these lesions in a separate manner (Bret and Coupez, Masciotta) and fall short in describing many of them (Hin-selmann, Mestwerdt et al.) because their interest is in potentially malignant lesions, and they disregard those considered benign beyond any doubt. The objection to this way of thinking is that apart from their intrinsic importance, many of the colposcopic appearances to be described will arouse suspicion if their colposcopic characteristics are not well known.

Dystrophies usually form an incorrectly defined and poorly classified group of colposcopic entities. The grouping which we favor, despite the diversity of its components, has the advantage of offering a common definition and a didactic classification founded on solid histologic background. This chapter provides a place for many lesions not heretofore described.

Various terms have been coined by colposcopists, not without the opposition of pathologists. An example is "deciduosis," but we retain it because of its graphic character.

Table 13. Anatomic Classification of Cervical Dystrophies

Epithelial dystrophies	Atrophic mucosa, with or without petechial vaginitis
	Dystrophic erosion
	Dystrophic leukoplakia
	Superficial deciduosis
Glandular dystrophies	Glandular cysts
	Endometriosis
Stromal dystrophies	Hypertrophic deciduosis
Vascular dystrophies	Vascular hypertrophy of diverse origin

55

ORIGIN

Sometimes cervical dystrophy is due to an endocrine disturbance. A hormonal deficit may cause an atrophic mucosa or an excess may cause deciduosis and hormonal vascular hypertrophy.

On other occasions the cause is ectopic tissue which cannot be assimilated by the cervical mucosa and which continues to function as if in its proper location. An example is endometriosis.

Dystrophy may be the consequence of genital dystopia (uterine prolapse) which changes the location of the cervix. In this situation the cervical mucosa may defend itself ("adaptation leukoplakia") or be severely damaged by the deficient tissue sustenance that the change causes (erosions and ulcerations).

Glandular sequelae of former re-epithelialization processes may be the origin of trophic problems, both in the recovering epithelium and in the vascular supply (glandular cysts).

Some local circulatory disturbances (stasis of pregnancy, sclerosis of the vascular wall in the menopause, destruction of the superficial vascular network as an aftermath of coagulation) may create some deficient nutritional conditions which, among other mucosal alterations, are accompanied by venous ectasia and adaptive vascular neoformation (vascular dystrophies).

Finally, it is possible that some trophic alterations of the cervicovaginal mucosa arise because of a vitamin deficiency or a toxic syndrome. In these cases, a complex systemic syndrome is added to the purely local alteration.

FREQUENCY

About 20 per cent of the cervices observed colposcopically show lesions of this nature, but most of these are associated with other well defined colposcopic pictures (Table 14).

COLPOSCOPIC APPEARANCES AND THEIR HISTOLOGIC CORRELATIONS

Having adopted an anatomic classification for our colposcopic description, we may examine both morphologic aspects jointly.

Epithelial Dystrophies

Atrophic Mucosa. When ovarian function ceases, whether spontaneously at the menopause or because of surgical castration or drug-induced failure of ovulation, the squamous mucosa of the cervix suffers progressive atrophy, which colposcopy reveals step by step. This dystrophy is made even more apparent because it is generally preceded by a short-lived enhancement of glandular and vascular sequelae of former re-epithelialization processes (Fig. 81). This phenomenon is clearly hyperestrogenic and may be the stimulus for reactivating old epithelial atypia.

Table 14.   Absolute and Relative Frequency of Dystrophies

		Per Cent of Total Colposcopies	Per Cent of all Dystrophies
Epithelial dystrophies	Atrophic mucosa	6.9	34.5
	Dystrophic erosion	0.7	3.5
	Dystrophic leukoplakia	0.9	4.5
	Superficial deciduosis	0.5	2.5
Glandular dystrophies	Glandular cysts	2.7	13.5
	Endometriosis	0.11	0.5
Stromal dystrophies	Hypertrophic deciduosis	4.8	24.0
Vascular dystrophies of diverse etiology		3.4	17.0

The incidence of atrophic mucosa is generally given as 6 to 10 per cent of colposcopic explorations, with the figure varying according to the patient's age (Table 15).

When menopause begins and estrogenic levels fall, the cervicovaginal mucosa rapidly becomes thinner, especially at the expense of the intermediate layer. From a colposcopic viewpoint, these modifications are expressed by a mucosa that is much paler than ordinarily, unusually smooth, and without elevations, since accidents of previous re-epithelialization have been erased by the process. The squamo-columnar border disappears in the interior of the cervical canal. Also missing is the typical glow of the original mucosa, which instead gives a characteristic impression of dryness (Fig. 80A).

The subepithelial vascular network, which is not very fine, is more visible than ordinarily, due not to any real increase in vascularity but rather to the extreme thinness of the epithelium.

It may be surprising that this mucosa, without any inkling of epithelial atypia, does not take up iodine when

Table 15. Incidence of Atrophic Mucosa

Fernández Laso et al. (1960)	1.6%
Guzmán et al. (1970)	2.2%
González Merlo (1966)	6.6%
Berger and Wenner-Mangen (1952)	10.0%
Our Series (1972)	6.9%

Lugol's solution is applied (Fig. 80B). However, the explanation is logical: atrophic mucosa is poor in glycogen because practically the whole intermediate layer that is the richest in glycogen is missing.

The notable fragility of the atrophic mucosa gives rise to two types of accidents:

1. Subepithelial hemorrhages of varied forms and sizes, caused all too frequently by the examiner himself when introducing the speculum. They occur because of the thinness of the epithelium and the sclerosis of the subjacent vessels (Mestwerdt). Their traumatic nature will be suspected because of their localization in relationship to the valves of the speculum (Fig. 82). Old hemorrhages are differentiated from recent ones by their vascular organization (Fig. 83). On occa-

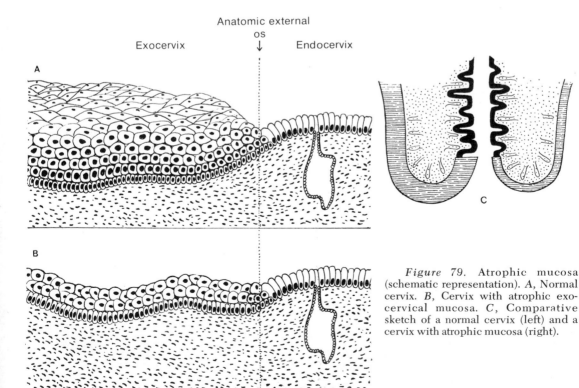

Anatomic external os

Exocervix   Endocervix

Figure 79. Atrophic mucosa (schematic representation). *A*, Normal cervix. *B*, Cervix with atrophic exocervical mucosa. *C*, Comparative sketch of a normal cervix (left) and a cervix with atrophic mucosa (right).

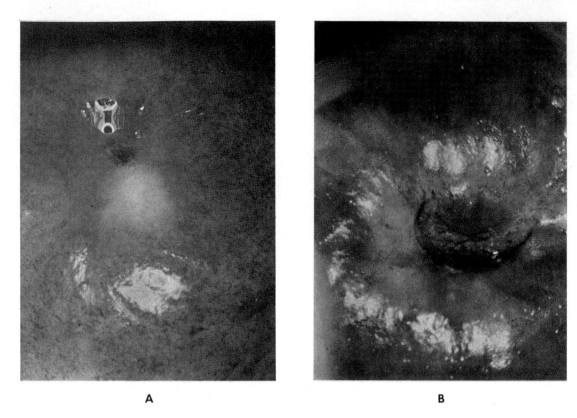

A   B

Figure 80. *A,* Atrophic mucosa after application of acetic acid. The paleness of the vaginal mucosa and the absence of high points is striking. *B,* Atrophic mucosa after application of Lugol's solution. Due to its lack of glycogen it takes up iodine poorly.

sion, pathologic examination will reveal a vasculitis with obliterating endarteritis.

2. Senile vaginitis, also called petechial vaginitis, is made up of red spots which are nothing more than innumerable petechiae disseminated along the cervix. Its distribution is capricious, but unrelated to the valves of the speculum, certifying its dystrophic-inflammatory origin (Fig. 84).

It is quite probable that the marked decrease in glycogen alters the vaginal chemistry, causing a local deterioration in its defenses. This could explain why atrophic mucosa is easily attacked by the bacteria which are normally present in the vagina. The impressive lymphocytic infiltration which is usually seen histologically in the stroma partly justifies the use of the term "vaginitis," objectionable in other aspects.

Some cases of vaginal bleeding which cause the menopausal woman to consult the gynecologist are due to these accidents involving the mucosa. However, in our experience, such hemorrhages do not cause more than 7 per cent of all postmenopausal vaginal bleeding. Such an explanation must not be considered until the patient has been subjected to an adequate endometrial evaluation (Abbas, Pelletier and Latour). Displacement of the "transitional zone" toward the interior of the endocervical canal (entopy) may also present serious difficulties in diagnosing neoplasia of this zone colposcopically.

Mucosal atrophy is progressive. Hence, in the early menopause, the most frequent colposcopic picture is still that of the typical re-epithelialization zone (35 per cent), followed by infectious vaginitis (12 per cent), and in third place atrophic mucosa (11 per cent) which is still unaccompanied by petechiae. In the "advanced climacterium," atrophic mucosa without petechiae is seen in 42 per cent of cases, a similar mucosa with pe-

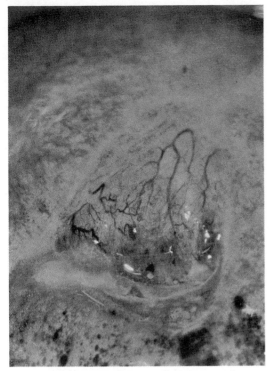

Figure 81. Besides atrophic mucosa, hypertrophy of the glandular and vascular elements is notable in a premenopausal woman.

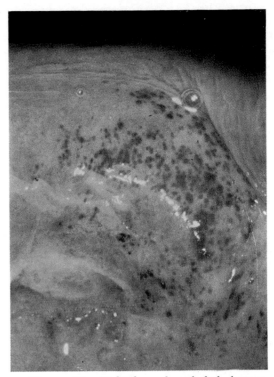

Figure 82. Multiple subepithelial hemorrhages that occupy the major portion of the exocervix.

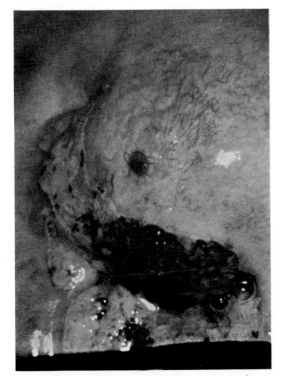

Figure 83. Old organized traumatic petechiae, in the shape of a spider angioma.

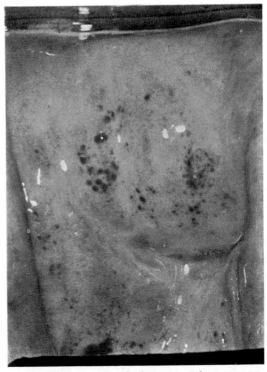

Figure 84. Petechial or senile vaginitis which coexists with some subepithelial hemorrhages, occurring in an intensely atrophic mucosa.

techiae in 10 per cent, and the remaining common images of the cervix reduced to less than 15 per cent. Lastly in the late or presenile climacterium, the predominant lesion is atrophic mucosa in its two variants, with petechiae (48 per cent) and without (18 per cent).

Histologically, the most outstanding feature, as we have already indicated, is the extreme thinness of the epithelium, especially at the expense of its intermediate layer, which may be absent entirely. The stroma becomes fibrous due to progressive degeneration of its elastic component, and there is always a certain degree of leukocytic infiltration, much more accentuated when a petechial vaginitis coexists (Fig. 85).

The papillae disappear slowly, so that years after the menopause, the columnar epithelium still shows faint undulations.

When small subepithelial hemorrhages have occurred, they appear on histologic preparations as small elevations of the cellular coating; these represent the residua of hemorrhagic vesicles which ultimately peel off the stroma (Fig. 86).

Special Forms of Atrophic Mucosa. There are three colposcopic forms of atrophic mucosa, with well defined characteristics, which separate them from the usual type.

ALABASTER MUCOSA. Its most obvious factor is the marbled appearance which it gives to the exocervical surface. Aside from its smoothness and absence of elevations, typical of the atrophic mucosa, its whitish lichenoid color is remarkable and justifies its comparison with marble or alabaster. Blood vessels are difficult to observe, and hemorrhagic accidents are rare. Biopsy reveals, along an extremely thin epithelium, a hyalinized stroma with an almost total absence of vascular structure (Fig. 87). Beneath it, a lymphocytic infiltration is usually found.

PACHYDERMAL MUCOSA. When atrophic mucosa is exposed for a long time to an inhospitable medium which distends and dehydrates it, as occurs with uterine prolapse, its superficial layers are thickened (reactive keratinization) as a defense mechanism. As this objective is only partly achieved, in addition to frequent erosions and ulcerations, a wrinkling of the epithelium is produced and partial separation from the underlying stroma occurs. Under the colposcope, this mucosa appears extraordinarily dry, wrinkled, and furrowed by creases, which are more or less parallel but do cross each other (Figs. 88 and 89).

ATROPHIC INFLAMMATORY MUCOSA. Atrophic mucosa, subjected to an intense inflammatory process, acquires a tomentose appearance in which smoothness is replaced by embossing, pale color by reddening, and the dryness by a blood-tinged discharge. Careful colposcopic observation shows marked vascular hyperplasia, with the presence of vascular papillae which resolve superficially in tiny extravasations. If doubt still exists after colposcopy, institute anti-inflammatory treatment and then repeat the examination.

Dystrophic Erosion. There are three types: the "erosion" that accompanies an intensely atrophic mucosa; the erosion associated with uterine prolapse; and the erosion without apparent traumatic cause, unquestionably benign, and coexisting with an apparently normal mucosa.

ATROPHIC EROSION. When the mucosa of the cervix is affected by accentuated atrophy, with abundant hemorrhagic subepithelial suffusion and petechial vaginitis, it is not rare that major or minor loss of epithelium is produced by simple placement of the speculum or even spontaneously. On occasion, erosion is limited to the site where an intense vaginitis existed or where a former episode of subepithelial hemorrhage occurred (Fig. 90). In these cases a denuded stroma is seen, with its traumatized vessels. The edges of the lesion are very clear, since remnants of the peeled off mucosa remain (Fig. 91). Erosions may be multiple (Fig. 92).

The speculum can easily cause "traumatic erosion," even without a very atrophic mucosa, when the cervix is off center, descended or fixed, and the instrument is difficult to place.

These erosions rarely tend to resolve spontaneously, resulting instead in adhesions between the two vaginal walls.

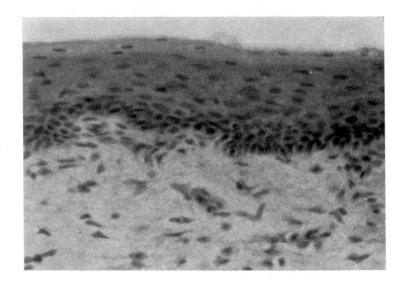

Figure 85. Histologic section of atrophic mucosa. The marked thinning of the epithelium is characteristic, with an almost complete disappearance of the intermediate layer.

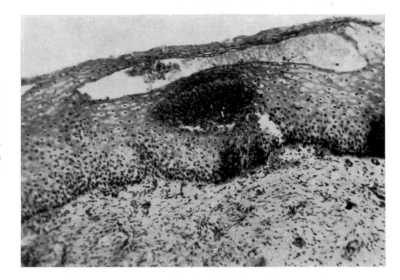

Figure 86. Histology of a-trophic mucosa affected by pete-chial vaginitis and subepithelial hemorrhages. Observe the pres-ence of a hemorrhagic vesicle (the central dark spot) and a serosan-guineous one above it. The stroma is affected by a leukocytic in-filtration.

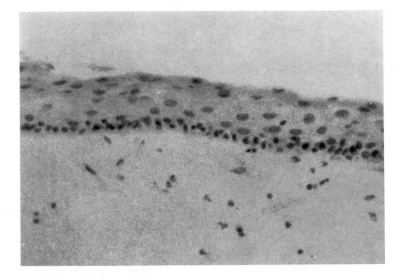

Figure 87. Histology of so-called "alabaster mucosa." Be-sides the extreme thinness of the epithelium, the most charac-teristic finding is hyalinization of the stroma, which almost totally lacks vessels.

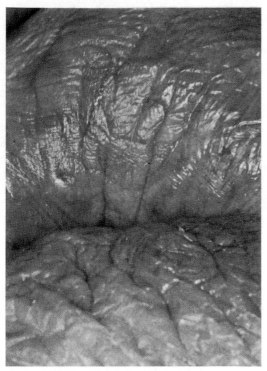

Figure 88. Pachydermal mucosa in uterine prolapse. Besides its notable sensation of dryness, this mucosa exhibits folds with radial orientation.

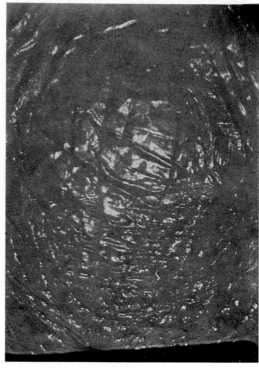

Figure 89. Wrinkled mucosa with phenomena of tissue dehydration, furrowed in a manner that resembles a brick pavement.

These then may be loosened violently as the result of vaginal exploration or coitus. This is the condition formerly called "adhesive" or "atretic vaginitis."

Colposcopy done at this time may lead one to suspect a malignant process, due to the irregularity of the lateral vaginal fornices, which ooze abundant blood and exhibit extensive erosions. The existence of anomalous vascular pathways (corkscrew type) of unequal caliber increase colposcopic doubt (Fig. 93). Bolten advised the application of a vaginal cream with estrogens for 8 to 15 days. Improvement in the appearance of the lesions verifies their dystrophic origin. The role of atrophy in the origin of this type of erosion is made clear when comparing the incidence of these lesions in women of reproductive age (1 per cent) and in senility (6 per cent).

EROSIONS COEXISTING WITH UTERINE PROLAPSE. The coexistence of mucosa in the process of atrophy with uterine prolapse increases the possibility of erosions and even extensive ulcerations, visible without the aid of colposcopy (Fig. 96). They are characterized by lack of bleeding and intense keratinization of the bordering epithelium (true keratinization due to adaptation to the medium), which causes the edges of the lesion to become more apparent (Fig. 97). In many cases they are authentic ulcerations, and when the basement membrane is ruptured, granular tissue is found by histology (Figs. 94 and 95). Around these areas of loss of substance, the mucosa is somewhat altered and may appear dry and wrinkled.

For many years it has been said that it is exceptional for cancer to coexist with these types of erosions. However, Stone and Mansell have demonstrated that malignant transformation occurs once in each 100 cases of prolapsed uterus subjected to persistent irritation. Mossetti and Russo give an even larger incidence

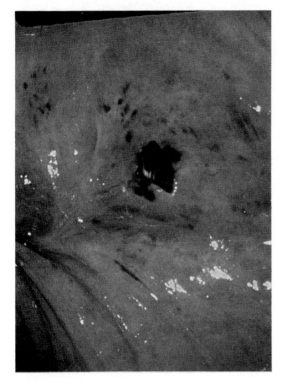

Figure 90. Atrophic erosion, on a mucosa with petechial and small subepithelial hemorrhages.

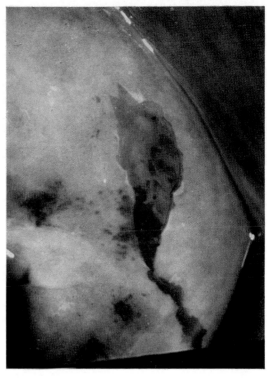

Figure 91. Traumatic dystrophic erosion. The edges are clearly seen, and the stroma shows numerous hemorrhages.

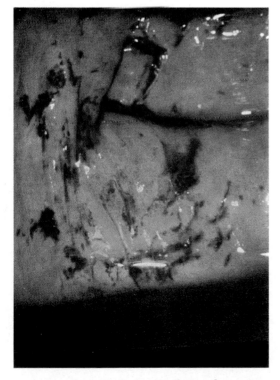

Figure 92. Multiple atrophic and traumatic erosions. Placing the speculum has caused erosions and subepithelial hemorrhages.

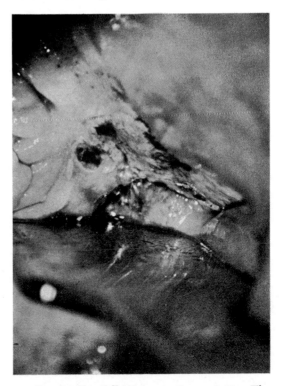

Figure 93. Adhesive, atretic vaginitis. The vaginal fornix with multiple erosions and ulcerations makes the presence of cancer likely.

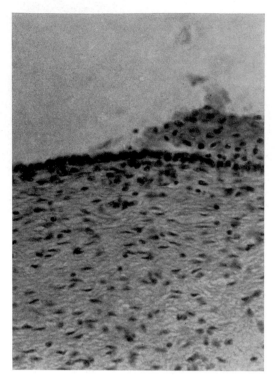

Figure 94. Histopathology of erosion. The stroma is not affected and the basement membrane is intact. Observe the epithelial edge.

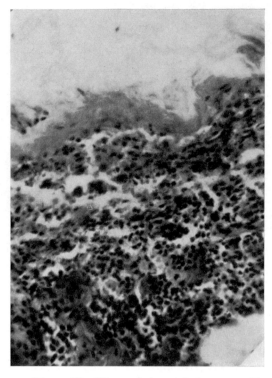

Figure 95. Histopathology of ulceration. Observe the existence of granulation tissue.

(9.7 per cent of their total number of cases of prolapse). We have published two cases of carcinoma in situ in ulcerated uterine prolapse in elderly women, and other authors have presented similar cases. The apparent rarity of this malignant transformation is probably due to incomplete studies of the operative specimen.

DYSTROPHIC EROSION WITH NORMAL MUCOSA. It is rare but not exceptional to see a fairly extensive and evident non-bleeding erosion, not located near the cervical os (which would make it suspicious), coexisting with a completely normal cervical mucosa (Fig. 98). Many times it presents the appearance of a simple "noncharacteristic red zone" until silver nitrate makes them evident. Then it can be seen that the erosion is not single, but multiple. There can be various causes of this condition, of which the most likely, in the absence of an infection or malignant process, is vitamin A deficiency. If, jointly with the vaginal mucosa, the buccal and tracheal mucosa

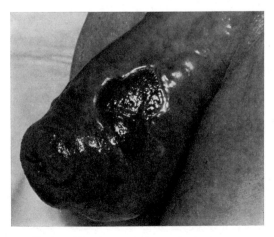

Figure 96. A cervicovaginal ulceration complicating total uterine prolapse.

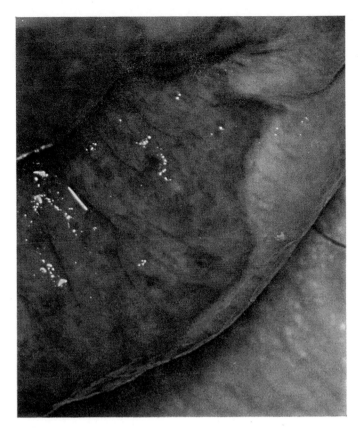

Figure 97. Ulceration associated with uterine prolapse. Besides the absence of bleeding, note the intense keratinization of the raised epithelium that sharply borders the ulceration.

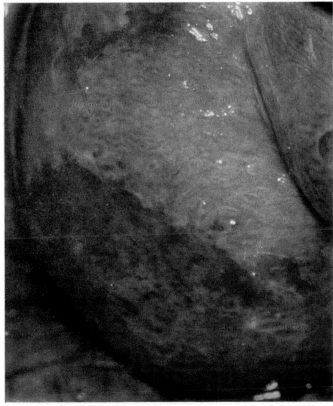

Figure 98. Dystrophic erosion which coexists with an apparently normal cervicovaginal mucosa. The lesion became evident only after application of acetic acid.

are affected, a toxic mechanism should be considered, and the condition is probably secondary to a drug allergy.

In these cases the epithelium comes away in large sheets. The vascular elements of the stroma are hypertrophied and hyperplastic, and it is not unusual to see an erythematous reaction around the lesion (Fig. 99). If the erosion is not seen in the acute phase, but rather days or weeks later, a typical collar may be seen around the process in a healing state.

Leukoplakia. The introduction of colposcopy has permitted better study of this lesion, which has long been known because it is visible to the naked eye. It is necessary to divorce the colposcopic concept from the histologic. The colposcopist speaks of "leukoplakia" or a "leukoplakic area" in the presence of a white spot, while the histologist requires the presence of a pathologic cornification (keratosis or parakeratosis) which increases the thickness of the superficial layers of the mucosa at the expense of the intermediate layers, which practically disappear (D'Alessandro and Bernardini).

According to its density as perceived at exploration, leukoplakia has been classified as delicate, simple, hypertrophic and verrucous (p. 135). The first two types usually form part of the "atypical re-epithelialization zone" (p. 146) and usually are not leukoplakias in the histologic meaning of the term. Their whitish aspect is due to a much heavier cellular or nuclear density of the epithelium. The other two types may belong to an "atypical transformation zone" (p. 164) with much superficial keratosis or, to the contrary, may represent a simple dystrophic lesion.

True leukoplakia of dystrophic origin is usually present as plaques of variable size, which are always visible, even without previous preparation. They are located in completely healthy mucosa, generally far from the cervical os. Occasionally, they are found in the region between the columnar and squamous epithelium, giving the appearance of an excessive keratinization of a stable atypical scar (p. 160). Rarely are they seen in the vagina.

The borders may be somewhat blurred, and in spite of the elevation of the lesion, it may have the neatness of a stable atypical scar. Its surface may be completely smooth or verrucous, with more or less deep furrows. Fundamental characteristics are an absence of any other superimposed patterns (if there are any, a dystrophic origin must be excluded) and a lack of vessels (Fig. 101). Leukoplakic lesions do not fix iodine (Fig. 100). Only rarely are dystrophic leukoplakic plaques seen in an "iceberg" form (Fig. 104).

An attempt to pull off these dystrophic lesions is followed by persistent bleeding from the base, which is formed by a papillar stroma.

Leukoplakia may be single or multiple. There is a variety called "cotton ball," characterized by the presence of a leukoplakic spotting, having marked elevation, above an extensive area of cervicovaginal mucosa. It really represents a leukoplakic papillomatosis (p. 202).

It is said that cervical secretion in these cases is lessened, and that dystrophic leukoplakia generally exists in a dry medium.

These leukoplakic dystrophies may be due to deficiencies in the neurovascular supply or to the presence of repeated trauma.

Despite the fact that leukoplakia of dystrophic origin is a totally benign lesion which tends to heal spontaneously if the cause disappears, it is convenient to perform a biopsy to avoid missing a diagnosis of an atypical transformation zone. The only exception is the leukoplakia of a prolapse; in this case, the proper approach is surgical correction of the problem, if possible by vaginal hysterectomy.

Histologically, besides the absence of dysplastic signs (regular basal membrane, sparse activity of the germinative layer of cells, well ordered stratified epithelium), superficial keratosis and parakeratosis are notable. This is the reason for the colposcopic appearance, not a true increase in cellular or nuclear density (Fig. 103).

Superficial Deciduosis. This dystrophy will be studied in Chapter 9; it is a decidual reaction of the covering epithelium, which has definite colposcopic characteristics.

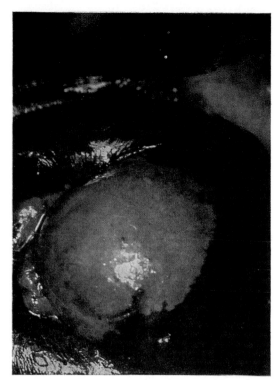

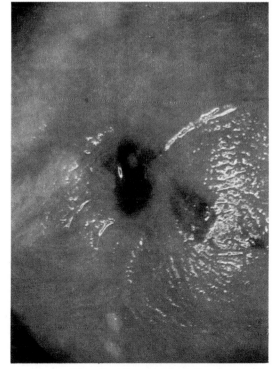

Figure 99. Old dystrophic erosion. The hyperplasia of the vascular elements of the stroma is noteworthy.

Figure 100. Dystrophic leukoplakia after application of Lugol's solution. The fact that this type of lesion does not take up iodine is confirmed.

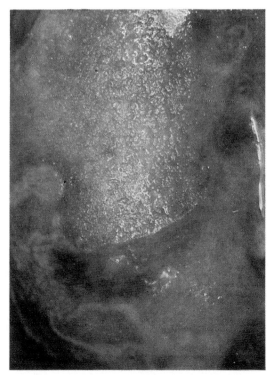

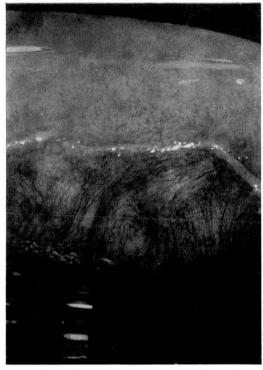

Figure 101. Dystrophic leukoplakia due to prolapse.

Figure 102. Postelectrocoagulation dystrophic leukoplakia.

Glandular Dystrophies

Two types of glandular dystrophies are recognized, according to whether the glandular alteration affects the normal mucosal epithelium of the cervix or is ectopic endometrial glandular tissue.

Glandular Cysts. These are very frequent in the irregular variety of typical re-epithelialization. A type of retention cyst with a larger volume than usual can cause modifications of the external appearance of the cervix. These cysts of the glandular elements are more or less deeply situated and are prevalent in the premenopausal woman, whose hormonal disturbance favors hyperplasia of any preexisting glandular residua.

From a colposcopic viewpoint, two varieties are distinguished:

SUPERFICIAL GLANDULAR CYST (ORDINARILY KNOWN AS NABOTHIAN FOLLICLE). The development of this retention cyst is superficial, and the thinning of the stratified mucosa which covers it is notable due to distention by its contents, making it possible to visualize the characteristics of the secretion (thick, clear, or opalescent mucus). Two or three vessels of large caliber invade it, with pseudoanastomosis of their branches forming a dense network. The whole has a characteristic yellowish color (Fig. 105).

DEEP GLANDULAR CYST. Between the encysted gland and the epithelial surface, there is a greater thickness of the stroma, which causes the cyst to be hidden, but its consequences are felt: distortion of the surface and even of the cervix as a whole. These cysts may be formed near the cervical os, deflecting it and causing stenosis of the canal. There are no characteristic colposcopic signs, but puncture of the cyst will make the diagnosis (Fig. 107).

Histologic study of these formations reveals in both varieties a large distended glandular cyst containing mucus (Fig. 106). The only difference is in topography. In the first type the cyst is located immediately under the covering epithelium, which even modifies itself to resist the pressure of the contents. In the second type, between the epithelium and the cyst there is a thick intact stroma

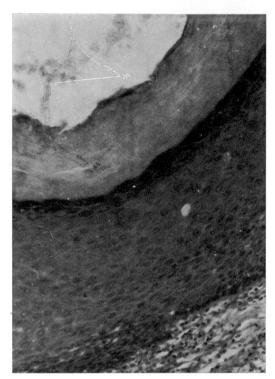

Figure 103. Histopathology of dystrophic leukoplakia due to prolapse. Superficial keratosis and parakeratosis are evident, but there are no other signs of dysplasia in the rest of the mucosa.

which protects the epithelium against cystic distention.

Endometriosis. The existence of ectopic endometrial tissue at the level of the cervix is relatively frequent following coagulation therapy (Bret, Branscomb, Coupez), and in women who have undergone cervical repair after delivery or curettage (Allan and Cowan). In contrast to statistics prepared by pathologists (Fluhmann, Williams, Overton, Murphy, Wolfe, etc.), we rarely see lesions of this type. The colposcopic incidence of endometriosis has been diversely estimated by different authors, the percentages varying between 0.1 and 0.4 (Table 16).

In our experience three forms are possible:

PSEUDOTUMOR FORM. A cyst the size of a medium or large nabothian follicle, but of a blue, violet, or brown color is

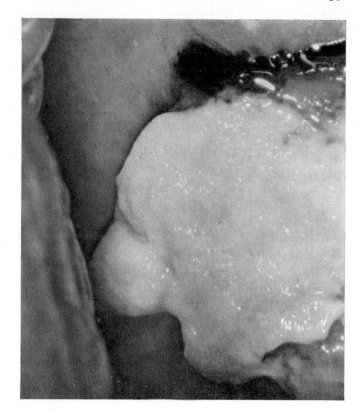

Figure 104. "Iceberg" leukoplakia. Its elevation and nacreous surface are characteristic.

Figure 105. Very vascularized superficial glandular cyst, close to the anatomic external os.

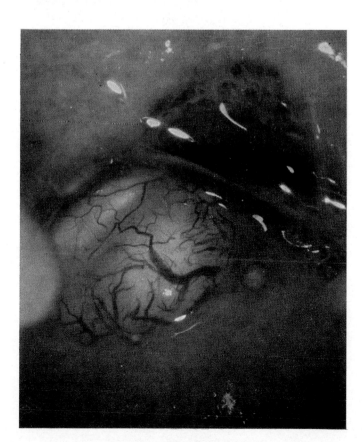

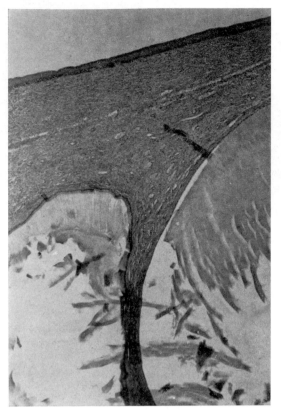 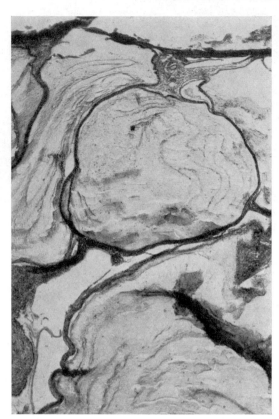

Figure 106. Histopathologic appearance of glandular cysts, containing mucus and buried under a layer of squamous epithelium of metaplastic origin.

seen (Fig. 108). There are some vessels in its surface, but always less abundant than in the mucoid cysts. Puncture of this cyst produces a liquid that looks like chocolate (Bret, Coupez, and Grepinet).

Jahier and Gautray have described formations of considerable size which they called "endometriomas" and which grow significantly during gestation. We have seen some cases of this nature (Fig. 109).

ULCERATED FORM. Quite probably these are caused by rupture of the chocolate cysts (Fig. 110). Identification of the absence of squamous epithelium on the surface is facilitated with Lugol's solution, or better yet with silver nitrate. They are distinguished from other types of ulceration because during menstruation they bleed considerably, and by the absence of infiltration around them (Fig. 111).

FLAT FORM. These are congested red plaques, as seen after treatment with acetic acid, which are generally situated around the cervical os and which become swollen and even bleed during the menses (Fig. 112). At other times, they may be nearly invisible and have a linear appearance. Most of these are sequelae of previous coagulation (Jahier and Gautray), and not infrequently they are multiple (Dilts and Greene).

The differential diagnosis includes hemorrhagic retention cysts (much deeper red color, more abundant superficial vessels), hemangiomas (absence of menstrual variations, multiple images), and some hypertrophic varieties of deciduosis (different color).

Histology confirms the diagnosis in 70 per cent of cases. The remainder represent either colposcopic errors or, as is more frequent (Gardner, Williams), in-

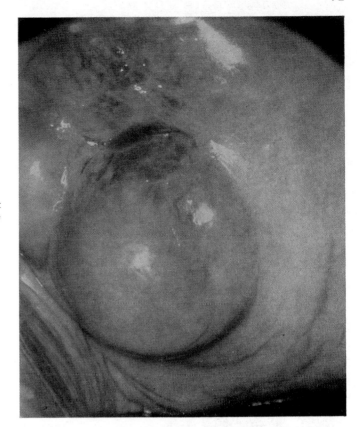

Figure 107. Deep glandular cyst which modifies the gross aspect of the cervix.

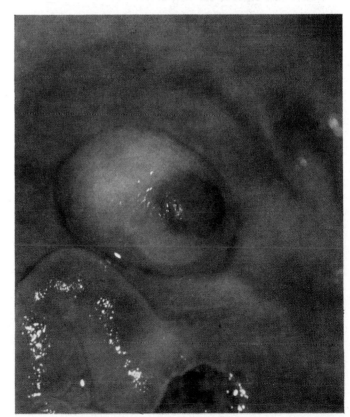

Figure 108. Pseudotumor endometriosis. A presumptive diagnosis is made on the basis of the purplish-blue color.

Table 16. Colposcopic Frequency of Cervical Endometriosis

	NO. OF COLPOSCOPIES	PERCENTAGE
Chali, Hermansson and Davison (1965)	3,265	0.11
Lagruta, Laguens and Quijano (1966)	3,141	0.12
Candia and Asua (1965)	2,945	0.13
Arenas et al. (1961)	?	0.20
diPaola and Vásquez (1958)	2,000	0.30
Aruta (1971)	4,000	0.40
Bret, Coupez and Grepinet (1965)	2,031	0.44
Our Series (1969)	10,000	0.11

correct biopsy procedure. Pressure of the punch biopsy forceps can rupture the cyst and empty its contents. Use of a rotating cutting biotome instrument is therefore recommended (Aruta). Examination of specimens obtained by careful biopsy of these formations shows the presence of glandular tissue of an endometrial type, whose appearance varies according to the time in the cycle and the width of the exocervical mucosa. Many times pseudocystic cavities are seen, filled with degenerated blood which arises from the functional activity of the ectopic endometrial epithelium. These cavities may communicate with the outside (by previous rupture), or be deeply located in the cervical wall, as occurs in endocervical endometriosis (Gardner).

Stromal Dystrophies

These dystrophic lesions are reviewed on page 238 in our discussion of the colposcopic appearances of the gravid cervix. As we see it, all of them are based histologically on the decidual transformation of the cellular components of the stroma.

Vascular Dystrophies

These disorders have in common a vascular hypertrophy caused by trophic or nutritional alterations of the cervix. They may occur in several circumstances:

(1) After cervical coagulation. Thickened vascular elements will be found at different levels around the cervical os. (Fig. 113). Because of this localization, they may be mistaken for endometriosis (Bret). The differential diagnosis is established by the absence of swelling during the menses, and also because along these vessels, the two other colposcopic appearances that characterize a cervix after coagulation will be seen: "rake-like" images and the presence of "re-epithelialization of hemorrhagic vesicles," which disappear some months after coagulation. This last colposcopic pattern has been histologically studied by Janata et al. It is also not unusual to see as an accompanying lesion the "superficial papillary elevation" of Hinselmann.

(2) During pregnancy. At this time real varices may appear. Changes in the blood supply during pregnancy cause vascular dilatation which generally does not cause diagnostic problems because, besides its evident etiology, it does not present other anomalies (Fig. 114).

(3) During the climacterium, both pre- and postmenopause. There are two causes: sclerotic alteration of the venous wall and steroid hormonal disturbances (Fig. 115). At this time a considerable amount of vascular thickening is seen, which is similar to the serpentine varicosities of the lower limbs.

(4) In association with alterations of steroid equilibrium, both exogenous and endogenous. Vascularity is increased in

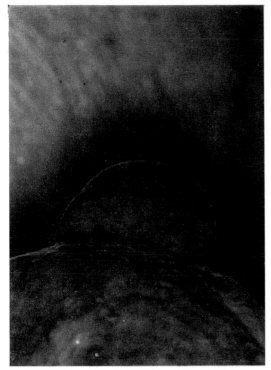

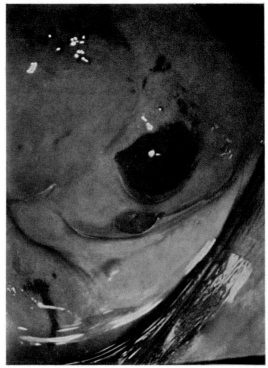

Figure 109. Endometrioma in a pregnant cervix. Its brownish color attracts attention.

Figure 110. Over a focus of an intact pseudotumor endometriosis, another larger ulcerated one is seen.

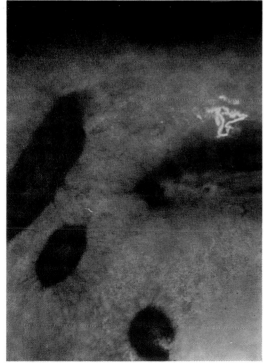

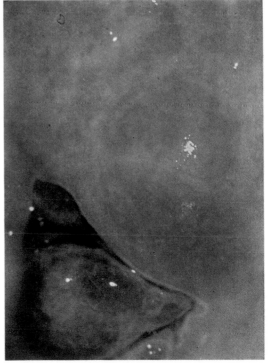

Figure 111. Ulcerative endometriosis. The large red zone is a true ulceration, but the other two are simple congestive spots.

Figure 112. Flat endometriosis in the premenstrual phase. At another time in the cycle it was less apparent.

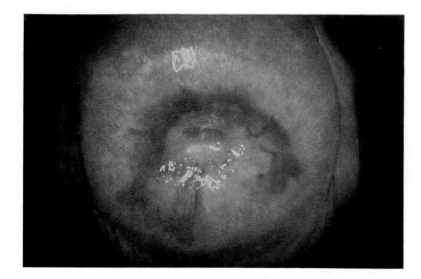

Figure 113. Vascular irregularities after electrocoagulation of an ectopy.

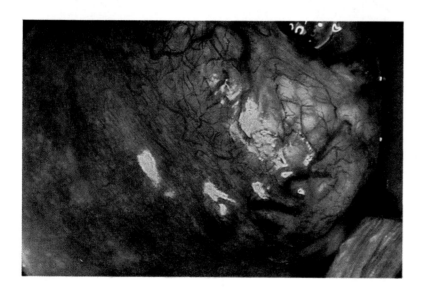

Figure 114. Vascular irregularities (phlebectasia) in a pregnant cervix.

practically all patients on more than six months of anovulatory therapy (Fig. 116), but in 35 per cent of these, thick vessels are seen (although normally oriented), as well as isolated vascular skeins in a zone of well determined typical re-epithelialization, and vessels of normal caliber that have adapted definitely pathologic forms (corkscrews, forks, etc.) (Table 17). Other authors have observed similar phenomena (Carbia et al.).

(5) When an exaggerated histologic proliferation exists. In these cases an "adaptative vascular hypertrophy" takes place, and the vessels, in order to provide a sufficient blood supply and to avoid necrosis, may adopt monstrous shapes. We will deal with this type of vascular alteration on page 215 when referring to malignant neoplastic images.

In all cases the result of a biopsy, considered in conjunction with the appearance of the vascular anomalies, determines the existence of diverse epithelial alterations, ranging from metaplastic phenomena of regeneration to epithelial

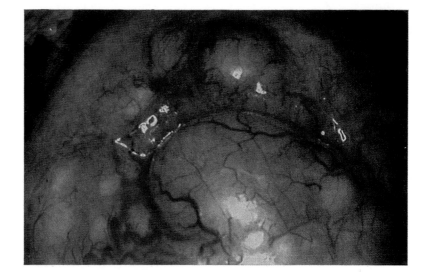

Fig. 115. Vascular irregularities in the cervix of a woman at the climacterium. This is a short-lived hypertrophy of old vascular changes.

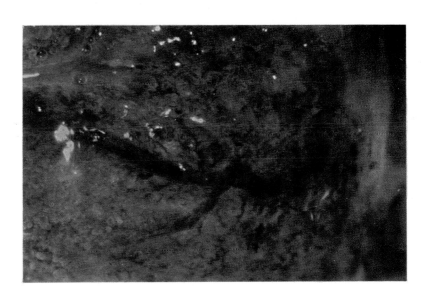

Figure 116. Vascular irregularities after prolonged use of anovulatory agents. The thickness of the vessels makes them resemble varices.

atrophy and a constant leukocytic infiltration of the stroma, especially accentuated around the vascular structures. Histologic study is obligatory when vascular anomalies compatible with malignant change are seen.

CYTOLOGIC CORRELATIONS

Logically, the only dystrophies which may have some cytologic identity are the epithelial ones. The others lack any desquamative expression, if they are really accompanied by an intact epithelium. Atrophic mucosa usually corresponds with Papanicolaou's intermediate smears (31.2 per cent of mucosa with incipient atrophy), parabasal smears (43.7 per cent of atrophic mucosa without petechiae), or frankly atrophic smears (95 per cent of atrophic mucosa with petechiae) (Fig. 117 and Table 18). From the point of view of this classification, "atrophic mucosa with petechial vaginitis" is

Table 17. Role of Anovulatory Agents in the Appearance of Dystrophic Vascular Anomalies

Incidence	
Expected percentage of vascular irregularities	3.8%
Percentage after anovulatory treatment (more than 6 months)	35.6%
According to the anovulatory agent used	
With classical anovulatory agents	52 %
With sequential anovulatory agents	48 %

accompanied by a high order of suspicious cytology (30 per cent of the smears). On the other hand, atrophic mucosa without petechial changes reveals only a 1.5 per cent incidence of Classes II-III and III (Table 19). Undoubtedly, the serious epithelial trophic disturbances producing the petechiae are responsible for the cellular alterations, but these do not imply any increased frequency of malignant changes.

Thanks to colposcopy it is not necessary to carry out conizations in these cases of suspicious cytology. Bolten recognized a marked decrease in this diagnostic operation after colposcopy is introduced in a given gynecologic service.

When the dystrophic erosion has atrophy as its cause, it is most often seen during the late climacterium and during senility. In 66.6 per cent of cases it is accompanied by totally atrophic smears, and in the remainder by smears of the parabasal type.

The rare dystrophic erosions of the nonclimacteric woman, since they coexist with normal cervicovaginal mucosa, do not have cytologic identity.

Just as in atrophic mucosa with petechial vaginitis, erosions are associated with an increased finding of Papanicolaou's Classes II-III smears (33 per cent of our cases).

Leukoplakia of dystrophic origin yields an inconsistent number of keratinized superficial cells, without nuclei and strongly eosinophilic, of a slightly smaller size than normal superficial cells (Fig. 118). In routine cervical scraping, this cell type is observed in less than 20 per cent of all smears, corresponding to patients with cervical keratosis or parakeratosis. In our experience the frequency of those cells increases when scraping is selectively done over a leukoplakic area. Then about 50 to 60 per cent of all smears show this cell type.

Superficial deciduosis (see p. 240) with its specific histologic correlation (decidual reaction of the covering epithelium) may be accompanied by some cytologic modifications which, in essence, consist of hydrophilic degeneration of the cytoplasm in some superficial and intermediate cells. Quite probably it is a special type of balloon-like degeneration (p. 236).

CLINICAL COURSE

Generally, the evolution of dystrophic lesions is uneventful, with a low incidence of malignant transformation. Some of these lesions recede spontaneously, as occurs after delivery with the deciduosis and vascular hypertrophy of pregnancy. Others recede only partially, examples being the hypertrophic glandu-

Table 18. Distribution of Cell Types Found in Papanicolaou Smears in Atrophic Mucosa

	WITHOUT PETECHIAE	WITH PETECHIAE
Superficial type	0.0%	0.0%
Intermediate type	31.2%	2.5%
Parabasal type	43.7%	2.5%
Atrophic type	16.0%	95.0%

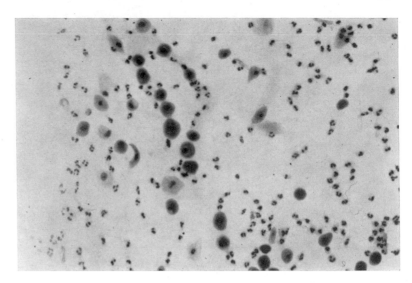

Figure 117. Cytologic smear of an atrophic mucosa. The most characteristic finding is the presence of abundant deep cells (basal and parabasal).

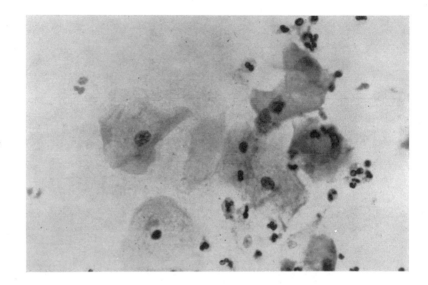

Figure 118. Cytologic smear of an extensive area of dystrophic cervical leukoplakia. The existence of keratinized anucleated superficial cells is typical.

lar sequelae of irregular re-epithelialization (retention cysts) and endometrial ectopies.

In fact, after the temporary endocrine crisis of the premenopause, all glandular dystrophies will wane due to the absence of the hormonal stimulus that maintained them. Those that originate from transient toxic or hyperallergenic causes will also disappear spontaneously.

Certain dystrophies will improve with re-establishment of tissue homeostasis. Examples are erosions caused by a deficit in vitamin A or the vascular irregularities associated with exogenous or endogenous steroid disturbance.

Some dystrophies will remain indefinitely if the causative factors persist. This is true of irritative or adaptive leukoplakia caused by a genital dystrophy (uterine prolapse or cervical elongation)

Table 19. Distribution of Papanicolaou Smear Results
in Atrophic Mucosa

	WITH PETECHIAE	WITHOUT PETECHIAE
Class I	26.5%	2.4%
Class II	71.8%	67.4%
Class II–III	1.5%	20.0%
Class III	0.0%	10.0%
Class IV	0.0%	0.1%

and also by the ulcerations caused by these same factors.

Finally, some lesions will undergo aggravation with augmentation of the endocrine deficit which initiated the process. An example is menopausal atrophic mucosa which, at the presenile climacterium, will acquire morphologic characteristics (petechial vaginitis, atrophic erosions) indicative of the deep trophic-nutritional disturbance.

MANAGEMENT

Nothing needs to be done for a colposcopically well defined dystrophy which, in addition to presenting almost no clinical manifestations, has a tendency to spontaneous regression. The most typical example is "deciduosis"; with a follow-up colposcopic examination 2 to 3 months after delivery, its complete disappearance is usually verified.

In the case of vascular irregularities of iatrogenic cause (such as anovulatory therapy) it is unnecessary to take therapeutic measures except to stop the medication until the picture improves substantially.

On the contrary, some epithelial dystrophies, which cause bloody discharges and irritative complaints, should be treated medically. Atrophic mucosa with or without petechial vaginitis and the dystrophic erosion found in some climacteric women are hypohormonal states with superimposed inflammation. They improve notably with vitamin A and estriol, given orally, intramuscularly, or

topically, along with topical anti-inflammatory agents (antibiotics, sulfonamides, corticoids, etc.).

The absence of estrogenic activity in the endometrium makes it permissible to administer large doses without causing uterine bleeding due to estrogen withdrawal.

A certain number of epithelial erosions, with normal surrounding mucosa, also improve with vitamin A.

Some dystrophies require surgical treatment to solve the underlying problem. This occurs with erosions and ulcerations associated with total uterine prolapse, and with the irritative leukoplakia of similar origin. In these cases the continued trauma suffered by the cervicovaginal mucosa may explain a certain tendency toward malignant change.

Finally, the opportunity for treatment of certain lesions will be determined by their clinical manifestations. This occurs with some glandular dystrophies. If a given nabothian follicle or endometrioma causes discomfort due to its size, because of concomitant descensus uteri, or simply because it has been noted by the patient, its volume may be reduced by evacuating its contents or by extirpation. Excision should probably be accompanied by a plastic operation to reestablish the architecture of the cervix, possibly deformed by the cyst.

Endometriosis, especially in its ulcerated form, may be accompanied by postcoital bleeding and bloody discharge. If these lesions are not accompanied by symptoms, they only require periodic control.

The vascular sequelae of coagulation

may be more serious. Another fulguration may be attempted, including the hypervascularized areas, but if vascular hypertrophy again appears, surgical conization is advised.

Ranney et al. advise against the use of any prophylactic antibiotic or sulfonamide vaginal creams after cervical cauterization, because they believe that ectopic endometrial implantation is possible only in a surface free of infection.

REFERENCES

Abbas, T. M.: Postmenopausal genital bleeding: An analysis of 180 cases. Med. Press, 244:250, 1960.

Allan, N., and Cowan, L. E.: Primary endometriosis of the cervical remnant following a Manchester repair operation. Obstet. Gynec., 22:253, 1963.

Aruta, J.: Diagnóstico colposcópico de la endometriosis cervical. Rev. Arg. Ginec. Obstet., 2:86, 1971.

Balagueró, L.: Endometriosis primaria del cuello uterino. Toko-Ginec. Práct., 24:523, 1965.

Baruffi, I., Brandão, H. J. S., and Valeri, V.: Über die Regeneration des Portioepithel nach Elektrokoagulation. Zbl. Gynäk., 88:199, 1966.

Bernoth, E., and Bettzieche, H.: Die verschorfte Portio vaginalis uteri (Ergebnisse klinischer und morphologischer Nachuntersuchungen). Zbl. Gynäk., 86:185, 1964.

Bolten, K. A.: Colposcopy, Histopathology, and Cytology: A correlation study. Thesis, University of Oklahoma Medical Center, 1965.

Bolten, K. A.: Practical colposcopy in early cervical and vaginal cancer. Clin. Obstet. Gynec., 10:808, 1967.

Bouda, J., and Dohnal, V.: Zur Frage der Krebsprophylaxe durch Elektrokoagulation bei Ektopie und Umwandlungszone. Geburtsh. u. Frauenheilk., 25:1186, 1965.

Branscomb, L.: Habitual premenstrual spotting following electrocauterization of the cervix: A newly observed phenomenon. Am. J. Obstet. Gynec., 79:16, 1960.

Bret, J., and Coupez, F.: Colposcopie. Paris, Masson et Cie., 1960.

Bret, J., and Coupez, F.: Le traitement des cervicites par électrocoagulation: Séquelles vasculaires et endométriose du col. Gynéc. Obstét., 64:483, 1965.

Bret, J., and Coupez, F.: Colposcopie. In Encyclopédie Médico-Chirurgicale, Paris, 60 B, 1969.

Bret, J., Coupez, F., and Grepinet, J.: Sur les endométrioses du col. Bull. Féd. Soc. Gynéc. Obstét., 17(Suppl. 5):652, 1965.

Candia, E., and Asua, P. A.: Soc. Arg. Pat. Cerv. Ut. y Colposc., Act. Cong., Buenos Aires, 1:289, 1965.

Carbia, E., Alvarado-Duran, A., and Lopez-Llera, M.: Colposcopic study of the uterine cervix during administration of ethynodiol diacetate with mestranol. Am. J. Obstet. Gynec., 102:1023, 1968.

Carrera, J. M., and Dexeus, S., Jr.: Estudio colposcópico de los cambios cervicales inducidos por anovulatorios orales. Progr. Obstet. Ginec., 14:1, 1971.

Chali, A., Hermansson, A., and Davison, J.: Soc. Arg. Pat. Cerv. Ut. y Colposc., Act. Cong., Buenos Aires, 1:313, 1965.

Coupez, F.: Endométriose du col utérin. Gynéc., 287, 1966.

D'Alessandro, P., and Bernardini, G.: Aspetti istologici di alcune lesioni colposcopiche. Quad. Clin. Obstet. Ginec., 18(Suppl.):1511, 1963.

deBrux, J.: Histopathologique Gynecologique. Paris, Masson et Cie., 1971.

Dexeus, S., Jr., Carrera, J. M., and Palacin, A.: Carcinoma in situ en la vejez. Bol. Asoc. Obst. Ginec. Acad. Cienc. Med., 1:303, 1966.

Dilts, P. V., Jr., and Greene, R. R.: Multiple areas of endometriosis of the ectocervix and vagina. Am. J. Obstet. Gynec., 91:292, 1965.

di Paola, G., and Vasquez Ferro, E.: Comentario sobre 2000 colposcopias. Bol. Soc. Obstet. Ginec. Buenos Aires, 37:140, 1958.

Ferrario, E.: Aspetti colposcopici dell'endometriosi della portio e della vagina. Clinica Ginec., 3:542, 1961.

Fluhmann, C. F.: The Cervix Uteri and Its Diseases. Philadelphia, W. B. Saunders Co., 1961.

Gardner, H. L.: Cervical endometriosis, a lesion of increasing importance. Am. J. Obstet. Gynec., 84:170, 1962.

Gompel, C.: Anatomie Pathologique Gynécologique et Obstétricale: Corrélations Anatomoclinique. Brussels, Éditions Arscia, 1963.

Hinselmann, H.: Einfuhrung in die Kolposkopie. Hamburg, Paul Hartung, 1933.

Jahier, H., Laffargue, P., Gautray, J. P., and Jahier, J.: Les endométriomes du col utérin. Gynéc. Obstét., 60:606, 1961.

Janata, J., Filip, O., and Kolář, F.: Die durch Elektrokoagulation hervorgerufenen Zervixveränderungen. Zbl. Gynäk., 85:1623, 1963.

Lagrutta, J., Laguens, R. P., and Quijano, F.: Cancer de Cuello Uterino: Estados Primarios. Buenos Aires, Editorial Intermedica, 1966.

Masciotta, A.: La Colposcopia nella Lotta Contro Il Cancro e nella Diagnosi Ginecologica. Bologna, Licinio Cappelli, 1954.

Masukawa, T.: Vaginal smears in women past 40 years of age, with emphasis on their remaining hormonal activity. Obstet. Gynec., 16:407, 1960.

Mestwerdt, G.: Atlas der Kolposkopie. Jena, Gustav Fischer, 1953.

Mossetti, C., and Russo, A.: Osservazioni sui rapporti fra carcinoma del collo dell'utero e prolasso. Minerva Ginec., 10:785, 1958.

Murphy, E. J., and Herbut, P. A.: The uterine cervix during pregnancy. Am. J. Obstet. Gynec., 59:384, 1950.

Novak, E. R., and Woodruff, J. D.: Novak's Gynecologic and Obstetric Pathology. 7th ed. Philadelphia, W. B. Saunders Co., 1974.

Overton, D. H., Jr., Wilson, R. B., and Dockerty,
M. B.: Primary endometriosis of the cervix. Am. J.
Obstet. Gynec., 79:768, 1960.

Pelletier, J.-P., and Latour, J.-P.-A.: Incidence du
cancer dans la ménopause. Union Méd. Canada,
89:33, 1960.

Ranney, B., and Chung, J. T.: Endometriosis of the
cervix uteri. Am. J. Obstet. Gynec., 64:1333, 1952.

Rigaill: Endometriose du col de l'uterus. Thesis,
Paris, 1968.

Stone, B. H., and Mansell, H.: Procidentia and
cervical cancer. Obstet. Gynec., 5:198, 1955.

Usandizaga, J. M., and Ballesteros, L.: Prolapso
uterino y carcinoma de cuello. Communicat. to
Fac. Med., Barcelona, 1965.

Williams, G. A.: Endometriosis of the cervix uteri—
a common disease. Am. J. Obstet. Gynec., 80:
734, 1960.

Wolfe, S. A., Mackles, A., and Greene, H. J.: Endometriosis of the cervix: Classification and analysis
of 17 cases. Am. J. Obstet. Gynec., 81:111, 1961.

Chapter Five

CERVICAL ECTOPY

DEFINITION

In colposcopic terminology, ectopy is the presence of endocervical mucosa outside of its normal boundaries, replacing to a greater or lesser extent the normal exocervical epithelium. This means that the normal stratified squamous epithelium of the vagina and exocervix has been replaced by the columnar, mucoid epithelium which normally covers the cervical canal (Fig. 119).

SYNONYMS

Ectopy. Ectopia. Ectropion. Pseudoerosion. Glandular pseudoerosion. First stage of healing. Cervical erosion. Papillary erosion. Follicular erosion. Erythroplasia.

In the gynecologic literature, the term ectropion frequently appears, so that many colposcopists consider it synonymous with ectopy. This equivalence should be applied only to eversion of the endocervical mucosa which is directed to the exterior of the canal, due either to an inflammatory swelling or to a cervical laceration that leaves it open. In ectopy, the endocervical epithelium invades the exocervix by superficial growth, while in ectropion the endocervical mucosa appears on the exterior of the canal because of purely mechanical distortion.

It is logical that, previous to the colposcopic era, clinical and pathologic terms were used to describe this lesion, which now seem incorrect. Hence, Robert Meyer called columnar colonization of the exocervix "pseudoerosion" or "first stage of healing," because he thought that through this mechanism the "true erosion" of the mucosa of the portio vaginalis of the cervix, caused by inflammation or trauma, was repaired. Although this interpretation cannot be completely disregarded, it is evident that, in the majority of cases, events occur in a different manner.

Undoubtedly the most appropriate term is ectopy, introduced by Hinselmann to replace the old and inadequate name of erosion. The condition does not represent a loss of epithelium, but rather replacement of one kind of epithelium by another. Such expressions as papillary erosion or follicular erosion, which refer to different microscopic aspects of the lesion, are also inappropriate.

The gynecologist not trained in colposcopy, when looking with the naked eye at a red zone surrounding the cervical os, might cause some confusion by using terms that imply the existence of well defined colposcopic pictures. Probably the term erythroplasia would be best in this case, because it means nothing more than a red area that should be subject to study.

ORIGIN

The genesis of ectopy is quite diverse; a "congenital" or "acquired" ectopy may appear during the course of postnatal life as a result of diverse pathologic circumstances.

Congenital Ectopy. To understand this possibility, it is necessary to recall some embryologic concepts, especially those popularized by Meyer.

Until the third month of intrauterine life, the genital apparatus is covered by a columnar type of epithelium which comes from the coelom, but around the fourth month, when the tunneling of the fused caudal portions of the Müllerian duct takes place in an ascending manner, the resulting vaginal cavity remains covered by squamous epithelium derived from the endoderm of the urogenital sinus.

By the fifth month of gestation, stratified epithelium not only has covered all of the vagina but has ascended into the interior of the cervical canal, establishing a "first limit" or "epithelial border" in the middle portion of the cervix.

Later, in the seventh month of intrauterine life, the columnar epithelium, now converted into mucus-producing tissue, advances caudally, shedding and replacing the squamous epithelium throughout the whole endocervix, and even colonizing part of the exocervix. In the establishment of this "second limit," the macerating effect of the mucus secreted by the epithelium and the effects

of maternal hormones need to be considered.

Near the end of gestation, the stratified epithelium again takes the initiative, encircling the columnar epithelium on the inside of the external cervical os and establishing at this level the so-called "third limit," which becomes the physiologic border between the two types of cervical epithelium.

Congenital ectopy occurs when the border of the columnar epithelium is not pushed back by the squamous epithelium of the vagina, with arrest of development so that the os ends at what we have called the "second limit." Undoubtedly, this is due to the effect of maternal or placental steroid hormones.

An alternative explanation consists in an attempt to interpret congenital ectopy as a prolapse of the cervical mucosa, due to a sliding displacement of the inner layers against the more stable and resistant external layers of the cervix, during the process of growth of the organ.

At birth, about 40 per cent of girls present an ectopy of this nature. During infancy, the "struggle of the epithelia" is again initiated, so that by the time of

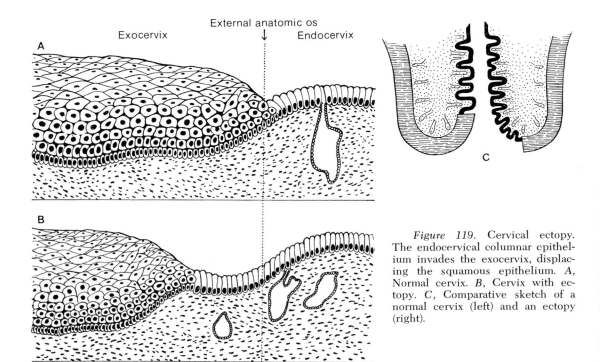

Figure 119. Cervical ectopy. The endocervical columnar epithelium invades the exocervix, displacing the squamous epithelium. *A,* Normal cervix. *B,* Cervix with ectopy. *C,* Comparative sketch of a normal cervix (left) and an ectopy (right).

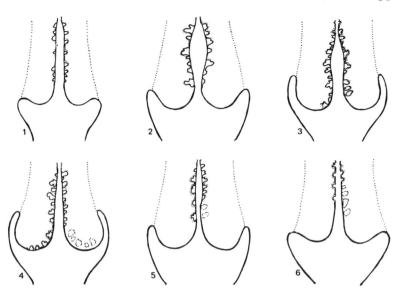

Figure 120. Borders of the squamous and columnar epithelia during the lifetime of a woman: *1,* childhood; *2,* young nullipara; *3,* multipara; *4,* pregnant; *5,* menopausal; *6,* in old age.

puberty only half of these ectopies persist. In the remainder, the flat stratified epithelium of the exocervix has pushed the cylindrical epithelium back to the physiologic limit, or even beyond to produce what is called an "entopy" (Fig. 120). Hamperl has demonstrated that, during sexual maturity, displacement of the external os is followed by an identical displacement of the internal os, so that the length of the endocervical mucosa remains constant (Fig. 121).

There is no histopathological proof that congenital ectopy results in ectopy in adult life (Hamperl), but a clinical fact is that about 19 per cent of young and virgin women have ectopy, and it is considered congenital in the absence of traumatic or inflammatory antecedents.

Acquired Ectopy. Multiple hypotheses that have been invoked to explain the appearance of ectopy in a woman with no previous history of congenital ectopy can be summarized under three headings.

INFLAMMATORY THEORY. Originating with Meyer, this theory is the one that has dominated the thinking on this topic for the last 50 years. It postulates that no acquired ectopy exists without a previous inflammation.

The theory is that the primary insult

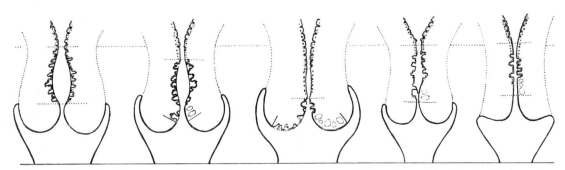

Figure 121. Displacements of the histologic external os are parallel to those of the histologic internal os, which indicates that, whatever their location, the length of the endocervical mucosa remains constant (After Hamperl et al.).

is an endocervicitis, producing alkaline and irritating mucus which macerates the flat stratified epithelium near the external cervical os, with its destruction as a logical consequence. Regeneration is interfered with by the same causes, but the resulting erosion or ulceration heals by caudal displacement of the endocervical epithelium, which occupies the denuded area. In support of this notion is the fact that vitality and growth potential of columnar epithelium is greater than that of the squamous epithelium, and it accommodates itself much better to inflammatory states. Meyer has called this columnar colonization the "first stage of healing." The definitive cure or "second stage of healing" takes place once the original inflammatory process has ceased. Then the stratified epithelium of the edges of the ectopy penetrates between the junctional stroma and the mucoid epithelium, replacing and necrotizing the latter. Slowly, the whole exocervix is re-epithelialized until the original boundary is restored.

With González-Merlo, we consider the inflammatory origin of ectopy to be debatable. In our own observations, this chain of events would not explain acquired ectopy in more than 2 to 3 per cent of cases. If true erosion were the obligatory precursor of ectopy, as Meyer believed, the colposcopic incidence of the former should be equal to that of the latter, whereas actually we see only a 1.8 per cent incidence of true erosion but a 38.9 per cent incidence of ectopy (separately or associated with a reparative complex). On the other hand, it is true that destruction by electrocoagulation of an area of flat epithelium near the external os is followed by its replacement not by columnar epithelium, but rather with the same squamous epithelium. The frequent inflammatory signs that accompany ectopy are not its cause but rather its consequence, in our view.

TRAUMATIC THEORY. Here the initiating event is eversion of the endocervical mucosa out of the limits of the external os, as a consequence of the trauma of childbirth. The columnar epithelium, prolapsed in this manner into the interior of the vaginal cavity, would be in an inhospitable medium, to which it would react with hypersecretion of mucus. This in turn would macerate the nearby squamous epithelium, which would separate and later be replaced by columnar epithelium. Consequently, what began as a traumatic ectropion would be followed by true ectopy due to epithelial colonization.

This hypothesis cannot be discarded. At least in some women the events just described do happen and our statistics confirm them. In the last trimester of pregnancy we observe a 47 per cent incidence of ectopy, while post partum the figure increases to 53 per cent. However, other authors (González-Merlo, Lang) have not corroborated these findings.

HORMONAL THEORY. The idea that certain states of hormonal excess may induce the appearance of ectopy is becoming more generally accepted. Due either to real growth of the columnar epithelium or to eversion of that tissue, there are a series of clinical circumstances that corroborate this hypothesis. Included are pregnancy, hyperluteinization, and the prolonged administration of steroid anovulatory agents.

During the progress of pregnancy, following the pattern of hormonal increase, the incidence of ectopy also increases significantly: from 21.6 per cent of women prior to pregnancy to 40 per cent in the first trimester, 46.6 per cent in the second, and 47 per cent in the third.

Hyperluteinization (spontaneous or caused by medication) also stimulates growth of columnar epithelium, with an apparent caudad sliding of the epithelial frontier. In 50 patients in whom a "hormonal pseudocyesis" was created by multiple progestational agents (because of sterility, infertility, genital hypoplasia, or other reasons) the existence of ectopy was confirmed in 72 per cent of cases, while at the beginning of the progestational therapy the figure was 26 per cent.

And finally, the prolonged administration of steroid compounds for suppression of ovulation has corroborated the importance of the hormonal factor in the genesis of ectopy. We have confirmed that anovulatory agents stimulate the appearance of extensive and hypertrophic ectopy (55 per cent of cases), which recalls the ectopy of gestation by its con-

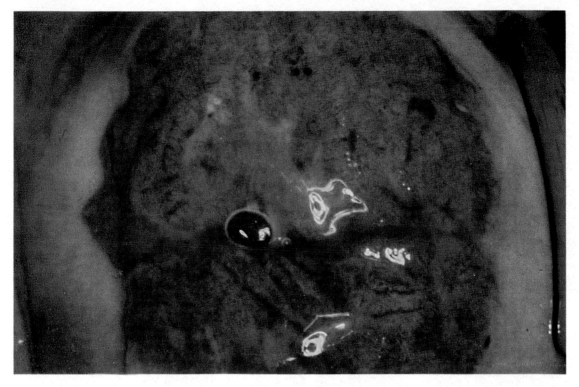

Figure 122. Ectopy, seen without preparation. Before the application of acetic acid, ectopy appears as a red spot with more or less precise edges. It is not possible to distinguish the papillary elements that define the lesion.

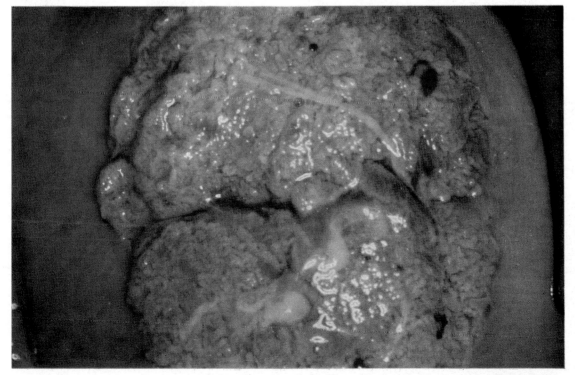

Figure 123. Ectopy after application of acetic acid, which facilitates the identification of the lesion by permitting observation of the characteristic cylindrical papillae. In this colpophotograph the typical "grape clusters" are seen.

gestion, vascularization and coarse granulation (Carrera and Dexeus, 1971). Also, Carbia et al. have observed this expansion of the ectopy.

As other investigators have indicated (Mateu-Aragonés, Hamperl and Kaufmann, and others), the incidence of ectopy varies during the lifetime of a woman, in accordance with her hormonal status. Its maximum incidence is found during the period of maximum ovarian activity. The incidence in our series was found to be 42 per cent of women of child-bearing age, while in the climacterium it is only 6.3 per cent. Ectopy in the menopause is always more discreet and less exuberant than in the young woman, and at this time it is not unusual to see true "entopies" (squamous metaplasia in the endocervix).

The presence of exuberant ectopy after the menopause should lead one to suspect a functional ovarian tumor (such as a granulosa cell tumor).

FREQUENCY

Ectopy is the most frequently observed colposcopic image, seen overall in 38.9 per cent of our cases. The highest incidence is in younger patients (under 30 years of age), in whom ovarian activity is accentuated (Mateu-Aragonés, Cano and others), while its incidence is rare after age 50.

The appearance of ectopy as a solitary lesion is relatively infrequent (12.2 per cent of our material). Its association with a typical reparative complex is seen in 20.2 per cent of cases, and ectopy with an atypical reparative complex represents 6.5 per cent of our cases. The figures listed by other authors are extraordinarily variable (Table 20).

COLPOSCOPIC APPEARANCES

Without any previous preparation, on direct colposcopy, ectopy appears as a simple red zone with an irregular surface and imprecise limits (Fig. 122). Its extent is variable, from a small circumoral strip to a large plaque which occupies the whole of the visible cervix.

Colposcopy will offer precise information for its identification after the acetic acid test, if the application of the acetic acid has been careful and has not caused bleeding which could impede vision. Then the papillae will be visible, and these are the principal elements of ectopy. They are small formations, adjacent to one another, of a pink color and translucent aspect, whose size varies according to environmental circumstances (Fig. 123). They have two characteristic shapes, a "grape-cluster" form resembling a racemose lesion, and a "gloved finger" form resembling an intermingling of digitations which press together and interlace with much disorder. The implantation point of the papillae is usually not visible. Their size is quite homogeneous (Fig. 124).

Covering the ectopy and agglutinating the innumerable papillae is an abundant amount of mucus, viscous and adherent, and sometimes of a gravel-like aspect, which is dissolved and removed only with difficulty by the acetic acid. This secretion, which is responsible for the numerous reflections seen on colpophotography, mostly comes from the glandular crypts, small holes seen between groups of papillae. These are the openings of glands located much deeper in the stroma. In the vicinity of the crypts small air bubbles are seen, dissolved in the residual mucus.

The ease with which an ectopy bleeds is due not to its great vascularity but to the fragility of the columnar epithelium. The vessels are actually scarce and only barely visible in the ordinary uninfected ectopy. Use of a green filter or special solutions does not improve visibility of the blood vessels.

Ectopy has a precise outer boundary with the squamous exocervical epithelium and an imprecise internal border with the normal endocervical mucosa. The only appreciable difference between these two columnar epithelia is the greater surface irregularity of the ectopy than of the endocervix, where the papillae are less marked. The external boundary may be extraordinarily regular,

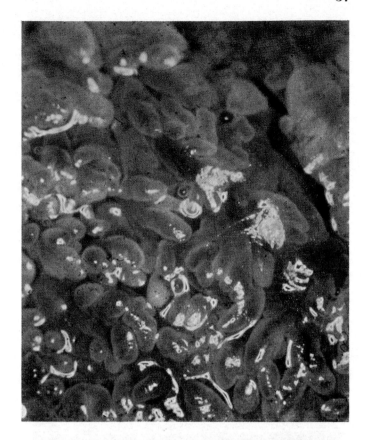

Figure 124. Colpophotograph at high magnification, in which the papillae of an ectopy are clearly seen. Even though the sizes are homogeneous, the shapes vary from the "grape cluster" papillae to that which resembles a "gloved finger." A widely opened glandular crypt is also seen.

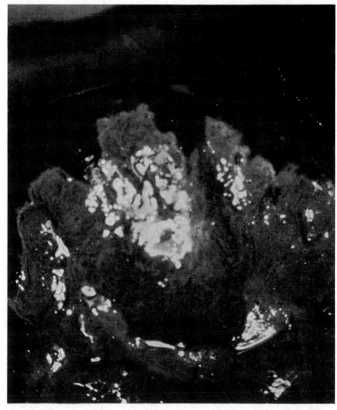

Figure 125. Ectopy seen after Schiller's test. The total iodine negativity of the ectopy is confirmed (the columnar epithelium lacks glycogen), which vividly contrasts with the good iodine fixation of the surrounding squamous epithelium.

Table 20.   Frequency of Ectopy

	ISOLATED	ASSOCIATED	TOTAL
Joussef (1957)	13.7%	–	–
Figuéro et al (1971)	–	–	19.7%
Berger and Wenner-Mangen (1952)	4.75%	17.25%	22.0%
Guzmán Llovet et al. (1967)	–	–	33.42%
González-Merlo (1966)	15.5%	19.7%	35.2%
Guerrero et al. (1957)	–	–	46.8%
Wilds (1962)	–	–	47.5%
Mateu-Aragonés (1971)	14.1%	50.2%	64.3%
Fernández Laso et al. (1960)	–	–	66.6%
Arenas et al. (1961)	–	–	67.4%
Our Series (1972)	12.2%	26.7%	38.9%

marked and definite, as in so-called "circinate ectopy," or notably diffuse and irregular, as "ectopy associated with active re-epithelialization" or "macerated ectopy."

Besides the constant and permanent elements described, in some cases there may be islets or flat epithelial plaques, of a pale color, ostensibly more fragile and slender than the normal squamous epithelium. They should be considered as metaplastic plaques.

Lacking in glycogen, the columnar tissue of the ectopy is totally iodine-negative and stands in clear contrast with the surrounding squamous epithelium, which fixes iodine perfectly (Fig. 125).

Varieties of Ectopy

From a purely morphologic viewpoint, it is possible to describe several types of ectopy according to its size, its constant elements, its superimposed elements, or the appearance of its outer edge.

According to Size. Ectopy may be classified as extensive if it invades more than 2/3 of the exocervix (Fig. 126), moderate if it occupies between 1/3 and 2/3, and small if it is limited to the central third. A variety of the latter is the so-called circumoral or minimal ectopy, which is merely a small strip of columnar epithelium which seems to flow through the anatomic external os.

Constant or Permanent Elements (Papillae and Glandular Crypts). Ectopy may adopt any of several shapes or arrangements, giving the overall appearance a distinct individuality.

PAPILLAE. Two types of ectopy are recognized according to the *size* of the papillae: "coarse granular ectopy" (the papillary ectopy or papillary erosion of the older literature), which may also be called macropapillary; "medium granular" or "fine granular ectopy" (or micropapillary), which the gynecologist calls simple ectopy (Fig. 127). A variety of coarse granular ectopy is "pseudopolypoid ectopy" (Fig. 128), in which the papillae are so large that it is possible to mistake them for small endocervical polyps. This occurs especially during gestation, giving rise to the entity known as "hypertrophic ectopy" of pregnancy (Fig. 130).

In accordance with the *shape* of the papillae, two types of ectopy may be distinguished: "racemose" ectopy, formed by innumerable rounded papillae grouped in bunches of 6 to 10 elements (Fig. 131), and "interlocked" ectopy formed by a multitude of "fingers" which intermingle in different directions (Fig. 126). In the latter type the papillae are disposed, in part or entirely, parallel to the surface, which affords better visualization of the vascular supply. The racemose variety is usual in acquired ectopy, while the other type is more frequently seen in the congenital instances.

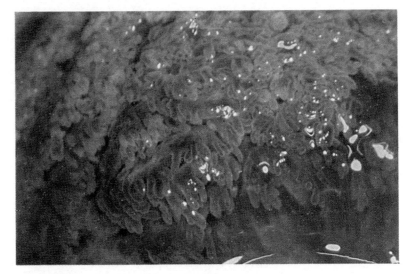

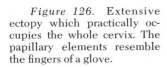

Figure 126. Extensive ectopy which practically occupies the whole cervix. The papillary elements resemble the fingers of a glove.

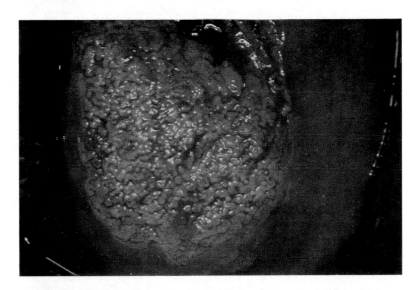

Figure 127. Micropapillary (or simple) ectopy, formed by finely granular papillary elements. Its uniformity, homogeneity and lack of elevations are striking features. Its borders are very precise.

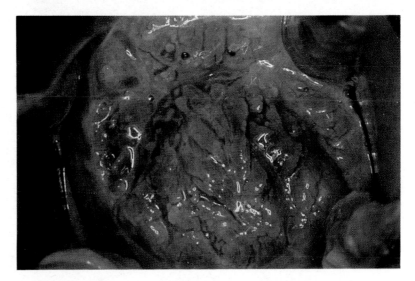

Figure 128. Pseudopolypoid ectopy. The coarse grains of the ectopy are agglutinated, creating larger elements which resemble the morphology of the endocervical polyp.

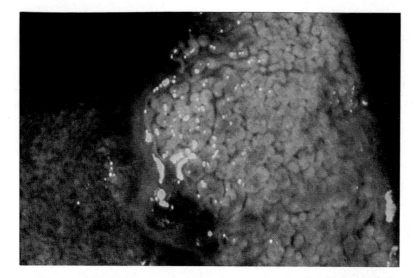

Figure 129. Ectopy in a postmenopausal woman. Two details attract attention: the uniformity and smoothness of the surface ("flat ectopy") and the color of white and purple ("ischemic ectopy").

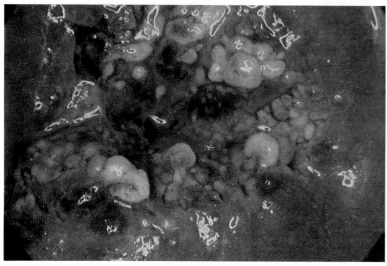

Figure 130. Coarse-granular ectopy on a pregnant cervix.

Another classification is possible by *color.* "Deciduous ectopy," seen in a considerable number of pregnant women, exhibits a more or less extensive whitish area formed by a given number of papillary elements which have exchanged the red color normal in ectopy for a white one which resembles polished crystal (p. 240). It is due to a transformation of the subjacent stroma, and for this reason it is known as "subcylindrical deciduosis" (Fig. 132).

During the climacterium, the few ectopies that are seen, besides being flat without any unevenness, adopt a characteristic violet-white color (Fig. 129).

According to the arrangement of the papillae, it is possible to identify two perfectly defined types of ectopy. The confluent type is characterized by the fact that the papillar elements are conjoined with one another. They do not appear in small bunches, but rather are tightly pressed together, making them difficult to distinguish individually (Fig. 133). This variety is most often seen post partum and less frequently in patients on anovulatory drugs. The other possibility is "interrupted" ectopy, characterized by a succession of crests, separated by breaks or valleys. The crests are formed by rows of two to four papillae, which are epithe-

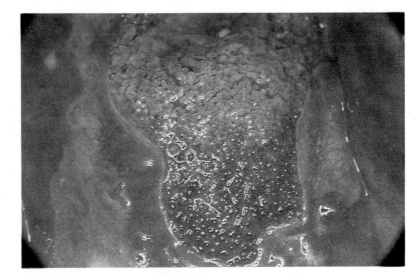

Figure 131. Flat ectopy formed by papillae in the shape of "grape clusters."

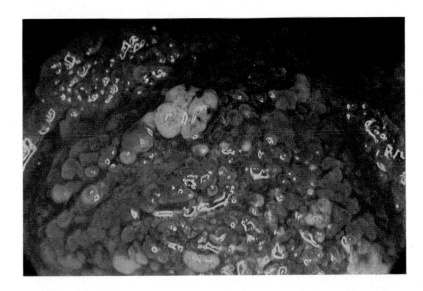

Figure 132. Decidual ectopy. Ample zones of ectopic endocervical epithelium, of whitish color which contrasts with the pink color of the usual ectopy.

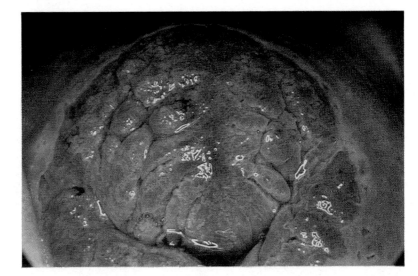

Figure 133. Confluent ectopy post partum. The papillary elements of the ectopy are pressed together, forming aggregates.

lialized, while in the breaks, rounded papillae are seen without epidermization or conglutination. This type of ectopy, which is frequently seen, almost always has a congenital origin and rarely heals spontaneously (Fig. 134). The columnar papillae that occupy the valleys are resistant to re-epithelialization because they are constantly macerated, while their glandular elements are deep in the stroma.

GLANDULAR ELEMENTS. Hyperplasia of the glandular elements of ectopic epithelium causes an increase in secretion, and some characteristic types of ectopy may then appear. With simple mucosal hypersecretion, we refer to "secreting ectopy" (Fig. 135). However, if edema of the chorion also exists along with general congestion, as occurs during gestation, we use the term "hypertrophic ectopy" because all elements of the lesion become exaggerated.

The ectopy of the remaining cervix after subtotal hysterectomy may secrete quite excessively.

Superimposed Elements. If these exist, they will change the colposcopic picture.

VASCULAR ECTOPY. The kind of ectopy that we consider normal in the exocervix is very poorly vascularized or not at all. However, in specific circumstances (inflammation, tissue proliferation), the ectopy becomes vascularized. Then, abundant vessels may be seen in the papillae, between them or over them, of diverse calibers, courses and paths.

The vessels that cross the surface of the ectopy are quite evident without preparation; however, after application of acetic acid, they become practically invisible within a few minutes. Hence a previous observation is necessary, and the examination must not be concluded before the effect of that reagent has ceased. Study of these blood vessels will permit the establishment of a correct diagnosis, because the presence of vascular atypia signifies malignant proliferation and not simple ectopy (Figs. 138 and 139). Formations with a vessel which ascends to the surface, and whose shape resembles a corkscrew, are especially suspicious (p. 216), In ectopy of pregnancy, the papillae may also be vascu-

larized, but the path of the capillary is a straight line. If vessels of unequal caliber are seen on the surface of an assumed ectopy, it should also be submitted for histopathologic study.

Confusion is possible, however. In our experience there is a case of a cervical epithelioma, which had a papillary appearance, being mistaken for a vascular ectopy. Confusion has also been described with adenocarcinoma of the endocervix with exocervical evolution. The differential diagnosis may be easy for the experienced colposcopist (p. 220), but we recognize that to the inexperienced, malignancy of a grossly obvious lesion may be much more apparent to the "naked eye" than when viewed through the eyepiece of the colposcope. In actuality, this problem pertains almost always to carcinomas in an overtly manifest and well defined state, whose diagnosis is easy merely by clinical examination.

INFLAMMATORY ECTOPY. This type of ectopy is characterized by coarse-granular or pseudopolypoid papillae, congestive and vascular, bathed by an especially adherent and sticky mucoid secretion which is not totally removed by acetic acid. It arises from hypertrophic glands that secrete continuously, macerating the surrounding epithelium, which is usually hyperemic and affected by vaginitis. The glandular crypts are ample and deep, because of the glandular irritation (Fig. 136). When the inflammation of the columnar epithelium is much accentuated, it is possible to see denuded epithelial zones, bleeding or necrotized (Fig. 140).

HEMORRHAGIC ECTOPY. So-called hemorrhagic ectopy does not have any real characterization. It can be the "flat ectopy" of a menopausal patient, which, being very fragile, bleeds with any minor trauma; or on the contrary it may be a "hypertrophic ectopy" of pregnancy, which bleeds easily because of its exuberant growth. "Inflammatory ectopy" also bleeds easily, and even spontaneously, without any traumatic insult. These patients have an abundant leukorrhea, which on occasion is spotted by small bloody tinges, or they may expel a maroon secretion.

Types of Boundaries. So-called

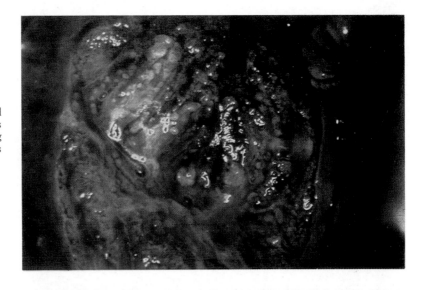

Figure 134. Interrupted ectopy. Even though this photograph was taken during pregnancy, the origin of this type of ectopy is congenital.

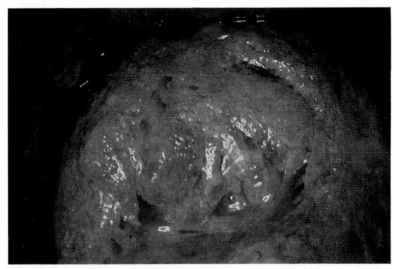

Figure 135. Secreting ectopy bathed by mucus from its own glandular elements, which are probably hyperplastic.

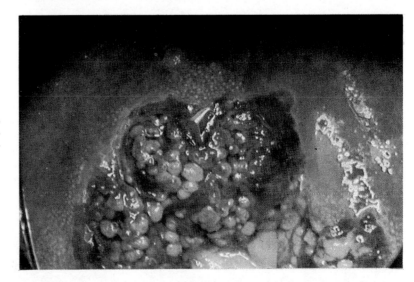

Figure 136. Slightly inflammatory ectopy of pregnancy, accompanied by striking papillary elevation.

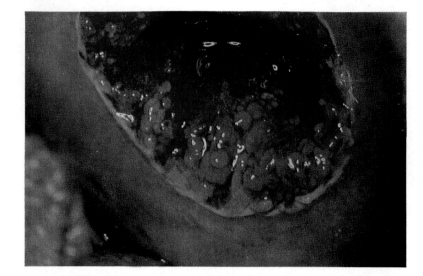

Figure 137. Circinate ectopy. The boundaries between the columnar and the squamous epithelia are precise.

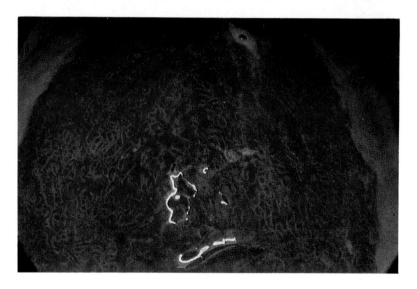

Figure 138. Ectopy of pregnancy formed by vascularized papillary elements, but without any atypical signs.

"circinate ectopy," whose interepithelial edges are extremely sharp (Fig. 137), is an ectopy that does not heal spontaneously, because its re-epithelialization, orthoplastic or metaplastic, is not produced by dystrophic causes. Usually it is a long-standing condition, of quite a few years evolution, which the patient tolerates well. But it may be of recent mechanical origin, as occurs at the beginning of a pregnancy. It is seldom seen in virgins, and such a case should arouse the attention of the colposcopist because of the apparent absence of causative factors.

In the periphery of these ectopies, frequent petechiae are seen, which point to a certain degree of epithelial dystrophy.

A totally different lesion is the "ectopy associated with re-epithelialization" (the regression ectropion of Bibiloni), which we will study in detail in Chapter 6. Moldings of squamous epithelium festoon the periphery of this ectopy, creating a zone in which it is difficult to state where the ectopy ends and where the newly formed squamous epithelium begins. On occasion, there is interference with re-epithelialization (due to gestation or inflammation) and then the periphery

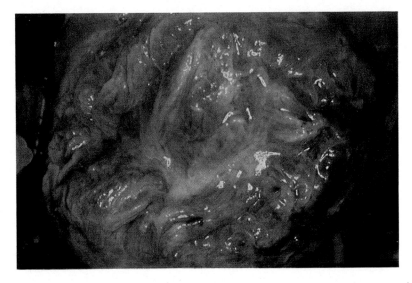

Figure 139. Ectopy in a woman six months pregnant. Vascularization increases the possibility of confusion with a malignant process. To be able to affirm that the lesion is benign it is necessary to look for intact papillae at the bottom of breaks or crypts.

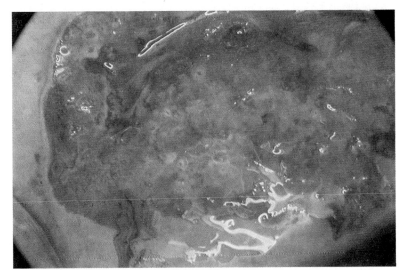

Figure 140. Macerating ectopy. The metaplastic exocervical mucosa appears reddened, edematous and covered by mucus.

of the ectopy is extraordinarily irregular. This is called "ectopy associated with interrupted re-epithelialization."

Lastly, there is a third variety which is important because it should occasionally arouse suspicion of a malignant process. This is the "macerating ectopy" already cited (Fig. 140). The edges are irregular and undergoing degeneration. Around the lesion some edematous, reddened plaques are seen, centered in a glandular opening, isolated within the stratified epithelium and secreting an abundant amount of mucus. The epithelium is macerated between these edematous plaques, and the subjacent stroma

may even be seen. The coexistence of erosive, edematous, and hemorrhagic plaques suggests an atypical transformation zone, even though localization in the periphery of an ectopy should instead suggest a simple mechanism of maceration. During pregnancy such an ectopy is frequently flanked by a remarkable papillary elevation (Fig. 136).

HISTOLOGIC CORRELATIONS

Under the microscope, ectopy is seen to be composed of numerous papillomatous formations which have the stroma as their base. The papillae have different appearances, depending upon whether they are studied by longitudinal or transverse sections. When the section is longitudinal, many contiguous papillae are seen, simple or with ramifications, with a more or less pedunculated implantation base, which establishes itself in the underlying connective tissue (Fig. 141).

In the case of congenital ectopy it is possible to show how the papillae are grouped in strips, separated by deep depressions, whose glandular elements are strongly anchored to the stroma. This does not occur in the acquired variety, where the papillae are disposed at regular intervals, nor in the pseudopolypoid type where, besides exhibiting marked congestion, edema, and inflammatory infiltration, the strips conglutinate to form easily visible entities (the pseudopolyps).

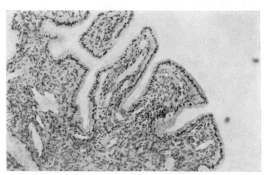

Figure 141. Longitudinal histologic section of a cervical ectopy. Several adjacent papillae are seen.

Individually each papilla is formed by a vascular core, covered by a single palisade layer of tall columnar cells. Its cytoplasm is basophilic, and the nuclei are dense and hyperchromatic, located at the base. With the alcian-PAS blue stain, the existence of this epithelium with

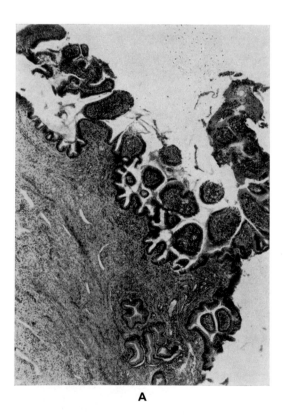

A

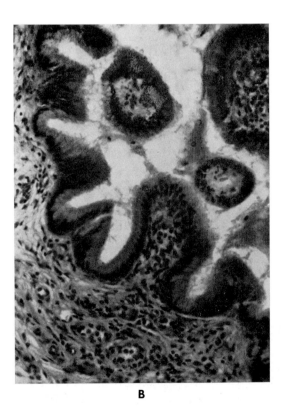

B

Figure 142. Transverse histologic section of an ectopy. *A,* At low magnification, the free extremities of several papillae are seen to adopt the shape of round elements of unequal caliber. *B,* An area of the first photomicrograph at higher magnification to demonstrate the vascular core of the papilla and its typical inflammatory infiltration.

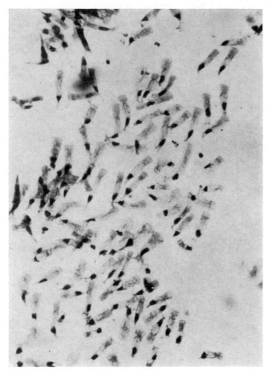

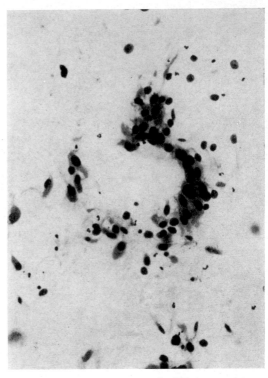

Figure 143. Polymorphous columnar cells, ciliated and secretory, desquamated by a patient who exhibits a large ectopy as the only colposcopic lesion.

Figure 144. Smear in which hypertrophic endocervical cells are seen, with notable anisocytosis. Hyperchromasia is evident.

large quantities of mucopolysaccharide acids is demonstrated. Vessels are not always visible, even though they are generally distinguishable at some point in their course to the surface. The stroma is almost constantly subject to an inflammatory lymphocytic infiltration.

Both the vessels and the inflammatory infiltration are significantly increased in inflammatory ectopy. The vessels are hypertrophied and adopt a less regular course, with the infiltration being more dense and extensive. Between the papillae, clustered glands are seen, sometimes in extremely large numbers.

In secreting ectopy, the glandular component increases both in number and size, with intensely dilated and almost cystic niches seen.

If the histologic section is transverse, some round, well individualized elements are seen, which are simply the free ends of the aforementioned papillae. In this projection the vascular axis is always

evident, as is also the inflammatory infiltration that encircles it (Fig. 142).

In both patterns clear mucus is observed, which superficially agglutinates the papillae.

CYTOLOGIC CORRELATIONS

The presence of endocervical epithelium in the vagina may cause columnar cells to appear on cytologic smears. Notwithstanding, this is not a common finding. In our series of ectopies, we found such cells in 8.8 per cent of nonpregnant women, 13 per cent of pregnant women, and 21 per cent of those on anovulatory agents (Table 21). The role played by the material used for sampling has been suggested as an explanation for the desquamation (Font Sastre). It is possible that the explanation for such a low incidence rests on a notable adherence of columnar cells to the basal membrane.

Table 21.   Percentage of Columnar Cells in
Smears of Ectopy

Pregnant	13 %
Nonpregnant	8.8%
Anovulatory treatment	21 %
Total	12.3%

When they appear on a specimen, they do so in groups which at times preserve their palisade arrangement. One does not often see a smear with abundant ciliated and secretory cells (Fig. 143). Individually the cells may be completely normal, or they may be moderately hypertrophic, with nuclear and cytoplasmic hyperchromia. On occasions the cytoplasm may appear eosinophilic. The cells often lose their customary shape and adopt a globular appearance, similar to the parabasal cells of the flat epithelium. However, identification is facilitated by the cytoplasm, which is more delicate and of unclear limits.

The hypertrophic aspect of these cells is especially apparent in women using anovulatory agents (Carrera, Palacin and Dexeus). In this case, the anisonucleosis and nuclear hyperchromasia may even make one suspect a malignancy (Fig. 144). These findings are justified by the presence of an adenomatous hyperplasia of the endocervix.

In regard to the classification of the smears according to Papanicolaou's grades, a high percentage of Class II is seen (33.6 per cent), which reflects the frequent inflammatory reactions of this lesion (Table 22). According to Herrera and Ruiz de la Hermosa, that incidence is significantly larger in papillary ectopy (coarse granular) than in the follicular (ectopy subjected to re-epithelialization) (p. 118).

Table 22.   Cytologic Correlation of Ectopy
When it Occurs as a Solitary Lesion

Class I	66.1%
Class II	33.6%
Class II-III	0.2%
Class III	0.0%
Class IV or V	0.05%

When ectopy is associated with inflammation, as is frequent, the smear appears dirty, with abundant mucus, granulocytes, and even histiocytes. The presence of red blood cells is not unusual, due to the vulnerability of the ectopic epithelium.

CLINICAL COURSE

The evolution of ectopy depends fundamentally on two factors: its etiology and the accompanying circumstances. In regard to the etiologic factor, it should be said that congenital ectopy does not tend to heal spontaneously, and in the absence of therapeutic intervention, it will persist for an indefinite period. On the contrary, acquired ectopy (traumatic, inflammatory, or hormonal) tends to undergo repair once the causative factor has disappeared, unless environmental factors interfere.

As environmental circumstances capable of impeding or slowing definitive cure of an ectopy, we can name inflammation, pregnancy, permanent hormonal imbalance, steroid treatment, abnormal tissue nutrition, alkaline vaginal pH, and permanent irritation of the epithelium.

As long as one or more of these unfavorable circumstances persists, cure of ectopy will be retarded. It is possible that at some time and in some zone, an attempt at re-epithelialization will be initiated but will soon be aborted, with the columnar epithelium holding its own once more. In practice, it is possible to observe ectopies which persist over many years, but whose boundaries are never constant. There is a permanent epithelial struggle, in harmony with hormonal changes or due to short-lived improvements of the trophic inflammatory conditions of the vaginal cavity.

If ectopy is repaired, thanks to the existence of optimal vaginal conditions or because of a therapeutic influence over the factors that impeded it, the repair may follow one of two different paths: typical re-epithelialization, which is associated with a "physiologic metaplasia," and atypical re-epithelialization, which usually corresponds to a metaplasia with

Table 23. Scheme of the Evolutionary Possibilities of Ectopy

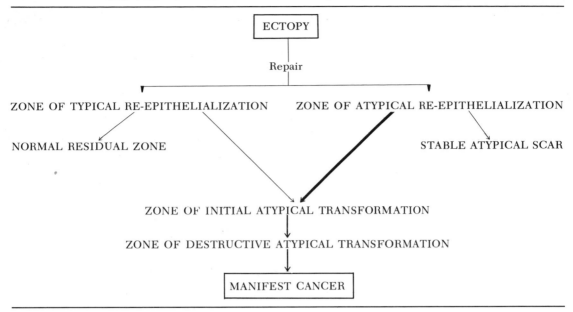

maturation disturbances ("moderate or slight dysplasia").

By virtue of both types of repair, the ectopy may heal totally, with the epithelial surface of the exocervix becoming progressively regular. On the other hand, in the course of either procedure, and especially in atypical re-epithelialization, healing problems may arise, and if they persist for many years, may accumulate a certain carcinogenic potential. An appropriate procedure for dealing with each type of ectopy is important.

In Table 23 the evolutionary possibilities of ectopy are diagrammed with special emphasis on the presumptive carcinogenic transformation of its reparative complex.

MANAGEMENT

Because ectopy is seen so frequently, it is tempting to consider it a normal and even physiologic pattern. However, the fact that its reparative evolution may produce potentially irreversible malignant lesions obliges us to regard it as pathologic.

The therapeutic approach depends greatly on the data offered by colposcopy. Only exceptionally does a common ectopy, in the process of normal re-epithelialization, produce symptoms which require therapeutic intervention despite a favorable colposcopic impression. More frequently, symptomatic ectopy presents colposcopic alterations which are thought to require therapeutic intervention, independent of the type and intensity of the complaints expressed by the patient (Table 24).

In the presence of congenital ectopy it is useless to await spontaneous healing or to try medical treatment. The ectopy should be destroyed by electrocoagulation, cryotherapy (Collins, Poloucek and others) or diathermic extirpation. Coagulation, if used, should be deep; otherwise it will fail. Remember that in the "valleys" the papillae are deeply implanted and the glandular elements are deep in the underlying stroma.

When ectopy is extensive, whether coarse-granular or of the "gloved finger" type, the likelihood of spontaneous re-epithelialization is remote, even in a favorable vaginal environment. Superficial coagulation seems to be the appropriate

Table 24.   Therapy of Ectopy

(1) Circumscribed ectopy with active edge of re-epithelialization (generally asymptomatic)	Stimulate re-epithelialization with estriol and topical treatment with vitamin A
(2) Possible congenital ectopy	Deep coagulation
(3) Ectopy due to anovulatory agents Asymptomatic Symptomatic	 No therapy required Discontinue anovulatory therapy and treat as in (1) or (4)
(4) Extensive ectopy without signs of re-epithelialization	Local and general treatment as in (1), with coagulation if this fails
(5) Ectopy and vaginitis	Treat the vaginitis; if the ectopy persists, treat as in (1) or (4)
(6) Ectopy and dysplastic lesion(s)	Cytologic investigation, with coagulation if negative
(7) Ectopy in an anatomically distorted cervix	Surgical treatment (conization with or without plastic surgery)
(8) Ectopy resistant to local and systemic treatment	Conization

Notes: Cervical coagulation should be done immediately after the menstrual period. In ectopies of pregnancy and the postpartum period, the natural evolution of the lesion should be observed without therapeutic intervention.

measure, except in pregnancy and the postpartum period. In our experience a cervix should never be cauterized until 3 to 4 months post partum, because many hypertrophic ectopies of pregnancy disappear in that period of time.

When coagulation is correctly done, total repair after cauterization takes place in 90 per cent of cases (Baruffi, Bernoth). During the 2 weeks after cauterization, the appearance of the cervix undergoing necrosis may be of such irregularity that it will lead the colposcopist not accustomed to such images, to think in terms of a malignant transformation process (Fig. 145B). There are whitish areas (representing tissue slough) at unequal levels, alternated with denuded zones (due to loosening of the slough) of sanguineous background, with hemorrhagic foci that dirty the field, and exuberant granulation tissue.

After another 2 weeks, the necrotic areas have totally disappeared and, in their place, a re-epithelialization process is seen. This originates in the periphery and advances toward the anatomic cervical os, covering the bleeding stroma left uncovered by the separation of the es-

char. The superimposed vascularization may be notably hypertrophic, without clear anomalies of its course in the part observed (Fig. 145C and D).

As a consequence of this reparative process, the new epithelium exhibits, for a time, some images that recall its origin: hemorrhagic vesicles which disappear 2 to 4 months after cauterization, leaving reddish depressions in their place (Fig. 145C); abundant vessels of regular course, but unequal widths and paths; and rake-like images (Fig. 145D). The latter are fine lines which radiate from the anatomical external os in the shape of a star. They are nothing more than very fine vessels, and are so called because they resemble the lines left by a rake on the ground. It is also not unusual to see more or less extensive papillary elevation in a radial arrangement (Fig. 148).

On some occasions there is a strongly keratinic reaction to electrocoagulation, with the development of a leukokeratotic plaque around a generally well vascularized residual ectopy, or endometriosis may appear as a sequel.

If the ectopy is inflammatory, extremely vascular, with glandular hyper-

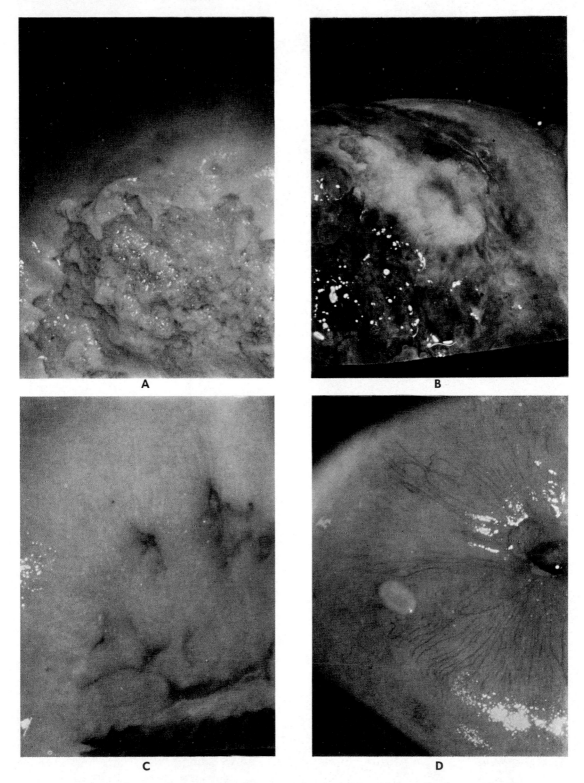

Figure 145. Evolution of ectopy after electrocoagulation. *A,* Part of the recently coagulated ectopy. *B,* After two weeks one sees alternating hemorrhagic zones with necrotic slough, which may induce one to suspect a malignant process. *C,* After seven weeks, the ectopy has disappeared, but patterns which resemble the early reparative epithelium are seen, and there are red areas which are nothing more than a residuum of the typical hemorrhagic vesicles of this process. *D,* At four months some fine "rakelike" vessels and a flat vesicle persist.

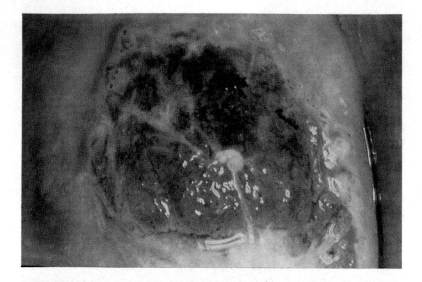

Figure 146. Infected ectopy before treatment. The presence of hemorrhagic and erosive zones may lead to a suspicion of malignancy.

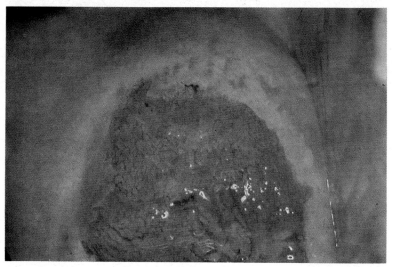

Figure 147. The same lesion, after adequate anti-inflammatory treatment. Its appearance has totally changed, and it is no longer an atypical lesion.

plasia and signs of peripheral maceration, the only correct approach is to implement anti-inflammatory therapy, using the vaginal route exclusively or combining oral and vaginal medications. Sulfonamide creams or suppositories give good results, as do antibiotics (chloramphenicol, oxytetracycline) by either route. The course of treatment should be sufficiently lengthy (20 days) to be effective (Figs. 146 and 147). When specific organisms can be identified by bacteriologic or cytologic examination, treatment to cure the ectopy should be delayed, until the vagina has been sterilized with the proper medication.

If the ectopy initiates its repair after disappearance of the additional inflammatory component, therapy is limited to adequate control or improvement of the vaginal trophism. Estriol may be used orally or intramuscularly at a dose of 1 mg daily. The intramuscular route is preferred when inflammatory ectopy coexists with trigonitis, which in our experience occurs in 20 per cent of cases. Other authors quote similar high figures (López, 19.04 per cent; Bueno Rodrigo, 37.8 per cent). Usually the 1 mg. dose given for 10 to 15 days is sufficient to resolve the secondary bladder infection and stimulate re-epithelialization of the

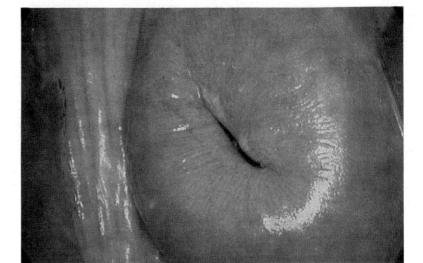

Figure 148. Keratinized "rake-like" patterns six months after electrocoagulation of an ectopy.

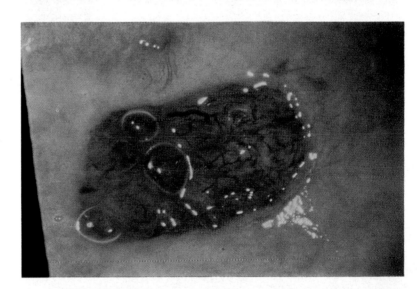

Figure 149. Circumoral residual ectopy after multiple coagulations.

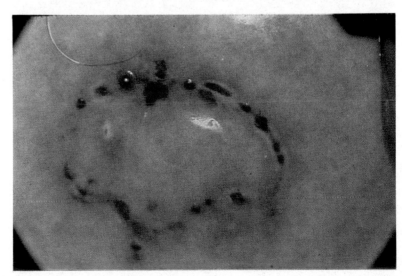

Figure 150. Cervical endometriosis as a sequel of coagulation.

ectopy. A single 80 mg dose of a depot estriol will produce continued activity for 2 months.

If there are no colposcopic signs of typical re-epithelialization after a month or two, the ectopy should be cauterized without further delay.

The appearance of the outer edges of the ectopy will often determine the procedure to be followed. If an area of typical and active re-epithelialization is seen in the periphery of the lesion, with abundant epithelial prolongations which progressively invade the zone of ectopy, in the center of which are some metaplastic plaques, the wisest thing is to do nothing. One should watch the healing process every 2 or 3 months and ensure that no interference appears (iatrogenic hormonal action, additional inflammation, etc.) which may disrupt the normal course of repair.

However, if the interepithelial limits are precise (circinate ectopy), or irregular but without any signs of young regenerative epithelium (ectopy without signs of re-epithelialization), it is wise to think about a deficient cervical trophism, which only responds inconsistently to estriol or ovarian cyclic regularization. It then becomes necessary to destroy the ectopic mucosa, when after a reasonable time (2 to 4 months) it persists without reparative signs.

If re-epithelialization of the ectopy is atypical, but cytologic examination is negative, we resort to adequate destruction of the ectopy and its anomalous re-epithelialization, except when we think that the observed patterns have an inflammatory origin, in which case local therapy is tried first. In the presence of suspicious cytologic findings, a histologic study of the atypical re-epithelialization will determine the proper means of management: coagulation if there is slight dysplasia, conization if it is severe.

The only objection to this approach is that if coagulation is effective, it displaces the squamocolumnar junction, with the result that if an atypical lesion reappears, it will be invisible at colposcopy (Bouda and Dohnal).

Some colposcopists are much more aggressive. In the presence of any ectopy in the course of atypical re-epithelialization, they practice selective biopsy, what-ever the cytological opinion, and whether the patient is pregnant or not (González-Merlo). We consider histologic study of the atypical re-epithelialization unnecessary if the lesion can be well characterized colposcopically. It would be different if the ectopy were a "zone of atypical transformation." We neither destroy nor biopsy the so-called "stable atypical scar" because it represents the final outcome of that abnormal re-epithelialization.

If the ectopy is resistant to all therapy (including coagulation), plastic surgery may be indicated, such as conization or amputation, with histologic study of the specimen. We have no experience with cryosurgery (Ostergard, Poloucek).

If it is possible to exclude malignant transformation of a lesion, there is no contraindication to doing a "hot conization" with an adequate electric scalpel, because destruction of the edges of the specimen is not an important inconvenience. On the contrary, if there is doubt regarding the exact nature of the lesion, it is better to undertake a "cold-knife" surgical conization or amputation, which will facilitate proper study of the excised specimen.

Recent statistics reveal that this type of ectopy suffers malignant transformation more often than the normal cervix. Li Ying et al. speak of an 8 per cent incidence of carcinoma and a 9.1 per cent incidence of precancerous lesions. The possibility has been raised that in these cases the phagocytic action of the leukocytes is inhibited for unknown reasons (Mardakhiashvili), predisposing to atypical cellular proliferation.

REFERENCES

Auerbach, S. H., and Pund, E. R.: Squamous metaplasia of the cervix uteri. Am. J. Obstet. Gynec., 49:207, 1945.

Baruffi, I., Brandão, H. J. S., and Valeri, V.: Über die Regeneration des Portioepithel nach Elektrokoagulation. Zbl. Gynäk., 88:199, 1966.

Bernoth, E., and Bettzieche, H.: Die verschorfte Portio vaginalis uteri (Ergebnisse klinischer und morphologischer Nachuntersuchungen). Zbl. Gynäk., 86:185, 1964.

Bouda, J., and Dohnal, V.: Zur Frage der Krebsprophylaxe durch Elektrokoagulation bei Ektopie und Unwandlungzone. Geburtsh. u. Frauenheilk., 25:1186, 1965.

Bret, J., and Coupez, F.: Colposcopy of ectopy, ectropion and epidermization. Acta Cytol., 5:83, 1961.

Bret, J., and Coupez, F.: Le traitement des cervicites par électrocoagulation: Séquelles vasculaires et endométriose du col. Gynéc. Obstét., 64:483, 1965.

Bueno Rodrigo, L.: Urologia Ginecológica. Madrid, Editorial Paz Montalvo, 1968.

Cano, A.: Colposcopia y colpofotografia de las lesiones benignas del cuello del utero. Toko-Ginec. Práct., 21:306, 1962.

Carbia, E., Alvarado-Duran, A., and Lopez-Llera, M.: Colposcopic study of the uterine cervix during administration of ethynodiol diacetate with mestranol. Am. J. Obstet. Gynec., 102:1023, 1968.

Carrera, J. M.: Control citológico de la hormonoterapia en ginecología. Revista Inform. Médico-Terapéutica, 44:333, 1969.

Carrera, J. M., and Dexeus, S., Jr.: Estudio colposcópico de los cambios cervicales inducidos por anovulatorios orales. Progr. Obstet. Ginec., 14:1, 1971.

Carrera, J. M., Palacín, A., and Dexeus, S., Jr.: Cambios morfológicos inducidos en el frotis vaginal por los anovulatorios orales. Acta Ginec., 19:869, 1968.

Collins, R. J., and Golab, A.: Cryosurgical treatment of uterine cervicitis: Preliminary report. Bull. Millard Fillmore Hospital, 13:47, 1966.

Collins, R. J., Golab, A., Pappas, H. J., and Poloucek, F. P.: Cryosurgery of the human uterine cervix. Obstet. Gynec., 30:660, 1967.

Corbeil, J., and Brunet, M. R.: L'érosion cervicale du post-partum. Union Méd. Canada, 92:1030, 1963.

Coupez, F.: La place de la colposcopie dans l'examen gynécologique actuel. Rev. Franç. Gynéc. Obstét., 65:209, 1970.

Fluhmann, C. F.: The Cervix Uteri and Its Diseases. Philadelphia, W. B. Saunders Co., 1961.

Fluhmann, C. F.: Management of so-called erosions of the cervix uteri. Clin. Obstet. Gynec., 6:344, 1963.

Font Sastre, V., and Alamany, R.: Estudio comparativo de dos tipos de espatula en citologia ginecologica. Progr. Obstet. Ginec., 12:143, 1969.

González-Merlo, J.: Colposcopia de las lesiones benignas del cuello uterino. Toko-Ginec. Práct., 20:220, 1961.

González-Merlo, J., Alonso, E., and Tarancón, A.: Ectopia del cuello uterino: Concepto y evolución. Hosp. Gen., 8:359, 1968.

Grünberger, V.: Die Ergebnisse von Routineuntersuchungen bei Erosionen der Portio. Arch. Gynäk., 189:368, 1957.

Hamperl, H.: Die angeborene Pseudoerosion der Portio und ihr Schicksal. Arch. Gynäk., 200:299, 1965.

Hamperl, H., and Kaufmann, C.: The cervix uteri at different ages. Obstet. Gynec., 14:621, 1959.

Herrera, E., and Ruiz de la Hermosa, A.: La colposcopia en las alteraciones cervicales benignas. Toko-Ginec. Práct., 21:310, 1962.

Hinselmann, H.: Colposcopy. Wuppertal-Elberfeld, Verlag W. Girardet, 1955.

Lang, W. R.: The cervical portio from menarche on: A colposcopic study. Ann. N.Y. Acad. Sci., 97:653, 1962.

Li Ying, et al.: Relationship between cervical erosion and cervical precancerous lesion or microinvasive carcinoma of erosive type of cervix uteri: A clinico-pathological study of 700 cases. Zhoughua Fu-Chauke Zazhi, 11:221, 1965.

López de la Osa, L.: Solución de penicilina bruta en la cervicitis. Toko-Ginec. Pract., 6:226, 1966.

Mardakhiashvili, Sh. I., and Taronshvili, R. S.: Phagocytic activity of leukocytes in indolent erosions and neoplastic processes of the uterine cervix and its changes under the influence of radium therapy. Akush. Ginek., 40:87, 1964.

Mateu Aragonés, J. M.: La exploración colposcópica en la práctica ginecológica: Lesiones benignas. Orbe Ginec. Obstet., 19, 1971.

Mestwerdt, G.: Enfermedades del hocico de tenca y del cuello uterino. In Schwalm and Döderlein (Eds.): Clinica Obstétrico-Ginecológica, Vol. 5, 1st Edit. Madrid, Editorial Alhambra, 1966.

Meyer, R.: Über Epidermoidalisierung (Ersatz des Schleimepithels durch Plattenepithel) an der Portio vaginalis uteri nach Erosion, an Cervicalpolypen und in der Cervicalschleimhaut. Zbl. Gynäk., 47:946, 1923.

Ostergard, D. R., Townsend, D. E., and Hirose, F. M.: Treatment of chronic cervicitis by cryotherapy. Am. J. Obstet. Gynec., 102:426, 1968.

Paloucek, F. P.: Communicat. to Symposium on Cryosurgery. U. Cal. Med. Center, March 11, 1967.

Rosenthal, A. H., and Hellman, L. M.: The epithelial changes in the fetal cervix, including the role of the "reserve cell." Am. J. Obstet. Gynec., 64:260, 1952.

Sands, R. X.: Cervical erosions in pregnancy. Obstet. Gynec., 2:414, 1953.

Zuckerman, S.: The histogenesis of tissues sensitive to oestrogens. Biol. Rev., 15:231, 1940.

Chapter Six

NORMAL RE-EPITHELIALIZATION OF ECTOPY

DEFINITION

Normal or typical re-epithelialization represents an effort of the flat squamous epithelium to replace the ectopic columnar epithelium gradually and to restore the epithelial limits that are considered normal (Fig. 151).

SYNONYMS

Zone of Typical Re-epithelialization. Transformation zone. Regular transformation zone. Normal transformation zone. Common transformation zone. Regeneration zone. Third cervical mucosa. Secondary original mucosa. Reconstruction zone. Reparation zone. Zone of normal scar readjustment. Cervical epidermization. Ascending epidermization. Sliding epidermization. Orthoplastic epidermization.

Hinselmann was the first to describe the reparative effort of the squamous epithelium, using the term *Umwandlungszone,* whose literal translation is transformation zone. This particular name, used by a multitude of foreign authors (Cramer, Mestwerdt, Coppleson, Lagrutta, and others) and Spanish ones (Mateu-Aragonés, Rodríguez-Soriano,

Gil-Vernet, and others), implies a mutation of shape or nature which really does not occur in the process under discussion. What does happen is the substitution of one epithelium for another. The term "transformation" might also suggest an unfavorable change, and it may induce the gynecologist not trained in colposcopy to think that he is facing an atypical lesion.*

The term "regeneration zone" does not seem correct either, because, as Masciotta states, if the term "transformation" is the excess of pessimism, that of "regeneration" is the excess of optimism. The mucosa originated as a consequence of the process of re-epithelialization is not exactly the same as the one that existed before, but rather a new mucosa which Barcellos and Nahoum call "third cervical mucosa" and other authors call "secondary original mucosa." It is characterized by the existence of glands in the deep layer and of squamous epithelium on the surface.

Even though in a broad sense one

---

*This logical explanation notwithstanding, the reader should be apprised of the nearly universal use of the term "transformation zone" in most current publications on this subject. — Ed.

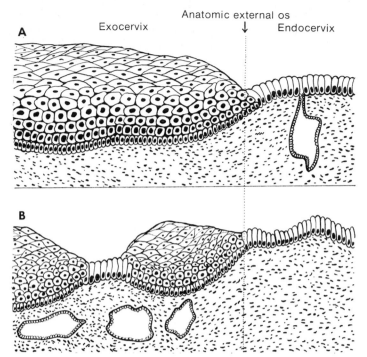

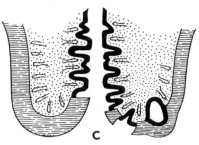

Figure 151. Typical re-epithelialization of ectopy. *A*, Normal cervix. *B*, Cervix with a zone of typical re-epithelialization. *C*, Comparative sketches of a normal cervix (left) and a zone of typical re-epithelialization (right).

could speak of a "reparation" zone, the term barely fits with the cervical changes we will study.

Bret and Coupez speak of a *zone de remaiement cicatriciel normal*, which literally could be translated as zone of normal scar readjustment. Use of the modifier "cicatricial" is not in accord with the facts.

Pathologists use the expression cervical epidermization, but the flat stratified epithelium of the vagina and exocer-

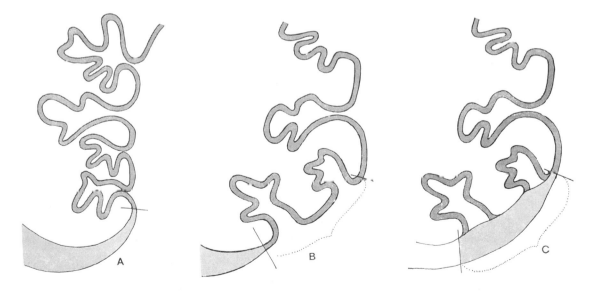

Figure 152. Mechanism of epidermization. *A*, Normal cervix. *B*, Displacement of the endocervical glandular columnar epithelium by the squamous epithelium of the endocervix has produced an ectopy. *C*, The ectopy has been "epidermized," the ectopic endocervical glands being covered by squamous epithelium which has grown from the periphery to the center in the second stage of healing (after Robert Meyer).

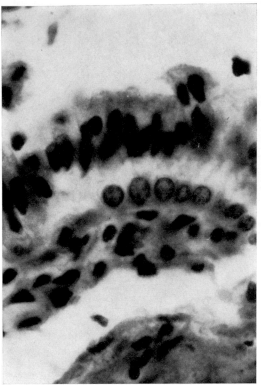

Figure 153. In a histologic section, reserve cells can be seen under the endocervical columnar epithelium. They are round, and each has a large nucleus.

vix is not equivalent to the epithelium of the epidermis.

Due to all these reasons we believe that the most appropriate term is typical re-epithelialization, used by González-Merlo, Calvo de Mora, and other authors and exactly expressing the histologic concept. However, there is a valid objection that this term could imply a prior lack of epithelium.

ORIGIN

For many years Meyer's idea has prevailed: that healing of ectopy was the consequence of growth of the squamous epithelium from the periphery to the center ("second stage of healing") (Fig. 152). This progression, in the form of tongues, would take place between the basement membrane and the columnar

epithelium of the surface, with the logical consequence of the shedding of the latter and its replacement by a flat stratified epithelium (orthoplastic epidermization). When this epithelium reaches the glandular orifices, it may act in two different ways: invade the gland, displacing the columnar epithelium and refilling the residual cavity, or continuing its surface growth, closing the glandular opening and causing a small retention cyst. This process, as Meyer recognized, is not continuous, but may be interrupted frequently by unfavorable circumstances which convert the re-epithelialization in a contest or epithelial struggle which may last for years.

This manner of interpreting the cervical reparative process is very suggestive, and even to modern colposcopists the ideas of Meyer have offered a viable explanation neither lacking in logic, nor failing to explain the morphologic details seen at the level of the "zone of typical re-epithelialization." However, it must be recognized that inexplicable aspects remain, such as the existence of plaques of squamous epithelium in the center of the ectopy, without any connection with the flat epithelium of the exocervix. Also, the presence of nests of stratified epithelium in some glands, which could not have arrived at that site by simple contiguous growth, cannot be entirely explained. It is not convincing to say that these could be remnants of squamous epithelium which resisted the pressure of the columnar epithelium in the course of the continuous epithelial struggle.

At present there is unanimous agreement that substitution of the columnar epithelium for the flat stratified type takes place by virtue of a process of indirect metaplasia, known also as physiologic metaplasia, squamous metaplasia, or prosoplasia. Even though the idea that "reserve cells" exist under the columnar epithelium with the capacity of being transformed into either columnar or squamous cells was suggested very early by authors such as Ruge and Veit (1878), the details of the metaplastic process were not well known until the investigations of Fluhmann and de Brux. Other authors, like Reid, have studied the histochemical aspects.

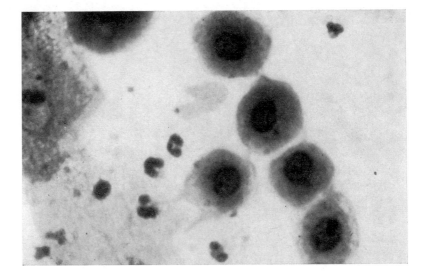

Figure 154. Cytologic smear in which a small group of reserve cells are seen. Observe the existence of the large nucleus and dense cytoplasm with some small vacuoles.

Origin of the Reserve Cells

The reserve cells, also called "metaplastic cells," "replacement cells," "subcolumnar cells," "infraepithelial cells," and "substitution cells," may theoretically have one of the following origins:

(1) From undifferentiated embryonic remnants, as assumed by Eichholz, which would remain for years under the columnar epithelium. More recently, Hellman and Rosenthal have presented this view.

(2) From squamous cells which had remained located in the basal layer of the columnar epithelium, in one of the frequent epithelial reversals of intrauterine life. This could take place at the establishment of the "second interepithelial border" around the seventh month (p. 82), when the columnar mucosa expels and replaces the squamous epithelium in the whole of the endocervix, even occupying part of the exocervix (Novak).

(3) From columnar cells of the ectopy itself, whether they are adult cells that survived a first stage of degeneration and which later divide by mitosis until they become differentiated as squamous epithelium (Kaufmann, Ruge), or simply basal columnar or squamous cells, which may be considered equipotent because they have a common embryonic origin (Fluhmann).

(4) Recently, the origin of the reserve cells has been suggested to be the cervical stroma (Song, Mestwerdt, Coppleson and Reid, and others).

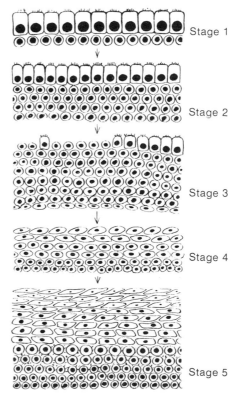

Figure 155. The stages of metaplasia, according to Fluhmann (explanation in text).

Whatever their origin, the reserve cells are an objective reality, because they are perfectly visible in many histologic samples (Fig. 153) and also in some cytologic smears (Fig. 154), and today there is no doubt regarding their role in the process of re-epithelialization of ectopy.

The reserve cells are round or oval, with a large nucleus that occupies the major portion of the cell, in such a manner that the cytoplasm is scarce but dense. Their size varies between 8 and 14 microns.

The reserve cells stain with silver nitrate but not with PAS, in contrast to the columnar cells which take up PAS but not silver nitrate. This fact may greatly contribute to identification of the reserve cells. Their resemblance to the basal cells of squamous exocervical epithelium in the female fetus is surprising.

Stages of Physiologic Metaplasia

Fluhmann has described five stages (Fig. 155):

(1) Appearance of the reserve cells, under the columnar epithelium.

(2) Proliferation and stratification of the reserve cells until there are 4 to 8 rows, preserving all the characteristics of the original cells. In this way the columnar cells are separated from the basement membrane.

(3) The columnar cells are separated; proliferation of the reserve cells ceases, and they begin to differentiate into squamous epithelium. By mistake they may continue proliferating, without differentiation, producing the appearance of dysplastic epithelium.

(4) Gradual differentiation and ordering of the newly formed epithelium. First a parabasal layer of hexagonal cells appears, which later elongate and then arrange themselves parallel to the surface. In this stage there is a small amount of glycogen, so that this epithelium stains faintly with PAS. This chromatic detail and the fact that the cells are still very compact make the contrast between the old and new squamous epithelium very notable.

(5) Appearance of squamous epithelium which histologically and functionally is practically normal.

The experienced histologist is capable of differentiating the two types of epithelium quite early.

Dynamic View of Metaplastic Repair

If environmental conditions are favorable, ectopy will be re-epithelialized, and its columnar epithelium replaced with flat stratified epithelium as a consequence of metaplasia with two possible origins. (1) Flat epithelial tongues progressively invade the ectopy from the outer edges. (2) A certain number of metaplastic plaques appear in the glandular mucosa, in the form of islets, initially dispersed and later grouped.

In a progressive manner, the squamous repair process from both starting points gains ground, until the epithelia from both origins are interlaced. Finally the whole exocervix is covered by a flat, squamous, normal epithelium. This process is considered as the normal route among the different possibilities of cervical repair.

Table 25.   Frequency of Typical Re-epithelialization

	ISOLATED	ASSOCIATED	TOTAL
Figuero et al. (1971)	—	—	22.9 %
Arenas et al. (1961)	—	—	30.6 %
Berger and Wenner-Mangen (1953)	20.75%	17.25%	38.0 %
Fernández Laso (1960)	—	—	40.0 %
González-Merlo (1966)	25.1 %	16.9 %	42.01%
Youssef (1957)	—	—	61.9 %
Mateu-Aragonés (1971)	15.17%	47.29%	62.46%
Our Series (1972)	12.4 %	20.2 %	32.6 %

FREQUENCY

After ectopy, colposcopic images associated with typical re-epithelialization are the ones most frequently observed, being not less than 32.6 per cent of all of our colposcopic diagnoses. In an important number of cases (20.2 per cent) there is evolutionary re-epithelialization, coexisting with a major or minor ectopy. In 12.4 per cent of cases re-epithelialization is diagnosed as a simple residual lesion. Figures found in the literature vary enormously (Table 25).

COLPOSCOPIC APPEARANCES

Typical re-epithelialization of ectopy takes place in three phases.

Initial Phase. Only at the outset is it possible to observe re-epithelialization originating from the edges of the ectopy. In this phase central metaplastic plaques are not yet seen.

Either in the whole periphery of the ectopy, or in only some areas, a very thin and transparent squamous epithelium appears, from which small extensions are directed radially to the center, sometimes accompanied by more or less fine vessels. On occasion, the epithelium is so thin that it gives the impression of a fine curtain covering a small portion of the ectopy, which shows through. This impression is erroneous because, as we know by histology, this metaplastic epithelium is not situated above the columnar epithelium, but beneath it until it sloughs.

The epithelial tongues are of different sizes and lengths. On occasion they adopt the shape of wide strips that slowly advance, forming a stable tissue. At other times they are slender branches which rapidly progress, interweaving

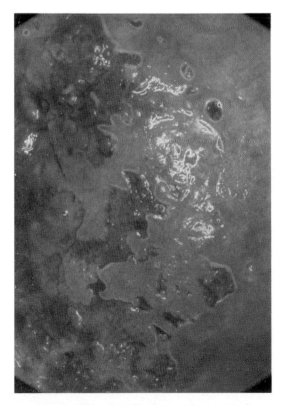

Figure 156. Initial phase of a typical re-epithelialization of an ectopy. Tongues of different sizes are seen, together with small islets of undamaged ectopy and some glandular orifices.

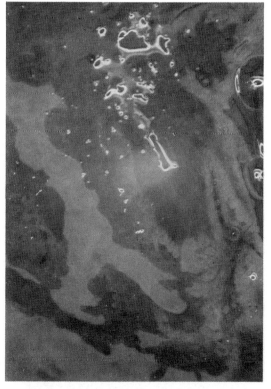

Figure 157. Interlacing of different tongue-like projections of re-epithelialization which give the cervix a "lacy" appearance. The fragility of these epithelial bands is evident.

one with another and leaving large islets of ectopy not epithelialized. These slender epithelial extensions are not visible unless the cervix is impregnated with acetic acid (Fig. 156). On occasion, the interweaving of bands of this newly formed squamous epithelium at different angles creates an overall picture not lacking in beauty, and resembling a lattice (Fig. 157).

When re-epithelialization is initiated rapidly due to favorable circumstances, the small glandular orifices of the columnar epithelium are usually not invaded to their utmost depths nor refilled. Rather the metaplasic epithelium jumps over them, obstructing the glandular opening and causing small retention cysts or "nabothian follicles," (p. 68) or bypasses the outlet, which remains intact (Fig. 158).

Advanced Phase. Also called "full evolution" by Bret and Coupez, this phase is characterized by the beginning of the central metaplastic process (Fig. 159) and by gradual maturation and differentiation of the recently formed squamous epithelium (Fig. 160). It is possible to observe three well defined zones:

CENTRAL CIRCUMORAL ZONE. Formed by ectopy without signs of re-epithelialization, which continues without transition into the endocervical mucosa.

INTERMEDIATE OR MIXED ZONE. Notably rich in admixtures of patterns, this is where the active process of re-epithelialization occurs. Several specific things may be seen.

(1) Metaplastic plaques of different shapes and sizes, depending on location and the degree of local resistance to their appearance. The epithelium of these plaques is similar at its edges to the newly formed epithelium, even though it does not present retention cysts, the glandular orifices are few or nonexistent, and these areas are brighter than the new epithelium (Fig. 159).

If the ectopy is not subject to an inflammatory process, its repair at the expense of the central metaplastic plaques may be very active, even more so than those proceeding from the edges of the lesion. The reason is that near the anatomic cervical os the pH is very low, permitting an easy disintegration of the columnar cells, which lose their lysosomes, making their replacement by metaplastic cells rather easy (Reid and Coppleson).

It seems beyond doubt that some ectopies heal exclusively from the effort of those central metaplastic plaques. The edges of the lesion adopt a circinate aspect until the end, with the result that until quite late in the process it is possible to see a considerable number of ectopic islets at this point, originated by the collision of the central reparative wave, with these fixed outer limits.

(2) The free edges of the peripheral tongues which are advancing toward their reunion with the central metaplastic plaques (Fig. 162). Their epithelium is not equally mature throughout its length. At the base, the iodine test is positive, which indicates that the cells contain glycogen; on the contrary, they do not fix iodine at the free edge (Fig. 163). Within these tongues, and especially the broader ones, a nabothian follicle is initiated at some point, signifying the deficient epidermization of a gland.

(3) Islands of ectopy, limited by the central plaques and peripheral extensions. On occasion, there are large fields of ectopy, whose papillae are intact. On other occasions a handful of papillae situated around a glandular crypt give the impression that the metaplastic process has suffered interference due to the abundant glandular secretion.

(4) Abundant vessels that course through the ectopy in all directions, but whose principal direction is toward the center.

PERIPHERAL ZONE. Here the characteristics of the initial phase, already described, are still seen, but are now undergoing progressive regularization. No islands of ectopy are seen, not even glandular orifices, even though the retention cysts formed at the outset persist. The pale and translucent epithelium has become thicker, its color being more pinkish, and it tends to look like normal squamous epithelium. If this does not occur, the most likely reason is that the vascularization is not normal.

Terminal Phase. The columnar epithelium of the ectopy has been completely replaced by squamous epithe-

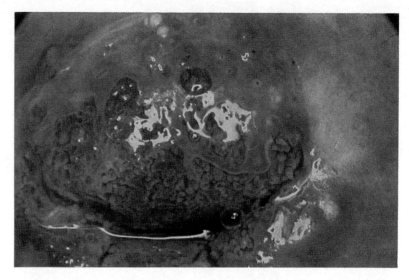

Figure 158. Re-epithelialization that occurs rapidly. Abundant islets of ectopy remain, and glandular orifices appear without covering.

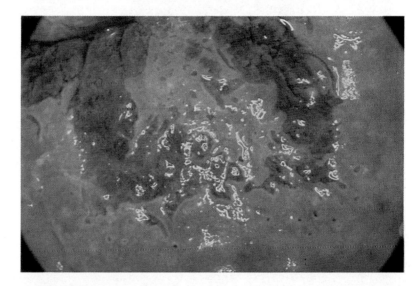

Figure 159. Central metaplastic plaque already connected to metaplastic epithelium coming from the edges of the ectopy.

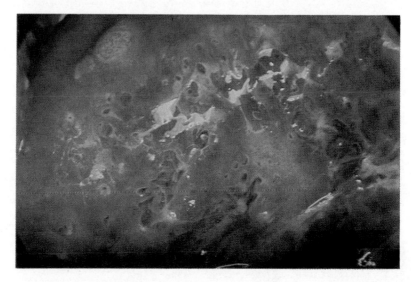

Figure 160. An advanced stage of typical re-epithelialization. The newly formed epithelium reaches the anatomic external os.

lium of metaplastic origin. However, this does not mean that the cervix has been totally restored to the appearance it had prior to the ectopy: there always remain sequelae, both glandular and vascular, which permit the expert in colposcopy to indicate the approximate limits of the old lesion.

We have proposed classifying this residual zone into two types, "regular" and "irregular," according to the appearance of the cervix. If the metaplastic repair is almost perfect, and the result nearly resembles the original mucosa, the residual zone is called regular. If there are numerous sequelae, seen under direct observation and without colposcopy, the residual zone is termed irregular and is suspicious.

To the contrary, Zinser speaks about "zones of open transformation" and "zones of closed transformation," considering that the glandular sequelae are formed by "fenced" images (red or white) and "islets of ectopy," or by tapered glands, closed by the reparative process ("drops of fat" "nabothian cysts," etc.). Lagrutta, Laguens and Quijano use identical nomenclature. This could really be a subclassification of our "irregular residual zone."

ZONE OF REGULAR TYPICAL RE-EPITHELIALIZATION. In this type the metaplastic epithelium has reached practically to the anatomic external os without leaving any islet of ectopy and with few glandular orifices visible in the zone previously occupied by the lesion. Such glandular orifices as do persist are not secretory and do not lead to maceration of the surrounding epithelium. Retention cysts are not found, or if present are practically invisible, because they have remained buried in the interior of the stroma and they no longer function. These characteristics justify the name of "secondary original mucosa," which has been applied on some occasions (Fig. 164).

Assurance that this epithelium is metaplastic and not original comes from its color, which remains less pink than the normal squamous epithelium, and the characteristic arborescent vascularization. There is a subepithelial vascular reticulum, which is clearly visible because the epithelium is always thinner than ordinarily, with a radial display and fine arborescent ramifications which cross each other. Its regular path, clearly seen and of uniform caliber, and its permanence in only one level, indicate that the picture is a benign one.

Generally the "regular" zone identifies a cervix free of infectious processes, or one which can defend itself properly when faced with inflammatory stimuli. Reid and Coppleson have insisted that besides the metaplastic re-epithelialization, a proliferation of the plasmocytes of the stroma is produced, with increased production of local antibodies and Russell's bodies.

ZONE OF IRREGULAR TYPICAL RE-EPITHELIALIZATION. In this case the sequelae are so numerous that to the naked eye, one does not know if the lesion is an extensive ectopy or a malignant process. Even with the colposcope, but without adequate preparation, doubt

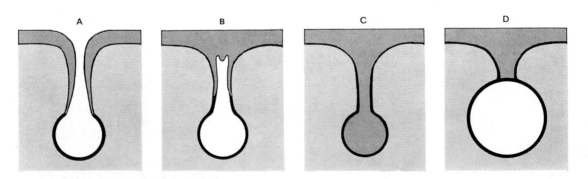

Figure 161. Sketch of the different disorders and sequelae of irregular typical re-epithelialization. *A*, White rings. *B*, Walled-in glandular orifice. *C*, Wax drops. *D*, Nabothian cyst.

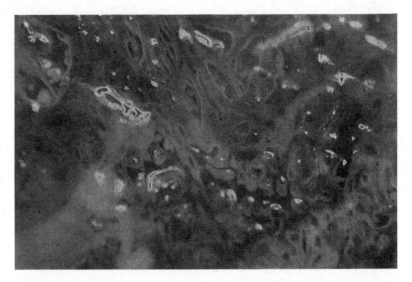

Figure 162. Detail of a typical re-epithelialization at high magnification. Beside the glandular crypts, encircled by granules of intact ectopy, metaplastic strips are seen that progressively reduce the extension of the columnar epithelium. Observe the thinness and delicacy of the new epithelium.

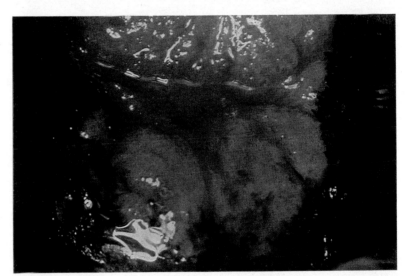

Figure 163. Typical re-epithelialization zone in an advanced phase, after Lugol's solution has been applied.

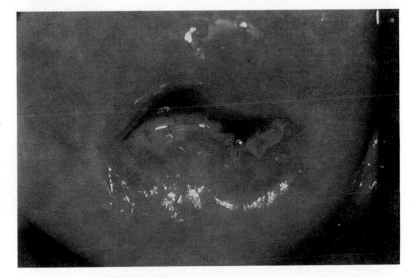

Figure 164. Zone of regular typical re-epithelialization.

may persist. Once the acetic acid test has been performed, the following sequelae are visible (Fig. 161).

Glandular Sequelae.

Islets of ectopy, which due to the presence of extensive glandular crypts have remained undamaged by the metaplastic attack. They usually secrete abundant mucus which keeps the squamous epithelium from growing because it macerates and destroys it. However, the papillae which are preserved are always paler than those of normal ectopy (Fig. 158).

Retention cysts or *nabothian follicles,* originated by the metaplastic epithelium when it closes the orifice of a gland without refilling it. The gland continues secreting mucus, which distends it and converts it into a cyst. The colposcopic appearance of these formations is typical: they appear as circumscribed swellings, of varying size up to the size of a nut, of white to yellowish color, with two or three vessels ramifying profusely on the surface (Figs. 165 and 166). Two or more nabothian cysts of small size may be found engulfed within a larger cystic process.

Nabothian follicles of considerable volume have a much whiter and denser color than the ordinary follicle due to the thickening of the epithelial layer, stimulated in its growth by the internal tension of the cyst.

On occasion intracystic bloody extravasation is produced, which makes the color change to reddish or bluish (hemorrhagic nabothian cyst). Frequently, the cause is traumatic. When the color is whitish and the follicle appears flat, differentiation from leukoplakia must be precise. The differences are basic: elevation, vascularization, and regularity of surface mark the nabothian follicle. Leukoplakia has little or no elevation and no vessels, and its surface usually has a nacreous or granular aspect.

"Wax drops," which are nothing more than glands completely refilled by

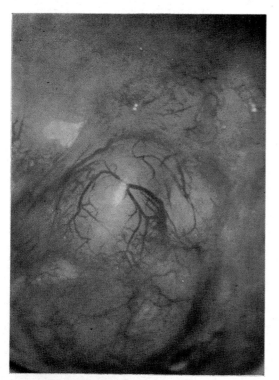

Figure 165. Retention cyst, with an exuberant vascularization, which also distorts the anterior lip of the cervix.

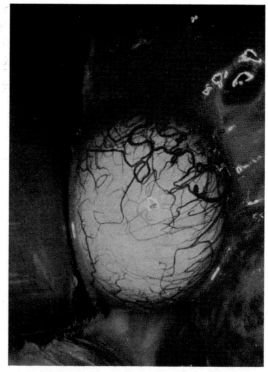

Figure 166. Nabothian cyst of unusual size, very striking due to its elevation and vascularization. It is an authentic mucous cyst.

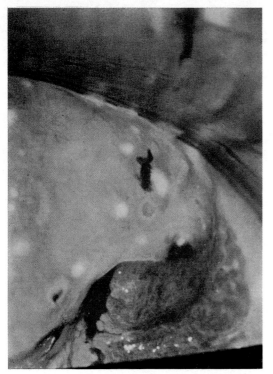

Figure 167. "Wax drops," sequelae of an irregular typical re-epithelialization. A small glandular crater is also seen.

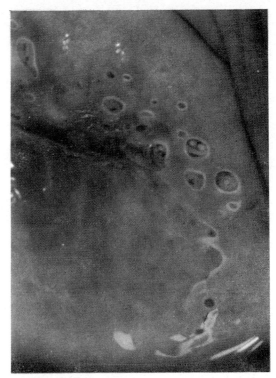

Figure 168. "White rings" forming part of an irregular typical re-epithelialization. Some glandular orifices exhibit papillary elements in their interior.

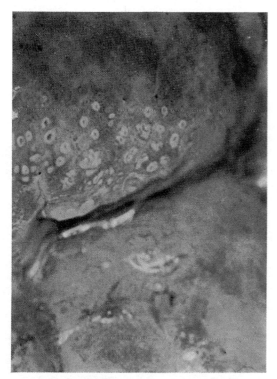

Figure 169. Cervix with many glandular orifices, markedly cornified. Their abundance justifies the term of "sieve cervix."

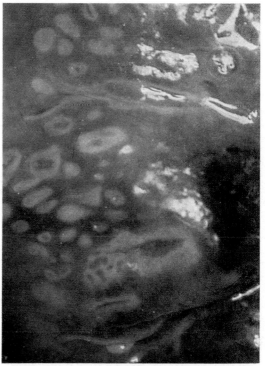

Figure 170. "White rings" which raise suspicion due to their wide diameter and visual intensity.

metaplastic epithelium ("glandular epidermization"). The additional thickness of the epithelium is responsible for its intense white color (Fig. 167). The existence of vessels excludes the possibility of leukoplakia. On occasion several drops unite, forming plaques which may become embossed.

"White rings" are point-like orifices limited by a whitish ring, sometimes quite wide (about five or six times the size of the orifice). Mestwerdt has called them "cornified orifices" (Fig. 168). On occasion a drop of clear mucous liquid flows and "drips" through the hole. This explains the frequent maceration of the tissue that forms the ring and also the persistence of glandular epithelium in its proximity.

The histopathologic explanation involves the partial re-epithelialization of the gland. Metaplastic epithelium has penetrated the glandular outlet, covering its walls, but without refilling or closing it.

On occasion the cervix may be totally perforated by orifices of this type, giving rise to the name "sieve-like" or "honeycomb-like" re-epithelialization zone (Fig. 169). As we will see in the next chapter (p. 167) this type of vascular sequela requires careful follow-up, because it can be the origin of an "atypical transformation zone" (Fig. 170).

Colposcopic signs that should make one suspect that the ordinary glandular sequelae of an irregular re-epithelialization are converting into extraordinary ones ("intraglandular dysplasia") are (1) persistence of the white cords and droplet images long after completion of the repair of the ectopy; (2) increase in the diameter of the white rings at successive examinations; (3) increase in the visual intensity of the rings, with or without augmentation in size; and (4) establishment of a superficial maceration zone around the white rings.

"Red cords" around the glandular orifices may be of two dimensions: small, if the glandular crypts are without epithelialization, and large, if they are formed by rupture of a retention cyst. It is possible to observe small craters bathed in mucus (Fig. 171).

Some of the glandular orifices, especially those circumscribed by a "red cord," may be provided with an evacuation channel, more or less prolonged and deep, with a reddish trench and macerated edges. When there are various orifices in this condition, the trenches will show a parallel arrangement. Exceptionally, an ectopic gland may be seen with two orifices and trenches that are disposed in opposite directions.

On occasion, re-epithelialization has been very laborious and there are successive metaplastic waves superimposed one on another. This explains why it is sometimes possible to observe a small glandular orifice within one of regular size. The small opening lies deeper and corresponds to an older epithelial layer.

Vascular Sequelae.

Vascular hypertrophy is associated with the regenerative process of the epithelium, because of an increased need for nutrition by the growing tissue. When the zone of typical re-epithelialization is regular, the principal vessels are oriented radially around the cervical os and exhibit fine arborescent ramifications.

In the irregular case, it is possible to observe benign vascular irregularities, which notably disturb the complete regularization of the cervix (Fig. 172). Possibly due to hormonal influences there may appear vascular dilatations that may be confused with true varices. These dilatations and the thinness of the newly formed epithelium explain the ease with which these cervices bleed. On other occasions, the vascular irregularities consist of a dense and tangled reticulum that tends to mask or hide some of the glandular sequelae (Fig. 173). The last branches of successive divisions are anastomosed, giving the aggregate an appearance that resembles a mosaic (p. 122 and 193). Nevertheless, detailed study of these vessels excludes the suspicion of malignancy, because besides being situated all at the same level, they present a regular caliber and orderly arrangement.

Other Varieties of Typical Re-epithelialization

Vesicular Re-epithelialization. Vesicles may be seen close together in

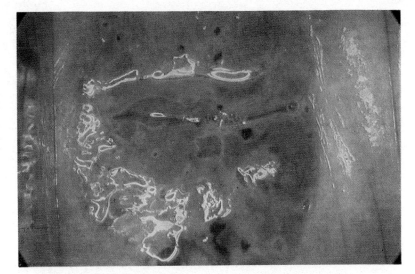

Figure 171. "Red rings" of different sizes, constituting a principal sequel of an irregular typical re-epithelialization.

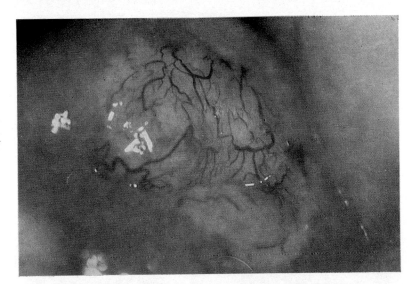

Figure 172. Vascular sequelae of a zone of irregular typical re-epithelialization, occupying the major portion of the anterior lip of the cervix.

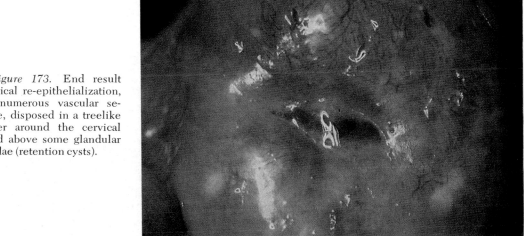

Figure 173. End result of typical re-epithelialization, with numerous vascular sequelae, disposed in a treelike manner around the cervical os and above some glandular sequelae (retention cysts).

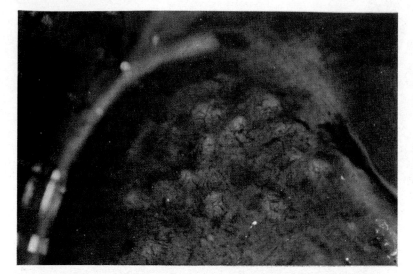

Figure 174. Microcystic typical re-epithelialization. The major portion of the cervix is occupied by minute retention cysts, very uniformly disposed. The endocervical mucosa is very reddened and has a striking vascular arborization, despite the small caliber of the vessels.

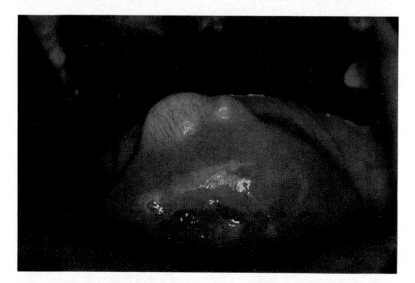

Figure 175. Vesicular typical re-epithelialization. On the anterior lip of the cervix a small honeycomb of vesicles of diverse sizes is seen.

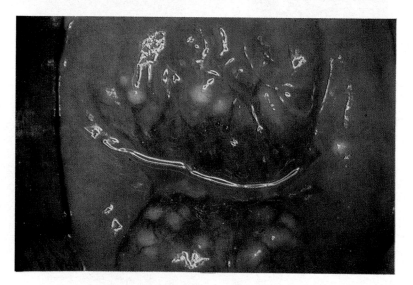

Figure 176. Uterine cervix perforated by retention cysts of small sizes, with a notable superficial vascular neoformation.

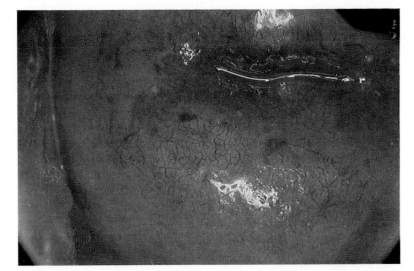

Figure 177. Zone of reticular typical re-epithelialization. The intertwining of the terminal vessels produce an image similar to that of a mosaic.

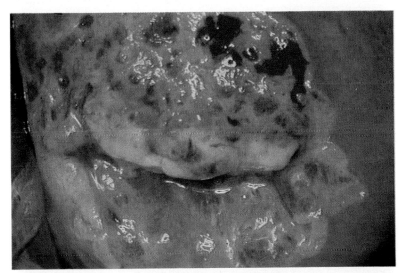

Figure 178. Inflammatory typical re-epithelialization. The existence of erosions, congestive and hemorrhagic zones, vascular irregularities, and images resembling vaginitis, alternating with wide areas of superficial maceration, may suggest a malignant process.

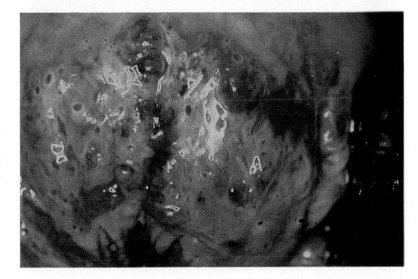

Figure 179. Macerated and infected zone of re-epithelialization, observed after the application of acetic acid. Extensive cervical areas adopt an edematous and whitish appearance. An infected secretion flows from the glandular orifices.

the periphery of an ectopy (Fig. 175). Their content, apparently liquid, is colorless and, as their epithelial covering is very thin, they stand out very little from the metaplastic mucosa. Sometimes the colposcopic picture resembles the rare "emphysematous vaginitis" (p. 40).

Perfect visibility of the vessels of the stroma through these vesicles calls attention to them. It seems as if their liquid content magnifies the size of the blood vessels.

Microcystic Re-epithelialization. This is the equivalent of the former term "follicular pseudoerosion." The whole cervix is full of small retention cysts, which to the naked eye appear as a multitude of yellow-whitish dots that perforate the exocervix (Fig. 174). Colposcopic observation demonstrates a very active vascular hypertrophy (Fig. 176).

Reticular Re-epithelialization. The entwined and pseudoanastomosed vessels of irregular re-epithelialization, if very intensive, may suggest a mosaic, especially if colposcopy is done without preparation (Hinselmann). Only adequate visualization of the vascularization, identifying its origin and course, will allow correction of the error (Fig. 177).

Inflammatory Re-epithelialization. As Bret and Coupez have said, secondary inflammation is practically constant at the level of the typical re-epithelialization, but when it becomes acute and affects re-epithelialization in its advanced phase, the resulting pictures may be very complex (Fig. 178). If the glands become infected, their mucus is transformed from clear to purulent, increasing epithelial maceration, which is common in the periphery of the open glandular orifices.

The infiltration of the stroma, the irregular vascularization, and the fragility of the recently formed epithelium, promptly cause the appearance of true erosion, which alternate with simple congestive or hemorrhagic zones. In some areas the stroma appears exposed and in others the residual columnar epithelium acquires a monstrous aspect. If to this appalling picture, we add the possibility of intermingled inflammatory lesions, it is easy to understand how a suspicious diagnosis can be arrived at in the presence of simple inflammatory re-epithelialization. Adequate anti-inflammatory treatment will rapidly wipe away these exuberant inflammatory images.

Pseudomosaic Re-epithelialization. This is a curious variety of typical re-epithelialization which may be very easily confused with an atypical one, because it simulates an image of superimposition identical to that identified as mosaic.

In the phase of initial re-epithelialization, when a young metaplastic epithelium replaces the columnar cells that cover the papillae of the ectopy, the papillary disposition takes some time to become regularized. The consequence is a colposcopic (and histologic) image analogous to that of mosaic, but more delicate (as delicate as the new epithelium), covering less area, and with poorly defined edges (contrary to the authentic "zone of atypical re-epithelialization," in which they are very precise). Another important difference is that the lines that separate the fields or "tiles" are in this case whitish, while in true mosaic they are reddish. These pathologic circumstances are especially found when a notable lymphocytic infiltration exists in the connective vascular axis which constitutes the papilla of the ectopy.

Macerated Re-epithelialization. Little has to be said in defining this variety. When glandular hyperplasia is very evident, and especially if the glands are infected, the squamous epithelium which surrounds them (including the remote ones) suffers the consequences of an altered moisture content and pH, with the logical consequence that its fragility increases and it erodes. The macerated areas take on an edematous, reddish appearance (white, after the application of acetic acid), with an exaggerated smoothness. These edematous plaques, which surround the hypersecreting glandular orifices, progressively unite until the major portion of the cervix becomes macerated. At this time the appearance of the lesion may be highly suspicious, and confusion with a cervix that contains a grave dysplasia is possible (Fig. 179).

The hormonal imbalances of the menstrual cycle and the outbreak of infections may perpetuate this state of affairs.

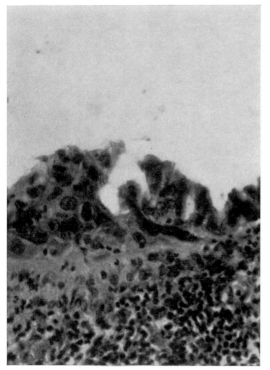

Figure 180. Histologic section of the intermediate zone of typical re-epithelialization, which shows metaplasia in its initial phases.

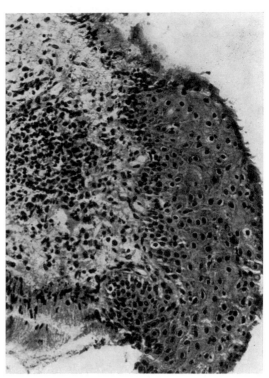

Figure 181. Histologic section corresponding to the periphery of a zone of typical re-epithelialization. Metaplasia in its final stage is observed.

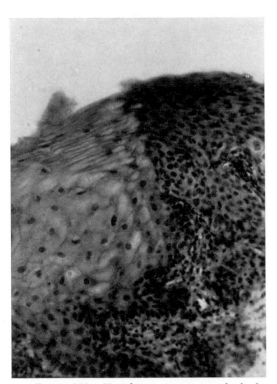

Figure 182. Histologic section in which the definite border between the original squamous epithelium and the metaplastic epithelium is observed.

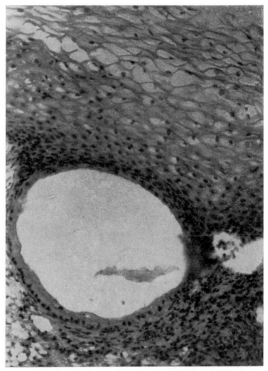

Figure 183. Histologic section of a small retention cyst located beneath a metaplastic squamous epithelium.

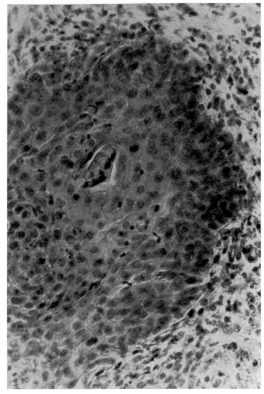

Figure 184. Total epidermization of a gland. The squamous epithelium has displaced or replaced all of the columnar epithelium of an endocervical gland. Only a small fragment in the center remains.

HISTOLOGIC CORRELATIONS

We have previously described the histogenesis of a zone of typical re-epithelialization, emphasizing the role of indirect metaplasia, starting from the reserve cells. On the other hand, when describing its colposcopic aspects, we have been correlating them with the histologic substrate. We now need only give a unified view of the newly formed epithelium in typical re-epithelialization.

Physiologic metaplastic epithelium may be seen during any phase of its formation, from the first stages, when the columnar epithelium of the surface has not completely sloughed (transitional zone), until maturation and complete differentiation (Figs. 180 and 181). The PAS stain permits a clear distinction between

Table 26. Histology of Evolving Typical Re-epithelialization

Physiologic metaplasia in its different phases	79.68%
Regular dysplasia	14.06%
Irregular dysplasia	0.0 %
Other benign diagnosis	1.68%
Carcinoma	1.56%

the two epithelial types. Some of the stages of the metaplasia may, undoubtedly, suggest the idea of cancer, especially while the epithelium remains undifferentiated and immature. Observation of the nuclei, which are completely normal, will prevent this error.

The overall appearance of the metaplastic epithelium will not be totally normal until much later. For this reason, the union between it and the squamous original epithelium usually forms an abrupt line (Schiller's physiologic line) (Fig. 182). The metaplastic epithelium, whatever its stage of maturity, is much thinner, denser, and darker in tone than the normal epithelium. The PAS stain accentuates these differences.

The stroma is usually occupied by a lymphocytic infiltration, due to the frequent inflammatory phenomena which accompany the reparative process. However, the most characteristic observation is the presence of glandular elements in different phases of epidermization, from the gland that has only its orifice obstructed, and which is developing into a retention cyst (Fig. 183), to the one whose opening is completely occupied by metaplastic tissue (Fig. 184).

On occasion, differentiation between partial epidermization and neoplastic invasion of a gland may be difficult. However, though the architectural characteristics of the smear may lead to such an

Table 27. Histology of Residual Typical Re-epithelialization

Physiologic metaplasia in its different phases	69.25%
Regular dysplasia	28.20%
Irregular dysplasia	2.54%

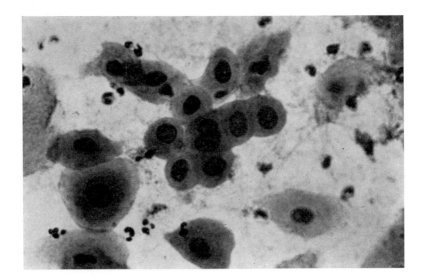

Figure 185. Cytologic smear in which a group of reserve cells is observed.

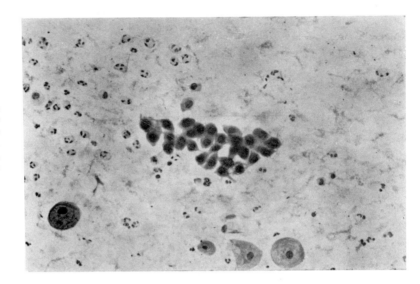

Figure 186. Reserve cells at low magnification. Compare their sizes with those of the other cells in the smear. Some of them are found with small typical cytoplasmic projections.

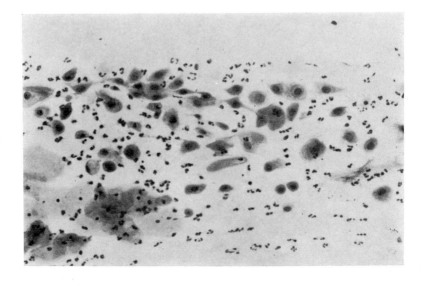

Figure 187. Cytologic smear showing cells of the reparative process.

Table 28.   Cytologic Correlation of
Evolving Typical Re-epithelialization

Class I	47.9%
Class II	50.0%
Class II-III	2.0%
Class III	0.0%
Class IV and V	0.03%

error on superficial observation, individual analysis of the cellular elements will clarify the impression.

We biopsy a lesion with this colposcopic image only on rare occasions (2.70 per cent of evolving zones, 2.77 per cent of regular residual zones, and 5.45 per cent of irregular residual zones), because we consider these benign. In 80 per cent of these biopsies the histologic picture is the one just described. The histopathologic diagnosis of dysplasia is not common. In the evolving phases of re-epithelialization dysplasia was found in only 14 per cent of cases, and in every one of these occasions it was mild (Table 26). However, the percentage increases significantly in irregular residual re-epithelialization (28.2 per cent show mild dysplasia and 2.56 per cent severe dysplasia), confirming the fact that, though the evolution of re-epithelialization is usually uneventful, in a small percentage of cases a neoplastic process may develop (Table 27).

CYTOLOGIC APPEARANCES

Unless the reparative metaplastic process is extensive and very active, cytologic smears have few characteristic signs (Table 28 and 29).

In the smears called "reparative" (10.7 per cent of all those obtained from evolving zones of typical re-epithelialization and 21.6 per cent of Papanicolaou's Class II smears obtained from the same material), the most significant element is the so-called "re-epithelialization cell" or "metaplastic cell." This is very characteristic, for its nucleus and cytoplasm both stain darkly. Its size is somewhat smaller than that of a normal parabasal cell and varies widely (Figs. 185 and 186).

The nucleus of such a cell is large and thick, situated either in the center of the cell or somewhat displaced to the periphery because of vacuoles or perinuclear halos which frequently occupy the cytoplasm. The latter is basophilic, and granulations are often observed. Typical of these cells is their oval, elongated shape, and the existence of small cytoplasmic projections which resemble the intercellular bridges of the deep thorny layer (Fig. 186).

Undoubtedly, re-epithelialization cells originate from the intense proliferation of the reserve cells which takes place during the metaplastic process.

Along with these cells, columnar elements may be seen, either more or less preserved or hyperplastic, as well as cytologic signs of the concomitant inflammation (leukocytes, plasmacytes, histiocytes, etc.). Mucus is abundant, and the squamous cells appear somewhat altered (perinuclear halos, vacuoles, discrete nuclear retraction, etc.). It is possible to observe inflammatory parabasal cells along with some reserve cells. Pure "desquamative-endocervical" extensions are rare, because the activity of the reparative process forces to the background the elements proceeding from the ectopy.

Table 29.   Cytologic Correlation of Residual Typical Re-epithelialization

	Total	Regular Zones	Irregular Zones
Class I	66.1%	68.1%	64.4%
Class II	32.0%	30.9%	32.9%
Class II-III	1.8 %	0.9%	2.5%
Class III	0.08%	—	0.14%
Class IV and V	—	—	—

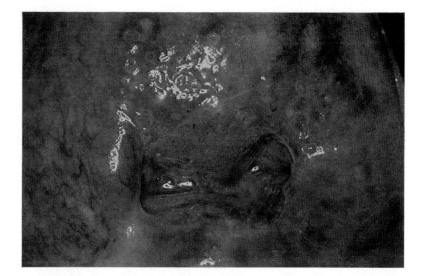

Figure 188. Typical re-epithelialization, which when seen requires only follow-up.

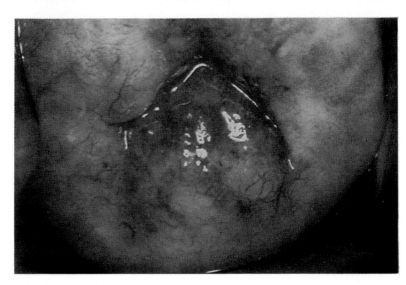

Figure 189. Typical re-epithelialization with vascular irregularities, which requires electrocoagulation.

CLINICAL COURSE

Statistics from the literature and our own series corroborate an idea in the mind of all colposcopists with sufficient experience: the regular zone of typical re-epithelialization, which has not suffered from periodic infections or hormonal imbalances that perpetuate an epithelial struggle, nor from mechanical traumatic interference, does not have any more tendency toward cancer formation than the original mucosa.

Something else must be said with respect to the irregular residual zone, the result of repeated epithelial upsets and subject to multiple adverse influences (especially inflammatory and hormonal) as a consequence of its fragility. In irregular epithelialization metaplastic phenomena are continual and alternate with destructive changes (maceration and inflammation). It is logical that at any given moment during these continuing cycles of destruction and reconstruction, appropriate circumstances may be produced so that physiologic metaplasia is disturbed in maturation and even in differentiation. Undoubtedly this is not the usual event, and cancer may develop in an irregular zone. This is to be expected in only a few cases, not more than 1.5 per cent. However, the possibility of dysplasia turning into cancer requires correct diagnosis and cautious management.

MANAGEMENT

In the initial phases of typical re-epithelialization, an expectant attitude must be adopted, observing the progress of the metaplastic process every two or three months and guarding against any pathologic circumstances which interfere with it, such as genital infection or unnecessary hormonal treatment. If difficulties are foreseen because of an inadequate vaginal environment (pH changes, concomitant vaginitis, incipient atrophy of the vaginal mucosa), it is necessary simultaneously to initiate adequate treatment to combat the inflammation, regularize the pH, or improve the tissue nutrition. In this respect, the good results obtained with estriol should be emphasized.

We take a similar approach to the advanced phases of re-epithelialization, when an infectious outbreak can easily overcome and destroy the restored epithelium, or worse, be the starting point of an irregular or inclusive atypical re-epithelialization.

Once the cervical re-epithelialization is complete, our action will depend on its appearance. If the exocervical coating has regained a practically normal appearance, and only a slightly pale coloration of the mucosa and an arborescent or "head of hair" vascularization suggest its metaplastic origin, it is unnecessary to do anything other than the obligatory annual check-up (Fig. 188).

However, with the disappearance of the ectopy, if a highly irregular re-epithelialization remains in its place, with multiple and extensive glandular and vascular sequelae which macerate the new epithelium and create a kind of medium for infectious processes, then the wisest approach is to destroy this deficient re-epithelialization (Fig. 189).

This has as its objective not only to prevent discomfort which could be caused by the irregular re-epithelialization (mucosal leukorrhea, periodic infections, suprapubic discomfort, possibility of extension of an infection toward the vesical trigone or the adnexa), but also to protect against possible development of cancer. It is not sufficient to destroy the epithelium by coagulation if an inflammatory process coexists. Sterilization to relieve infection is obligatory with topical sulfonamides or antibiotics as well as cortisone. This simple treatment often produces considerable improvement in the appearance of the cervix. Even so, sequelae will persist. Conization or surgical amputation may have to be done if the re-epithelialization zone is very old and the epithelial struggle has been prolonged, because there may be cervical hypertrophy as well as deep growth of the hyperplastic glands into the stroma. Conization with electrocautery or cryocoagulation may be used (see Management of Ectopy, p. 99).

Each zone of typical re-epithelialization that coagulated should be reexamined regularly until few glandular or vascular sequelae remain and the exocervical covering is practically normal. It may also be necessary to correct an ovarian steroid disturbance. The occasional success of treatment with androgens, once popular, may have been based on compensation for hyperestrogenism.

REFERENCES

Auerbach, S. H., and Pund, E. R.: Squamous metaplasia of the cervix uteri. Am. J. Obstet. Gynec., 49:207, 1945.

Barcellos, J. M., and Nahoum, J. C.: Cuello uterino: Notas de nomenclatura; Concepto de cuello normal y de tercera mucosa. Acta Ginec., 16:315, 1965.

Bret, J., and Coupez, F.: Colposcopie. Paris, Masson et Cie., 1960.

Bret, J., and Coupez, F.: Colposcopy of ectopy, ectropion and epidermization. Acta Cytol., 5:83, 1961.

Calvo de Mora, S. and Tubio, J.: Screening colposcópico en veintitrés mil enfermas ginecológicas. Communicat. to VII Cong. Nacional de Citologia, Seville, 1971.

Carmichael, R., and Jeaffreson, B. L.: Basal cells in the epithelium of the human cervical canal. J. Path. Bact., 49:63, 1939.

Coppleson, M.: The value of colposcopy in the detection of preclinical carcinoma of the cervix. J. Obstet. Gynaec. Brit. Comm., 67:11, 1960.

Coppleson, M.: Colposcopy, cervical carcinoma in situ and the gynaecologist: Based on experience with the method in 200 cases of carcinoma in situ. J. Obstet. Gynaec. Brit. Comm., 71:854, 1964.

Coppleson, M., and Reid, B. L.: Preclinical Carcinoma of the Cervix Uteri: Its Origin, Nature and Management. Oxford, Pergamon Press, 1967.

Cramer, H.: Die Kolposkopie in der Praxis. Stuttgart, Georg Thieme Verlag, 1956.

de Brux, J.: Morfología histológica y diagnóstico de las displasias y de los carcinomas "in situ" del cuello uterino. Progr. Obstet. Ginec., 7:19, 1964.

de Brux, J., and Dupre-Froment, J.: Papel de la citologia en el diagnóstico diferencial de las displasias, del epitelio activo de regeneración y del carcinoma "in situ" del cuello uterino. Acta Ginec., 14:1, 1963.

Eichholz, P.: Experimentelle Untersuchungen über die Epithelmetaplasie. Inaug. Diss., Königsberg, 1902.

Fluhmann, C. F.: Epidermidalization of the cervix uteri and its relation to malignancy. Am. J. Obstet. Gynec., 15:1, 1928.

Fluhmann, C. F.: The Cervix Uteri and Its Diseases. Philadelphia, W. B. Saunders Co., 1961.

Geschickter, C. F., and Fernandez, F.: Epidermidalization of the cervix. Ann. N.Y. Acad. Sci., 97:638, 1962.

Gil-Vernet, E., Balagueró, L., Gil-Vernet, E., and Ibáñez, R.: Valor clínico de los diferentes medios de exploración en el diagnóstico precoz del carcinoma de cuello. Communicat. to Sec. Esp. Asoc. Mund. Prev. del Cáncer Ginec., Málaga-Torremolinos, 1966.

González-Merlo, J., Vilar, E., Sánchez, J. and Silva, V.: Siete años de campaña colposcópica. Communicat. to Sec. Esp. Asoc. Mund. Prev. del Cáncer Ginec., Málaga-Torremolinos, 1966.

Green, G. H.: Cervical cytology and carcinoma in situ. J. Obstet. Gynaec. Brit. Comm., 72:13, 1965.

Hellman, L. M., Rosenthal, A. H., Kistner, R. W., and Gordon, R.: Some factors influencing the proliferation of the reserve cells in the human cervix. Am. J. Obstet. Gynec., 67:899, 1954.

Hinselmann, H.: Die Essigsäureprobe ein Bestandteil der erweiterten Kolposkopie. Deutsche Med. Wschr., 64:40, 1938.

Hinselmann, H.: Estado Actual de la Colposcopia. In Antoine, T. (ed.): Ginecologia. Buenos Aires, Edit. Mundi, 1956.

Kaufmann, C., and Ober, K. G.: The morphological changes of the cervix uteri with age and their significance in the early diagnosis of carcinoma of the cervix. In Wolstenholme, G. E. W. (ed.): Cancer of the Cervix. Ciba Foundation, Boston, Little, Brown and Co., 61, 1959.

Lagrutta, J., Laguens, R. P., and Quijano, F.: Cancer de Cuello Uterino: Estudios Primarios. Buenos Aires, Editorial Intermedica, 1966.

Lang, W. R.: Colposcopy—neglected method of cervical evaluation. J.A.M.A., 166:893, 1958.

Linhartová, A., and Štafl, A.: Morphologische Befunde an der Umwandlungszone der Portio vaginalis uteri. Arch. Gynäk., 200:590, 1965.

Masciotta, A.: La Colposcopia nella Lotta Contro Il Cancro e nella Diagnosi Ginecologica. Bologna, Licinio Cappelli, 1954.

Mateu-Aragonés, J. M.: Contribución al estudio de la exploración colposcópica: Importanicia de las modificaciones vasculares en la valoración de las imágenes colposcópicas atípicas. Rev. Esp. Obstet. Ginec., 24:141, 1965.

Mateu-Aragonés, J. M.: Clasificación de las imagenes vasculares y su importancia práctica. Rev. Clin. Inst. Matern., 18:281, 1967.

Meyer, R.: Über Epidermoidalisierung (Ersatz des Schleimépithels durch Plattenepithel) an der Portio vaginalis uteri nach Erosion, an Cervicalpolypen und in der Cervicalschleimhaut. Zbl. Gynäk., 47:946, 1923.

Novak, E.: The pathologic diagnosis of early cervical and corporeal cancer with special reference to the differentiation from pseudomalignant inflammatory lesions. Am. J. Obstet. Gynec., 18:449, 1929.

Reid, B. L., and Blackwell, P. M.: Physiological metaplasia on the human cervix uteri: Some histo- and cyto-chemical observations. Aust. N. Z. J. Obstet. Gynaec., 4:62, 1964.

Reid, B. L., and Coppleson, M.: Physiological metaplasia on the human cervix uteri: A colposcopic and histological correlative study of the earliest stages. Aust. N. Z. J. Obstet. Gynaec., 4:62, 1964.

Rodríguez-Soriano, J. A., and Benasco Naval, C.: La citologia tipo III y su correlacion colposcopica. Acta Ginec., 19:823, 1968.

Ruge, C., and Veit, J.: Der Krebs der Gebärmutter. Z. Geburtsh. Gynäk., 7:138, 1882.

Song, J.: The Human Uterus: Morphogenesis and Embryological Basis for Cancer. Springfield, Ill., Charles C Thomas, 1964.

Stegner, H. E.: Elektronenoptischen Untersuchungen bei der indirekten Metaplasie des Zervixepithel. Zbl. Gynäk., 91:762, 1969.

Wada, T., and Imamura, Y.: Metaplastic epithelial changes in the cervix of pregnant uterus. Clin. Gynec. Obstet., 15:505, 1961.

Zinser, H. K.: Colposcopy of ectopy, ectropion and epidermization. Acta Cytol., 5:86, 1961.

Zuckerman, S.: The histogenesis of tissues sensitive to oestrogens. Biol. Rev., 15:231, 1940.

Chapter Seven

DYSPLASTIC CERVIX

Cervical dysplasia continues to be one of the most debated topics in histopathology as well as in cytology and colposcopy. Until recent years, the word dysplasia (Ober, 1942) was considered synonymous to precancer. However, at present, the term is considered to be a non-neoplastic alteration of the cervix. As would be expected, this change has created problems; to follow this definition exactly, we would have to include among dysplastic lesions those far from malignancy, such as vaginitis and dystrophies. Such a grouping would be unduly exaggerated and not useful, so that, in practice, under the generic term dyspla-

sia are grouped all cervical lesions which, without being malignant, could have or attain some relationship to cancer.

One of the principal points of discussion is the possible relationship between cervical dysplasia and carcinoma in situ. Hence, while some pathologists speak about carcinogenesis of dysplasia (Willis, Peterson, Richart, Varga), because they attribute to that lesion the role of an intraepithelial precancer, others consider that the dysplasias should be catalogued as benign lesions, neatly separated from in situ cancer (de Brux, Rawson, and Knoblich). For the latter, "precancerous

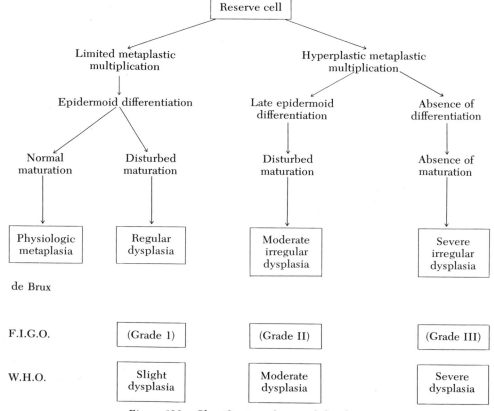

Figure 190. Classification of cervical dysplasia.

dysplasia" would not be anything else than cancer, more or less masked.

An attempt at harmonizing these disparities is found in the classification of dysplasias as "regular" and "irregular" (de Brux) or, as the WHO has suggested, as "slight," "moderate," and "severe" (Figure 190).

Regular or slight dysplasia would have very little to do with cancer, because it would create only a minor disturbance in epithelial maturation. On the contrary, irregular dysplasia (moderate or severe) could evolve, under certain special conditions, toward a clearly malignant epithelium. Some authors believe that these are potentially precancerous, because the epithelial disturbance they reflect involves not only maturation but also differentiation. Many pathologists find it difficult to differentiate a severe dysplasia from an in situ carcinoma.

Dysplastic cervix corresponds to the colposcopic images designated by Hinselmann as "matrix areas," and within this category, reference was made to patterns such as "leukoplakia," "ground structure," and "mosaic structure." The great authority of Hinselmann has resulted in the persistence of this classification, unmodified until 1949 when Glattharr introduced a fourth kind of atypical epithelium, the so-called "zone of atypical transformation," which is described as a lesion apparently unrelated to the matrix areas. At almost the same time, added to this list of atypical images were two colposcopic entities, true erosion and vascular irregularities.

The frequency of this aggregate of atypical colposcopic images or lesions (the expression "atypical epithelium" in colposcopy seems to us unfortunate) varies widely in the literature (see p. 10), but is most often stated to be between 10 and 20 per cent.

This simplistic and scarcely dynamic view of cervical dysplastic pathology has one strong drawback. If we biopsy all of the patterns of ground structure, mosaic, leukoplakia, erosion, and vascular irregularities that we see (as is usually advised), the frequency of biopsy would be high (near 20 per cent), but the number of truly dysplastic or frankly malignant lesions found would be small (around 2 per cent), undoubtedly not justifying the enormous effort that such an extensive histologic study would represent. Moreover, if this were done, colposcopy will come to be demeaned in spite of the logical and reasonable part it can play in arriving at an actual and prospective prognosis.

Mestwerdt says, with reason, that the relative ease with which "matrix areas" are identified by the colposcopist has caused an overemphasis upon these lesions and an inadequate amount of attention to the accompanying circumstances.

In an effort to state precisely which atypical images require biopsy and which do not, many authors (Dzioba, Busch, Martin-Laval and Dajoux, etc.) have attempted to establish a methodical arrangement of the atypical colposcopic appearances and the prognostic grades.

Table 30. Correlation Between the Diverse Classifications of Dysplastic Colposcopic Lesions

Rocha and Teixeira (1959)	Dzioba (1960)	Busch (1965)	Martin-Laval and Dajoux (1970)	Coppleson, Pixley and Reid (1971)	Our Series (1972)
Group I (Picture of moderate atypia)	Grade I	Class III	Grades III and IV	Grade I	Atypical re-epithelialization
	Grade II			Grade II	Beginning atypical transformation
Group II (Picture of severe atypia)		Class IV	Grade V		
	Grade III			Grade III	Destructive atypical transformation

Coppleson, Pixley and Reid were responsible for the latest of these endeavors, which included all the colposcopic pictures depending on metaplastic change in three grades. According to these authors, grade I corresponds histologically with slight dysplasia; grade II with moderate and severe dysplasia and, in exceptional cases, with preclinical carcinoma; and grade III corresponds with in situ and preclinical invasive carcinomas.

These contributions, attempting to classify in harmonious form all the atypical or dysplastic findings, are praiseworthy, but it is evident that they have increased the extraordinary terminologic confusion that already exists (see Table 30). To us it seems contradictory that, when trying to substitute the cytologic classification of Papanicolaou for more descriptive denominations, they attempt to introduce such hazy individual terminology into colposcopy.

These objections to the prognostic grades and the evident mistrust inspired in some schools by any attempt to establish a more exact correspondence between colposcopic and histologic appearances explain why many colposcopists obstinately cling to the classic terminology and unequivocally recommend biopsy for all atypical images or lesions.

At present, after having performed more than 30,000 colposcopic examinations in our hospital and private practice, we believe that the pathology of the dysplastic cervix cannot be followed by being studied through the classic prism. We think, after correlating the colposcopic, cytologic, and histologic findings in a significant number of cases, that it is necessary to keep in mind two habitually overlooked facts:

(1) The terms "image" and "lesion" are not interchangeable. This distinction, well established by Coupez (1968) and progressively expanded in the colposcopic literature, requires that the more elementary colposcopic appearances (images) not be confused with the nosologic pictures (lesions) that they help to elucidate. The images, which have a significance similar to that of the so-called "obvious lesions" in dermatology, have no importance except as they help define the lesion of which they form

a part. Thus, each lesion is made up of a variable number of images or primary elements, some of which can be practically specific for it, but which in some way admit of being confused with it.

These concepts are as valid for the typical appearances of the uterine cervix as they are for the atypical. Moreover, some images can indiscriminately form part of both typical and atypical lesions. Such is the case with erosion and vascular irregularities, and also with leukoplakia.

(2) There are some "aggravating" and other "attenuating" signs that allow the lesion to be interpreted as arising from certain determined elemental images. Some years ago we indicated as aggravating signs: the visualization of the lesion without prior preparation, the presence of vascular irregularities accompanying the remaining primary images, and the variegated mixture of them. They have somewhat the same meaning as the "warning signs" proposed by the Zurich school and by Palmer. As attenuating signs we noted the existence of a concomitant inflammation, clear borders of the lesion, and the presence of pregnancy. With attention to these signs and others of a morphologic nature that we will study in the following chapters, it is possible to diagnose not only images, a thing of very limited importance, but also lesions, a fact that will permit us to establish a prognosis and decide the management.

As atypical elementary images or colposcopic appearances would have to be considered: leukoplakia, ground structure, mosaic, vascular irregularities and erosion.

One or more of these images (usually two or more) can form a lesion endowed with legitimate individuality whose overall appearance will depend on those aggravating or attenuating signs and on a series of morphologic peculiarities specific for the lesion itself and for its biologic nature.

According to our experience two lesions or dysplastic entities are well distinguished colposcopically and have a very distinct pathogenetic and evolutionary significance: zone of atypical re-epithelialization and zone of atypical transformation.

The zone of atypical re-epithelialization is likely to correspond histo-logically with a moderate or trifling dysplasia. Its alterations are therefore limited to disturbances of epithelial maturation. Only in exceptional cases can they mask a carcinoma.

The zone of atypical transformation, on the contrary, has a high degree of malignancy, not only potential but actual-ly inherent. Its most usual histologic translation is irregular dysplasia (moder-ate or severe) and carcinoma in situ. It signifies that it contains alterations not only of maturation but also of differenti-ation. In only a small percentage of cases will biopsy demonstrate a trifling dys-plasia.

From this histologic correlation, which we will expound in greater detail later, can be deduced the importance of diagnosing lesions and not only images.

Ground structure, mosaic, or erosion can correspond, as elemental aspects that they are, with anything from a meta-plasia discretely disturbed in its matura-tion to an invasive carcinoma. And thence the recommendation of the colposcopists who follow the classic nomenclature that all atypical colposcopic images should be biopsied.

The two lesions indicated should, on the contrary, have a more fixed histologic correspondence. It is not that each of them can be considered as pathog-nomonic or a definite histologic lesion. To pretend that would be absurd, now that colposcopy has oriented us toward the architecture of the tissue and its vessels; it only provides us with indirect signs about the cell type. What has hap-pened is that when an expert colpos-copist takes a biopsy of a zone of atypical re-epithelialization, he knows that *very probably, but not always,* histologic examination will inform him about a dysplasia that is trifling or at most moderate. And when he does the same with a zone of atypical transformation, he expects to find a cancer in *approxi-mately* half the cases. In the remainder, histologic examination can give another diagnosis. For this reason, and taking for granted that cytologic examination can be done simultaneously, it is possible to abstain from biopsy in many cases of atypical re-epithelialization (for example, during pregnancy); biopsy should always be performed in atypical transformation.

This view of colposcopy, manifestly more extensive, dynamic and prospec-tive, tends not to introduce elements of confusion or complication into the terminology. On the contrary, the simpli-fication is noteworthy; all the innumer-able diagnoses of atypical "epithelia" and "images" are included in *two* legitimate, well defined pictures.

To facilitate comprehension in this chapter, we will describe first the elementary *images*, putting special emphasis on leukokeratosis (leuko-plakia, mosaic, ground structure). Final-ly, we will take up the *lesions*, describing successively their origin, their colpo-scopic diagnosis, their evolution, and the eventual management we recommend in each case.

Table 31.   Malignant Potential of the Matrix Areas of Hinselmann

	LEUKOPLAKIA	GROUND STRUCTURE	MOSAIC
Berger and Wenner-Mangen (1950)	12%	3.4%	8.9%
Burghardt and Bajardi (1954)	17.7%	12.6%	18.9%
Limburg (1956)	9.4	9.9	13.2
Bajardi (1961)	8	—	—
Wilds (1962)	27	7.6	4.3
Grismondi (1966)	3.1	—	—
González-Merlo (1966)	3.32	10.43	5.37
Zamarriego et al. (1966)	3.1	5.8	10
Guzmán Llovet (1967)	1.97	9.09	12.12
Villalba et al. (1968)	17	13	11
Gil Vernet et al. (1969)	5.8	11.26	7.1
Our Series (1972)	4.9	8	7.1

ATYPICAL IMAGES

Of the five traditional atypical images—leukoplakia, ground structure, mosaic, erosion, and vascular irregularities—we will study separately only the first three. The basic reason is that the last two, which as we have mentioned elsewhere, can form part of as many atypical lesions as typical ones, are studied in detail in other chapters of this work. Benign aspects of inflammatory erosions are described on page 42, dystrophic erosions on page 60, and vascular irregularities that also are of dystrophic origin are on page 72. In order to relate erosions and vascular irregularities of dysplastic origin, we take them up in minute detail at the time we study the colposcopic appearances of the "zone of atypical transformation," from which they are practically inseparable (pp. 172, 173, 176).

LEUKOKERATOSIS AND SUPERIMPOSED PATTERNS

These three images, called by Hinselmann "atypical epithelia" or "matrix areas," have in common the formation of areas of stratified squamous epithelium, of clearly different structure from the normal (Hinselmann), which are seen to persist (Mestwerdt) without showing any concurrent hormonal or inflammatory influence (Palmer), and which behave generally as iodine-negative zones, with more or less defined borders. There may be only one, or several may coexist.

In the modern literature, the terminology used by Hinselmann has been replaced by more adequate names and these colposcopic appearances are now called leukokeratotic patterns or lesions (Schiller, Bret and Coupez), endowed or not with superimposed images of ground structure and mosaic. This terminology has the advantage of being merely descriptive and not implying any judgment of the origin or potential of the observed image.

Leukoplakia. Hinselmann placed within this category all the areas of the cervix which show a white color at magnified colposcopy. For each leukoplakia observed by the naked eye, ten are diagnosed by colposcopy, because many zones that are red without preparation acquire a whitish color after the application of acetic acid. This criterion is very different from the histological one, which recognizes as leukoplakia only that mucosa with pathologic keratotic changes (Fig. 191).

In our series the frequency of leukoplakia is 1.9 per cent, a notably low figure by comparison with that of other authors, who probably apply more liberal criteria. Generally the incidence is given as between 2 and 6 per cent (Table 32).

Early colposcopists, interested almost exclusively in malignant or potentially malignant cervical pathology, attached considerable importance to leukoplakia. At present, and recognizing that some carcinomas may be covered by a plaque of keratosis or parakeratosis, it is evident that this is not the rule. Schiller says, with reason, that colposcopic leukoplakia should not be considered as a specific lesion, but rather as a generic concept that encompasses all kinds of epithelial anomalies, from the most innocent to the more serious. For this reason, the colposcopist should look for other signs which will induce him to perform a biopsy if they are present, or not if they are absent. Otherwise, leukoplakia will remain, in Rodriguez-Soriano's term, a "colposcopic deceiver."

The white spots of true leukoplakia or leukoplakiform zones appear isolated or in groups, in the periphery of an ectopy, forming part of a re-epithelialization zone, or isolated in the healthy exocervical epithelium. Less frequently they adopt a circular arrangement around the cervical os. On the surface, which is always lacking in vessels, one might see some superimposed ground structure or mosaic. The extent of leukoplakia varies from a minute, almost imperceptible zone to one that occupies the major portion of the exocervix.

According to the intensity of its color and the characteristics of its surface, different colposcopic varieties may be distinguished.

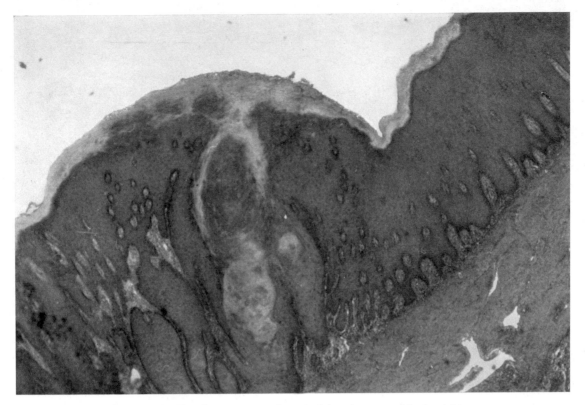

Figure 191. Histologic section of atypical (carcinomatous) leukoplakia.

DELICATE FORM. Totally invisible at first, and having a reddish color on direct colposcopy, this type becomes evident after the acetic acid test. It does not correspond to leukoplakia in the histologic sense, because its whitish appearance depends more on its cellular density than on the existence of true superficial keratosis (Fig. 193).

SIMPLE FORM. It is visible upon direct colposcopy, but not to the naked eye. It has a more intense color than the delicate form, and in the same way it does not usually represent keratinization but rather epithelial hyperplasia (Fig. 194). Schiller's test confirms the absence of glycogen (Fig. 195).

These two varieties become apparent because of the intense illumination of the colposcope. The whitish color derives from the increased superficial cellular density and is caused by reflection of the light rays. As Masciotta suggests, a useful means for differentiating these "leukoplakiform patterns" from "true leukoplakia" is to interpose a green filter.

HYPERTROPHIC FORM. This form is visible to the naked eye. Its surface is smooth, but the size of the lesion gives it an apparent prominence over the rest of the cervical mucosa. Its optical density is much more accentuated than in the others, and its color and appearance resemble those of mother-of-pearl. This form represents true superficial hyperkeratosis (Figs. 197 to 199), and although in some cases it may be accompanied by carcinoma, in the majority of cases its histologic substrate is a regular superficial dysplasia classifiable among the so-called "cervical dystrophies" (p. 66).

VERRUCOUS FORM. Also called papillary due to the irregularity of its surface, with elevations and depressions and even true furrows that cross from one part to the other (Figs. 200 and 201), this form reveals an intense epithelial proliferation, and most authors attribute to it a high degree of malignancy (Palmer,

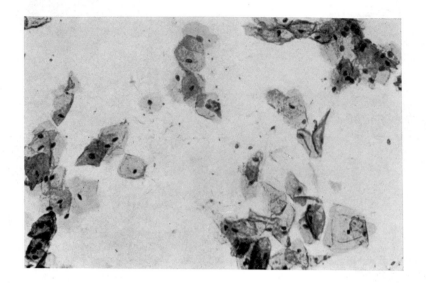

Figure 192. Cytologic smear of leukoplakia, Superficial cells predominate, some having nuclei.

Mestwerdt and Wespi, Henderson and Buck).

There are also some special colposcopic forms of leukoplakia, one consisting of clearly limited zones, with angular and well marked edges, that are somewhat elevated above the surface of the cervix (Fig. 196). This has been called "limestone" or "curdled milk" leukoplakia. Another finding is "islets" of leukoplakia separated by vascular irregularities and phenomena of epithelial injury such as erosions or hyperemic foci. The prognosis is bad, especially if this is found within the endocervical canal as frequently occurs.

Leukoplakia does not generally present differential diagnostic problems.

Only exceptionally is it possible to confuse it with (1) pseudomembranous monilial plaques, formed by fibrin, necrotic epithelial remnants, tiny buds, and inflammatory cells; (2) plaques of thick, hard cervical mucus; or (3) retention cysts with a very thick and dense epithelial lining (due to the pressure of the contents), which adopt a whitish mother-of-pearl appearance. In the first two cases careful cleaning of the cervix with acetic acid usually is sufficient to bring into view the plaques of mucus or discharge, avoiding the error. In the case of retention cysts, the presence of vessels on the surface and the fixation of iodine by the recovering epithelium, exclude leukoplakia.

(Text continued on page 140)

Table 32. Frequency of Leukoplakia

	PER CENT OF ATYPICAL IMAGES	PER CENT OF TOTAL COLPOSCOPIES
Mateu-Aragonés (1971)	12.54	1.00
Wilds (1962)	–	1.40
Figuero et al. (1971)	26.50	2.20
Hernández Alcàntara et al. (1971)	32.49	2.50
Arenas et al. (1961)	–	2.60
Guerrero et al. (1957)	38.70	3.10
Zamarriego (1966)	25.40	3.20
Bonilla (1965)	–	3.80
González-Merlo (1966)	31.50	5.90
Berger and Wenner-Mangen (1959)	–	6.20
Mossetti and Russo (1962)	–	10.60
Grismondi (1966)	–	12.40
Our Series	12.1	1.90

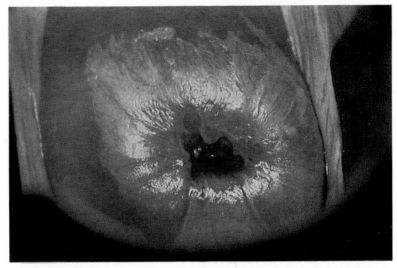

Figure 193. Slight leuko-plakia after acetic acid. This image forms part of a broader lesion (atypical re-epithelialization) which completely encircles an ectopy.

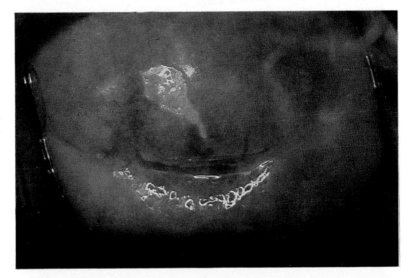

Figure 194. Simple leukoplakia which despite its marked visual intensity was not visible to the naked eye.

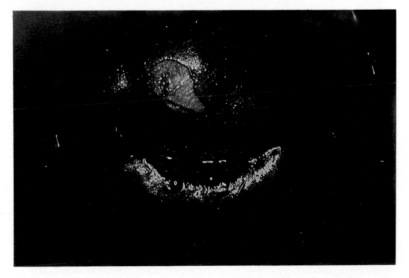

Figure 195. The same simple leukoplakia of the preceding picture after Schiller's test.

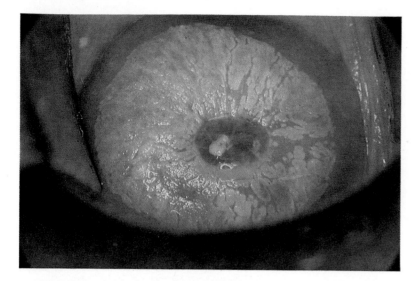

Figure 196. Leukoplakia in "limestone" formation practically occupying the whole exocervix.

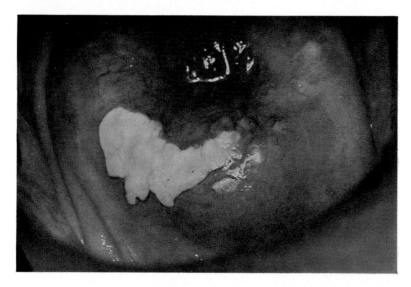

Figure 197. Leukoplakic plaque in "iceberg" form, notably elevated above the surface of the cervix. Its intense whiteness is striking. Even though not totally smooth, its surface lacks irregularities or suspicious disturbances.

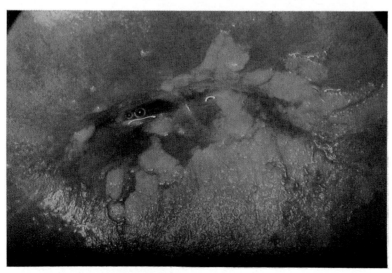

Figure 198. Extensive leukoplakic area with a slightly irregular surface. Since the lesion is partly within the cervical canal, a histologic study should be performed.

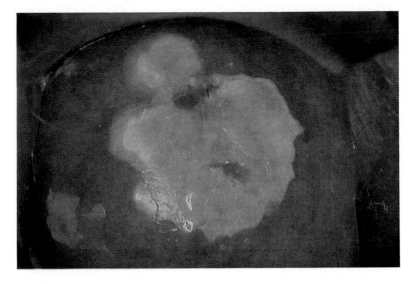

Figure 199. Large leuko-plakiform spot occupying much of the exocervix. The periphery is diffuse in some points, but its surface is regular. Cytology: Class II. Biopsy: regular dysplasia.

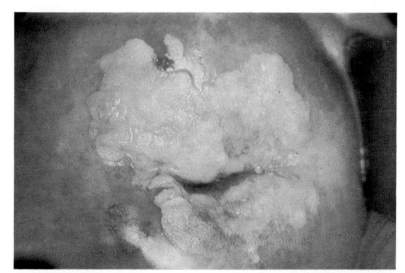

Figure 200. Extensive circumoral leukoplakia, of verrucous type, which attracts attention due to the irregularity of its surface (divided in parcels). Despite the absence of suspicious congestive, erosive or ulcerated zones, the colposcopist recommended a cytologic smear and histologic study. The results were: Endocervical cytologic smear: Class III. Exocervical biopsy: regular dysplasia.

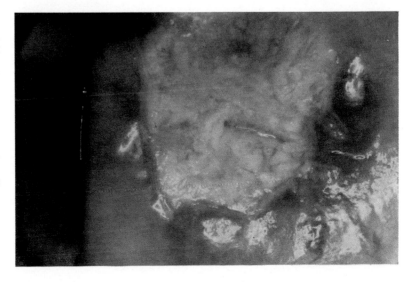

Figure 201. The image is similar to the preceding, but presents some important colposcopic differences. In the first place strongly congestive zones are seen around a leukoplakic plaque with diffuse edges, which almost seals the cervical orifice. Whereas in the patient shown in Figure 200, iodine negativity after Schiller's test was limited to the leukoplakia, in this patient it equally affected the peripheral congestive zone. Cytology: Class IV. Biopsy: in situ epithelial carcinoma.

Ground Structure. In the first texts on colposcopy this was also called the base of leukoplakia ("Grund" in German), because on occasions it appears when a plaque of leukoplakia is shedded. However, this qualification is not exact, because this mechanism of appearance is exceptional.

As an isolated or predominant lesion we have observed it in 2.7 per cent of our cases (Table 33). Most authors have given similar figures; however, Mossetti and Russo give an incidence of 0.2 per cent, while others such as Berger et al. have diagnosed this lesion in not less than 7 per cent of their cases.

Ground structure appears as red dots of high optical density, which stand out clearly over a whitish background that represents a more or less apparent plaque of leukoplakia. The distribution, size, and density of the dots is variable. Examination with the green filter permits recognition of the vascular origin of the red dots and the identification of one or more capillaries of more or less normal arrangement.

From a histologic viewpoint, ground structure usually corresponds to epithelial hyperplasia with acanthosis. The increased depth of the epithelium, which forms very evident crests, implies that some connective papillae, provided with vessels, remain very near the epithelial surface. These junctional-vascular papillae are those seen by colposcopy as red dots (Fig. 202).

Two colposcopic variants exist, whose prognostic significance is very different. The simple form is so called because the red dots show no elevation above the surrounding mucosa. It usually corresponds to a "zone of atypical re-epithelialization" (Fig. 203). The papillary form is characterized by the presence of round elevations, with the red dot being observed at the apex of each (and which at times may be identified as a corkscrew vessel). Kos, Mikolas, and Lane, by virtue of a combined colposcopic and histologic study, demonstrated that in this variety there exists only one elongated capillary loop.

Two or more of these elevations or papillae form small compartments, separated by reddish furrows. At the center of

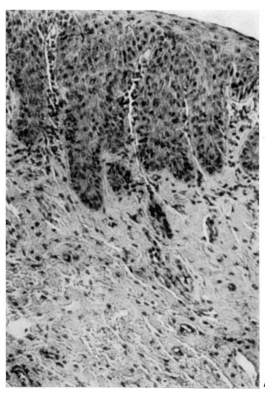

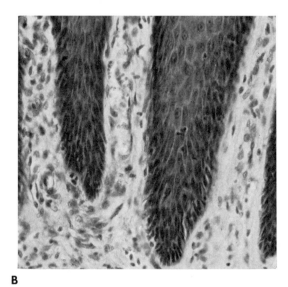

Figure 202. Histology of ground structure. *A,* Epithelial crests (in acanthosis) and connective vascular papillae which reach near the surface. *B,* Detail at a higher magnification of the epithelial crests sinking into the stroma.

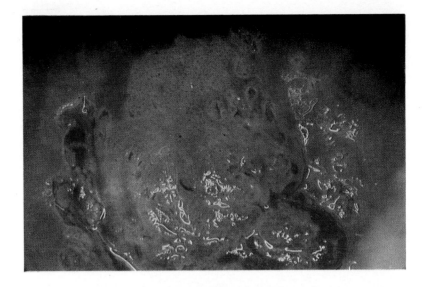

Figure 203. Simple form of ground structure. The red dots, notably regular and uniform, stand out above the exocervical surface.

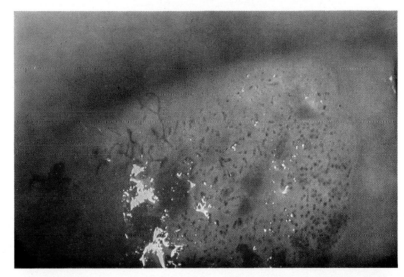

Figure 204. Papillary ground structure. Each dot becomes prominent above the exocervical mucosa. The image is very apparent and forms part of an atypical transformation zone.

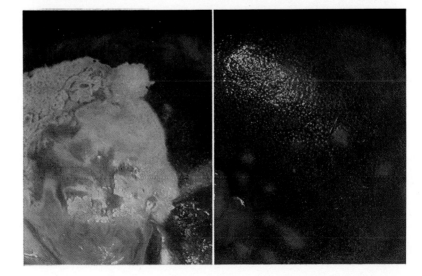

Figure 205. Differential colposcopic diagnosis between ground structure and red-punctate vaginitis, with the help of Schiller's test. *A*, Ground structure is totally iodine-negative, and the dots cannot be identified. *B*, The vaginitis takes up iodine except for the red dots, which for this reason stand out against the rest of the mucosa.

Table 33. Frequency of Ground Structure

	Per Cent of all Atypical Images	Per Cent of Total Colposcopies
Mossetti and Russo (1962)	—	0.20
Figuero et al. (1971)	9.8	0.80
Hernández Alcántara et al. (1971)	16.35	1.20
Mateu-Aragonés (1971)	15.41	1.22
Bonilla (1965)	—	1.60
Wilds (1962)	—	1.70
Zamarriego (1966)		
Guerrero et al. (1957)	23.8	1.90
Arenas et al. (1961)	—	2.20
González Merlo (1966)	15.02	2.86
Berger and Wenner-Mangen (1953)	—	7.00
Our Series (1972)	17.6	2.75

the lesion, the papillary elevations are especially thick, becoming less apparent near the periphery, where they tend to mix with other images. This variety usually coexists with other lesions (mosaic, verrucous leukoplakia, or erosions), forming part of a "zone of atypical transformation" (Fig. 204).

Ground structure may require differential diagnosis from other lesions, as follows.

RED-PUNCTATE VAGINITIS. Even a trained colposcopist may have some doubts in a given case. Schiller's test solves the dilemma, because uniform coloring of the area, with only the red dots appearing as iodine-negative, points to vaginitis. On the contrary, if the whole area resists fixation of iodine, the likely diagnosis is ground structure (Fig. 205).

PETECHIAL VAGINITIS. Here Schiller's test may not be as conclusive, because the atrophic mucosa that accompanies petechial vaginitis is often iodine-negative. The morphologic details of the red dots (larger and less uniform in petechial vaginitis) and the coexistence of other dystrophic lesions (starlike subepithelial hemorrhages, blanket-like hemorrhages, etc.) will be useful points in avoiding diagnostic errors.

HINSELMANN'S PAPILLARY ELEVATION. This diagnosis is generally difficult to mistake because the dots are white, but in exceptional cases there could be errors when the capillary element has undergone hypertrophy. Besides the morphologic and topographic differences, the Lugol test may also be capable of establishing the diagnosis.

Mosaic. This is undoubtedly the "matrix area" most frequently observed, found in 3.2 per cent of our cases. Despite the fact that other authors have given larger percentages, most colposcopic statistics offer figures between 0.6 and 3 per cent (Table 34).

Mosaic structure looks like a brick pavement, or a chessboard, formed by small square or polygonal tiles, of whitish color, separated by thin or interrupted reddish lines. The background, just as in ground structure, tends to be leukoplakia or leukoplakiform zone (keratinized mosaic). If this whitish platform is missing the term used is nonkeratinized mosaic.

Histologically, this lesion looks like ground structure, the only difference being that the crests of flat epithelium which sink into the stroma are broader and, therefore, the vascular connective papillae, acting as fine intercalated thin walls, having a fine vascular network, delimit much wider fields (Fig. 206).

From a colposcopic viewpoint it is possible to distinguish various forms:

In the *simple* or *flat form*, the "tiles" are not elevated and the lesion is delicate and only barely visible. Generally, this is part of an "atypical re-epithelialization" (Fig. 207).

The *acuminate* form is distinguished from the simple form by the fact that the "tiles" are elevated and the lines separating them constitute true furrows. Sometimes the fields are depressed instead (inverted mosaic). This is the characteristic form in "atypical transformation" (Figs. 210 and 211).

There is also the *regular* form, in which the size and shape of all the plots are approximately the same, and the *irregular* or *bizarre* form, whose aspect is polymorphous, including fields of diverse sizes and shapes in the same zone (Fig. 209). The regular form usually corresponds to slightly dysplastic re-epithelialization, while the irregular one is more frequently observed in strongly atypical lesions.

A variety of the latter is the so called "geographical" mosaic structure, in which the intermediate spaces may be undamaged, or present phenomena of epithelial reaction.

It is convenient to differentiate the mosaic structure just described from the so-called pseudomosaic, lesions of very diverse origin, but lacking dysplastic significance.

Pseudomosaic in a recent zone of typical re-epithelialization originates from the extension of the squamous metaplastic epithelium over the remnants of an ectopy whose connective vascular base persists in the form of papillae for a certain period (Fig. 208). Through the newly formed, delicate and whitish epithelium, the "grapes" of the old ec-

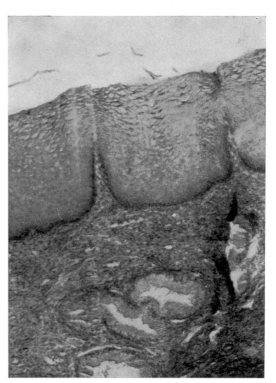

Figure 206. Histologic section of colposcopic mosaic. The epithelial crests are much wider than in ground structure.

topy become visible, and the colposcopic picture takes on a pseudomosaic appearance. The difference is that in this case the lines that separate the "tiles" are whitish and not reddish, and that their edges are less defined. This picture has been seen particularly in younger patients in whom an inflammatory state also existed (p. 122).

In vascular pseudomosaic (Hinselmann's zone of reticular transformation) the exocervical vessels have a reticular arrangement. Careful colposcopic observation avoids diagnostic error (p. 122).

In the healing stage of a diffuse red-punctate vaginitis, there appear, within the context of so-called geographic vaginitis, more or less geometric images which suggest a mosaic (p. 39). This is known as inflammatory pseudomosaic.

Microerosive pseudomosaic is an image which is reminiscent of "inverted mosaic," originated by the presence of multiple and small epithelial erosions. We have already referred to it on page 33.

(*Text continued on page 146*)

Table 34. Frequency of Mosaic

	PER CENT OF ATYPICAL IMAGES	PER CENT OF TOTAL COLPOS-COPIES
Figuero et al. (1971)	7.7	0.6
Guerrero et al. (1957)	12.5	1.0
Arenas et al. (1961)	–	1.3
Hernández Alcántara (1971)	21.31	1.6
Bonilla (1965)	–	1.7
Mateu-Aragonés (1971)	21.44	1.7
Zamarriego et al. (1966)	15.8	2.0
Wilds (1962)	–	3.0
González-Merlo (1966)	21.9	4.16
Mossetti and Russo (1962)	–	5.5
Our Series (1972)	20.5	3.2

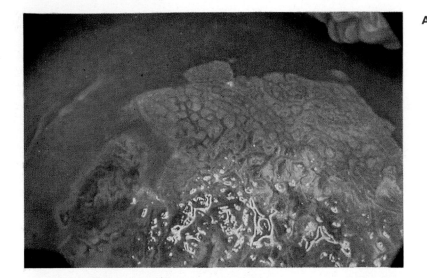

A

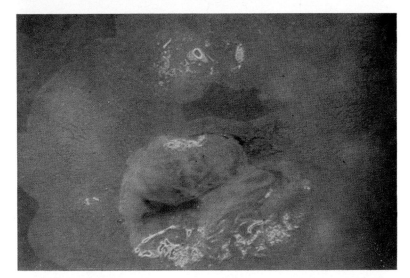

B

Figure 207. *A*, Simple mosaic with precise edges and zones of different visual density. The mosaic does not stand out and the segments are quite regular. It forms part of an atypical re-epithelialization *B*, Flat mosaic, very extensive and situated at the edge of an ectopy that has practically disappeared. This is an invisible lesion without preparation, and its appearance is not suspicious.

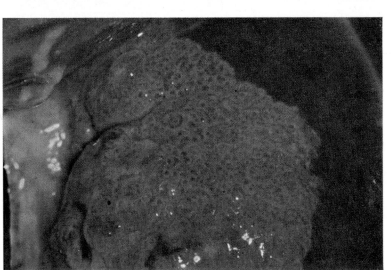

Figure 208. Large zone of pseudomosaic structure. The segments are outlined by white and not red lines.

Figure 209. Simple mosaic structure which alternates with zones of ground structure. Congestive areas are also seen. The limits of the lesion are not clear. Histologic study is imperative.

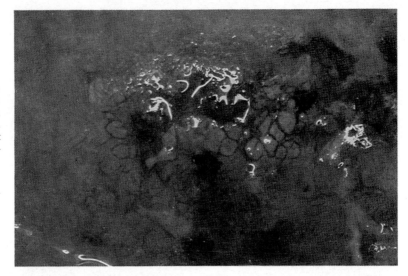

Figure 210. Elevated mosaic structure. It is an extensive lesion with elevations and with large segments separated by well defined furrows. Its external limits are relatively sharp. No red zones exist. Biopsy: moderate dysplasia.

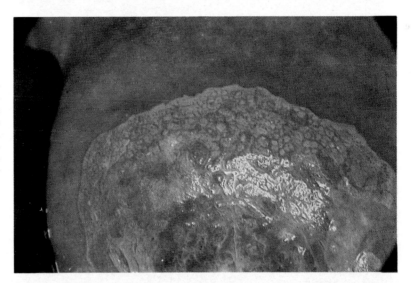

Figure 211. Acuminate, well keratinized mosaic alternating with atypical red zones (erosions and ulcerations), which are reducing its size. The lesion does not have well defined limits. Biopsy: microcarcinoma.

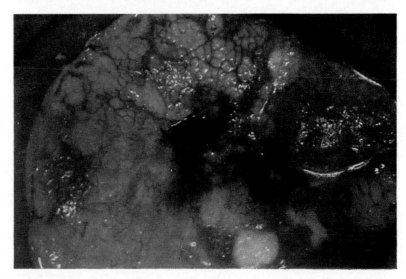

ATYPICAL RE-EPITHELIALIZATION

DEFINITION

The zone of atypical re-epithelialization is an abnormal, dysplastic form of healing of ectopy. Just as with typical re-epithelialization, its origin is a metaplastic process, in whose course a deviation of maturation has taken place that results in the appearance of squamous epithelium, devoid of glycogen (Fig. 212).

SYNONYMS

Atypical Re-epithelialization. Atypical epidermization. Doubtful colposcopic lesions. Leukokeratotic atypical epithelium. Dysplastic re-epithelialization. Class III colposcopic patterns. Grade I atypical transformation.

Bret and Coupez, to whom the conceptual individualization of this lesion is due in part, called it *epidermisation atypique,* as opposed to *epidermisation normale* or typical. However, the term epidermization seems to us unfortunate at present, because it suggests some similarity between squamous cervical epithelium and the epidermis.

The same authors formerly used the term doubtful colposcopic lesions, grouping in that category all patterns of questionable malignancy, as opposed to those of much more serious appearance which are almost always clearly malignant. At present this expression is not in use because of the more precise colposcopic terminology that has been devised.

Leukokeratotic atypical epithelium, besides its terminological inaccuracy (in colposcopy epithelia are not described, but rather patterns or lesions), leads to confusion because it alludes to a morphologic appearance which is common to it and other lesions that have a greater evolutionary potential.

Busch et al. classified colposcopic images in five classes, similar to Papanicolaou's cytologic classification. Class III corresponds to a cervix bearing leukokeratotic images, without vascular atypia, well defined and without differentiation of levels, which up to a certain point may be considered synonymous with the dysplastic lesion whose study we have just begun. Martin-Laval and Dajoux adopted a similar system. We believe that such nomenclatures, besides being not very expressive, are much too esoteric and are prone to errors of interpretation. Nor do we find advantages in the classification of atypical transformation zones into three grades (Coppleson and Reid), because in our judgment this confuses images as different as typical re-epithelialization (grade I), atypical re-epithelialization (grade II), and atypical transformation (grade III). The difference between these colposcopic entities is not, as we have already indicated, only one of grade.

For many reasons we feel that the expression atypical re-epithelialization, or dysplastic re-epithelialization, is the most adequate to define the lesion we are about to study. In addition to reflecting its reparative origin, and so relating it to typical re-epithelialization, as well as establishing its dysplastic significance, the term separates this image from so-called "atypical transformation," of greatly different diagnostic and prognostic significance.

ORIGIN OF ATYPICAL RE-EPITHELIALIZATION

The cause or group of causes which, at a given moment, may disrupt the met-

Table 35. Type of Cervical Re-epithelialization and Degree of Vaginal Inflammation

	GRADE I	GRADE II	GRADE III	GRADE IV
Typical re-epithelialization	56%	39%	5%	0%
Atypical re-epithelialization	14%	62%	20%	4%

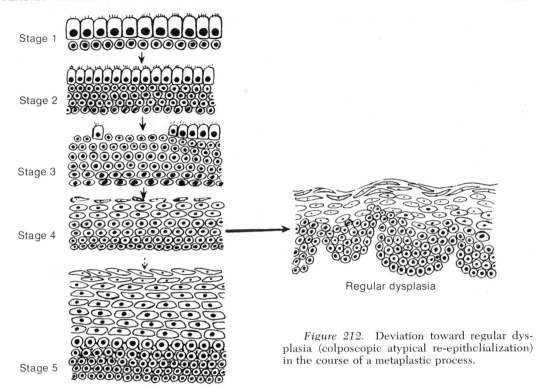

Stage 1

Stage 2

Stage 3

Stage 4

Stage 5

Regular dysplasia

Figure 212. Deviation toward regular dysplasia (colposcopic atypical re-epithelialization) in the course of a metaplastic process.

aplastic process and cause anomalies of maturation in the reparative epithelium are still hypothetical. Among the factors so far suggested, we may cite the following.

Hormonal Imbalance. Fluhmann and Song consider this the most important stimulus for dysplastic re-epithelialization. They base this conclusion on the rarity of cervical atypia in both young girls and women of advanced age, and on the postpartum disappearance of cervical atypia diagnosed during pregnancy. Our experience in this respect is mostly negative. During long-term use of anovulatory methods of all types, we observed an increase in the incidence of hypertrophic ectopy, zones of typical irregular re-epithelialization, vascular hyperplasia, and vaginitis, but not in dysplastic scars. Hormones seem to us to influence the cervical metaplasic process only marginally, preventing or interfering with it but not altering it.

Inflammation. To us and to other colposcopists (González-Merlo), inflammation is an evident cause of atypical re-epithelialization. The statistical evidence is a larger incidence of infection accompanying atypical rather than typical re-epithelialization (Table 35). We have also observed ectopy accompanied by atypical re-epithelialization in many women who have been recently violated. There is no doubt that infection is the factor that explains it, just as in "honeymoon cystitis." Later these zones of atypical re-epithelialization will disappear, absorbed by a strictly normal metaplastic process.

It is difficult to relate atypical re-epithelialization with factors such as age, parity, and gynecologic history.

FREQUENCY

Atypical re-epithelialization is, without doubt, the most frequent atypical lesion. In our series it represents 12.6 per cent of all colposcopic observations and not less than 96 per cent of atypical images. Comparison of these figures with those offered by other authors is not easy. The concept of atypical re-epithelialization is so recent that most statistics still continue to employ the classic matrix areas of Hinselmann, to which are added vascular irregularities and true erosion as if they were independent phenomena. In these circumstances it is risky to attempt to establish a parallelism between our atypical re-epithelialization — histologically and prognostically well defined — and those images lacking in all morphological and prognostic equivalence.

Only by exclusion, subtracting from the total frequency of atypical colposcopic pictures the zones of atypical transformation and the exophytic images, is it possible to calculate approximately the percentages of atypical re-epithelialization obtained by other authors, which in general fall between 8 and 15 per cent.

COLPOSCOPIC APPEARANCES

Just as in typical re-epithelialization, it is possible to recognize three phases in the development of this lesion: initial, advanced and terminal.

Initial Phase. In some part of the periphery of the ectopy (less frequently around the entire lesion), small wedges or tongues of metaplastic epithelium are suddenly formed. From the first moment they have an appearance that is different from the normal. The color of this epithelium is whitish, its surface is less smooth, and above all what attracts attention is the presence of some superimposed images caused by the vessels of the stroma. When these reach the surface, filled with papillae of different sizes and at different distances from one another, they create the appearance of ground structure (red spots) or mosaic (geometric shapes) on the surface of the new epithelium.

Atypical re-epithelialization in its initial phases also differs from the typical form in that, although its internal margins are unclear, by contrast its external limit is well defined, and it is separated from normal mucosa by a precise border. It is exactly in this area where the metaplastic epithelium is whiter and keratotic, contrasting with the mature epithelium of

the rest of the cervix. The acetic acid test makes these boundaries stand out (Fig. 213).

The tongues or wedges may be of different sizes, but wide strips predominate over thin ones; metaplastic furrows can be seen only on few occasions, whereas they are rather frequent in typical re-epithelialization. The direction of these wedges is always toward the heart of the ectopy.

Schiller's test demonstrates that both ectopy in the course of re-epithelialization and the metaplastic epithelium, typical or atypical, fail to take up iodine (Fig. 215). But it demonstrates the sharp borders of the atypical zone as opposed to those of the typical zone, which are more diffuse.

Advanced Phase. Two facts clearly differentiate this from the homologous stage of typical re-epithelialization: the absence of central metaplastic plaques and the persistence of the alteration of the maturation process in the progressing epithelium. Just as in the typical re-epithelialization, it is possible to describe three zones. There is a *circumoral central* zone, which has not yet been affected by the physiologic or pathologic repair process and which is still ectopic (Fig. 214). Even though attempts have been made to find a relationship between the characteristics of the ectopy (size, shape, appearance of the papillae, etc.) and the presence of dysplastic re-epithelialization, none has been found.

An *intermediate* zone is characterized by the following morphologic details:

(1) Absence of metaplastic plaques in the interior of the ectopy (Fig. 216). If such plaques are observed, they correspond to a parallel process of typical re-epithelialization and do not belong to the atypical repair process. On rare occasions we have seen that these "physiologic" plaques connect at some point with the peripheral atypical zone.

(2) In the course of re-epithelialization, the projections originating on the edges of the ectopy do not leave glandular orifices partially opened. Dysplastic epidermization colonizes all the glandular formations. If glandular openings are ever seen, they are surrounded by a

(*Text continued on page 152*)

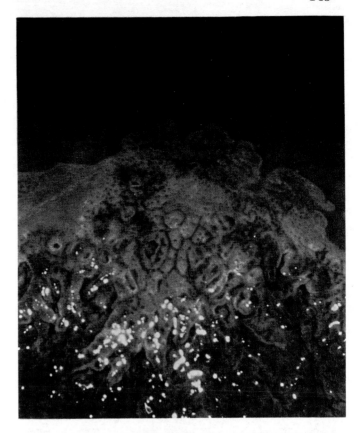

Figure 213. Atypical re-epithelialization in its initial phases. This colpophotograph, obtained after application of acetic acid, demonstrates a zone which begins suddenly at the edge of an ectopy. Its external edge is well defined and its progression is toward the anatomic os, toward which it reaches without central metaplastic plaques and without leaving opened grandular orifices. Retention cysts are not seen. There are striking superimposed images of ground and mosaic structure.

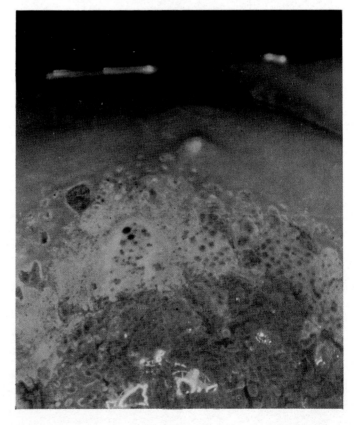

Figure 214. Central part of a zone of atypical re-epithelialization. Alongside the ectopy, strips of whitish epithelium are seen, with superimposed images of ground or mosaic structure. Glandular orifices are seen, which form part of the parallel typical re-epithelialization. The papillae of the ectopy are completely normal.

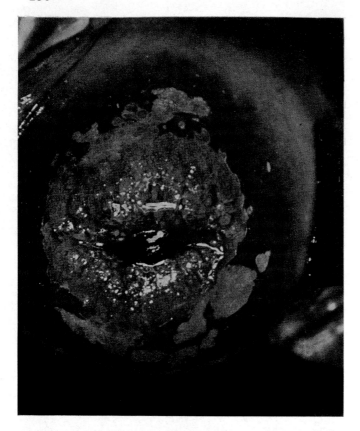

Figure 215. Atypical re-epithelialization subjected to Schiller's test. Neither the typical nor the atypical zone fixes the iodine, because they both lack glycogen, but even so it is possible to establish differences between the two kinds of re-epithelialization, because while the edges of the atypical zone are very well defined, those of the typical zone are somewhat diffuse.

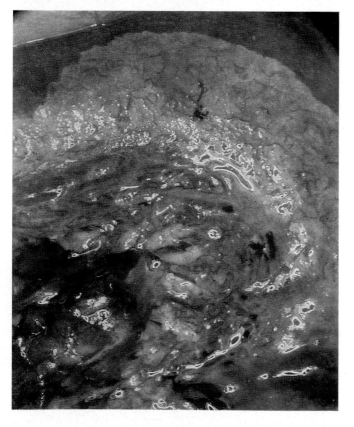

Figure 216. Circumferential atypical re-epithelialization, which has covered approximately two-thirds of a previous ectopy. Observe that central metaplastic plaques do not exist. Acetic acid brings into view the sharpness of the edges of the lesion as well as a superimposed image of mosaic.

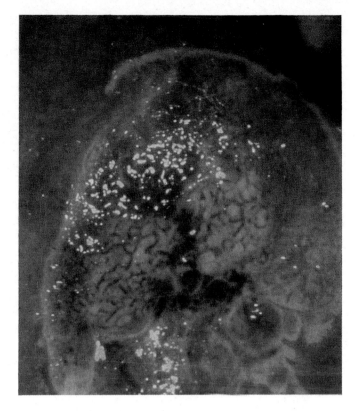

Figure 217. Atypical re-epithelialization (mosaic) which has covered almost all of a circumoral ectopy. Observe that unlike the typical re-epithelialization, there are no open glandular orifices or any nabothian cysts. The limits of the lesion are precise.

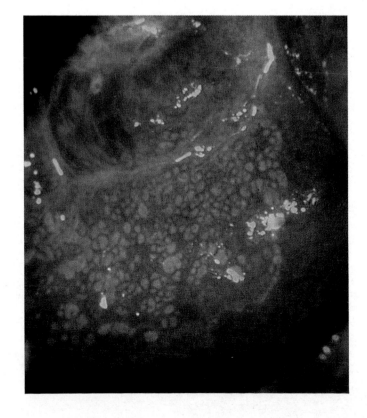

Figure 218. Atypical re-epithelialization, with a striking mosaic image, which has almost totally replaced a cervical ectopy. One single glandular orifice is seen, notably cornified, in a zone lacking superimposed images. Possibly this sector was epidermized in part by a typical metaplastic process.

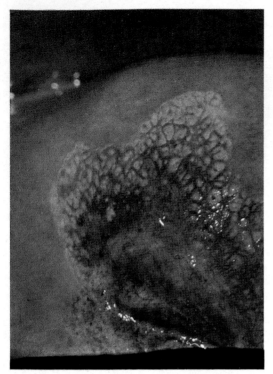

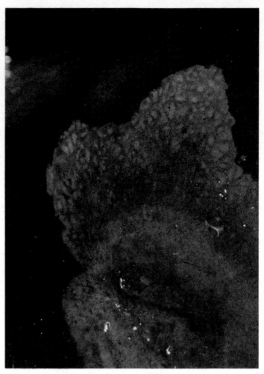

Figure 219. After the application of acetic acid, the periphery of this zone of atypical re-epithelialization has a greater visual density than the center of the lesion. This is why the outer limits of such a lesion are always well defined.

Figure 220. With Schiller's test, the absence of glycogen in this zone is clearly demonstrated. The interepithelial limit is very sharp.

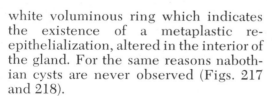

white voluminous ring which indicates the existence of a metaplastic re-epithelialization, altered in the interior of the gland. For the same reasons nabothian cysts are never observed (Figs. 217 and 218).

(3) Generally a dysplastic reparative process evolves jointly with a normoplastic one. The extent and borders of the atypical zone will depend not only on its own evolutional potential, but also on that of the parallel typical zone. The competition that will be established between both forms of repair will determine the general appearance of the cervix (Figs. 221 and 222). If initially the atypical zone affects a very small sector of the periphery of the ectopy, the rest of which is occupied by a very active typical re-epithelialization, the most probable result is that the atypical epithelium is in effect drowned by the typical. It does not reach the cervical os, but instead remains as an isolated plaque. On the other hand, if the marginal sector of the ectopy that is subjected to atypical re-epithelialization

is very wide, then the atypical zone may easily reach the os, even if it is shrinking progressively. Bret and Coupez showed that most atypical zones are to be found at the 12 and 6 o'clock positions.

(4) The boundary between the atypical zone and the physiologic metaplastic epithelium of the typical zone are always well defined, because the visual density of the lesion is greater at the periphery than in the center. Beyond these boundaries, there is no surrounding reaction whatsoever.

(5) In the sector of the ectopy where the atypical zone progresses, there are no islets without re-epithelialization.

(6) The plaques of atypical re-epithelialization that advance present on their surface the same images of superimposition that were seen in the initial phase of the process. Generally these appear flat. If ground and mosaic pictures coexist, the two images are not usually mixed in a disorderly manner, but rather are distributed in different sectors of the plaque. The absence of evident vascular

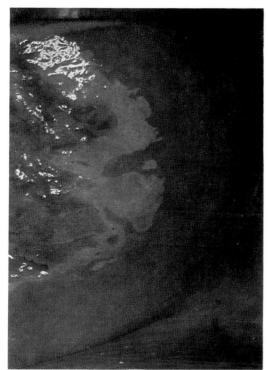

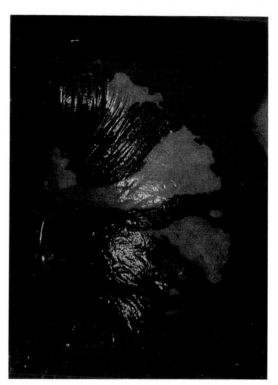

Figure 221. Typical and atypical re-epithelialization, advancing together. Two sectors of the atypical zone extend on both sides of the 3 o'clock position.

Figure 222. Seven months later, after Schiller's test, a new zone of atypical re-epithelialization is observed in the same patient as in Figure 221.

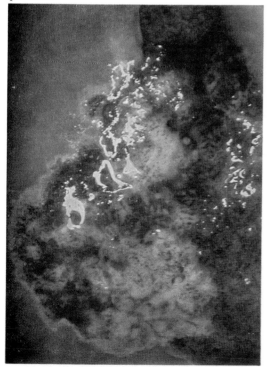

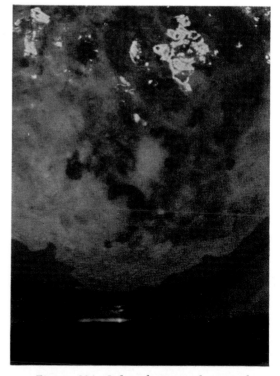

Figure 223. Infected zone of atypical re-epithelialization. The coexistence of leukokeratotic images, and congestive and erosive changes of inflammatory origin make this lesion a suspicious one.

Figure 224. Infected zone of atypical re-epithelialization, easily mistaken for a zone of atypical transformation. To avoid an error, anti-inflammatory treatment should be instituted.

irregularities in the interior or at the periphery of these strips is noteworthy.

Peripheral zone. Unlike the homologous zone of the typical re-epithelialization, here the newly formed epithelium tends not to regularize itself or to progressively assimilate the strictly normal epithelium of the cervix. On the contrary, it seems that as the dysplastic reparative process advances, its differences from the old squamous epithelium become better defined. Lugol's solution clearly demonstrates the absence of glycogen in this zone, even though much time has elapsed since its formation (Figs. 219 and 220).

Terminal Phase. The ectopy has almost totally disappeared, wiped out by the simultaneous development of both types of re-epithelialization, if not necessarily of equal intensity (Figs. 221 and 222). If the disappearance of the ectopy is total, the lesion is given the name "stable atypical scar," whose characteristics we will describe later.

The following morphologic details are a guide to conduct.

EXTENT OF THE ATYPICAL ZONE. If the final size of the zone of atypical re-epithelialization is small and the typical form predominates, the·process should be listed in principle as benign, especially if it becomes evident that the healthy areas are progressively absorbing the atypical plaques. At the other extreme is the so-called "circumferential atypical re-epithelialization" which includes the full outline of the ectopy (Fig. 225).

PROXIMITY TO THE CERVICAL OS. If the atypical zone is far from the os, with an ample strip of physiologic metaplastic epithelium between them, the lesion may be considered as nonsuspicious. On the contrary, contact with the orifice and especially the disappearance of the atypical zone in the interior of the endocervix should prompt a more profound study (Fig. 226).

IRREGULAR APPEARANCE. The existence of vascular irregularities and congestive or erosive zones, jointly with classical superimposed images, may be produced by inflammation, which bestows an apparent seriousness upon a totally benign lesion. If doubt persists after exhaustive colposcopic verification, the proper course is to give anti-inflammatory treatment. Failure of such measures should point toward the suspicion of malignancy (Figs. 223 and 224).

In our experience 35 to 40 per cent of zones of atypical transformation diagnosed at the first examination are actually zones of atypical re-epithelialization with infection. The colposcopist who has erred in this respect on several occasions learns not to be hasty in the diagnosis.

DEGREE OF KERATINIZATION. After a triple examination—directly, after the acetic acid test, and after Schiller's test—a terminal zone of atypical re-epithelialization should be judged benign if it does not become evident until after the last test, which simply indicates an absence of glycogen in the superficial layers. On the other hand, its visualization by direct colposcopy carries a poor prognosis. After application of acetic acid, the degree of keratinization may be evaluated by the·visual density of the lesion.

HISTOLOGY OF ATYPICAL RE-EPITHELIALIZATION

Study of a zone of atypical re-epithelialization or a stable atypical scar may reveal a spectrum of histologic pictures ranging from normal metaplastic epithelium to carcinoma in situ, even though in most cases the diagnosis is "regular" or "mild" dysplasia. In our material this kind of dysplasia was observed in 78.7 per cent of atypical re-epithelialization zones and in 85.3 per cent of stable atypical scars. Thus we consider regular or mild dysplasia as the habitual histologic substrate of atypical re-epithelialization (Tables 36 and 39).

Table 36. Histologic Correlation of Atypical Re-epithelialization

Physiologic metaplasia	18.18%
Regular dysplasia	78.78%
Irregular dysplasia	1.89%
In situ carcinoma	1.13%
Invasive carcinoma	0%

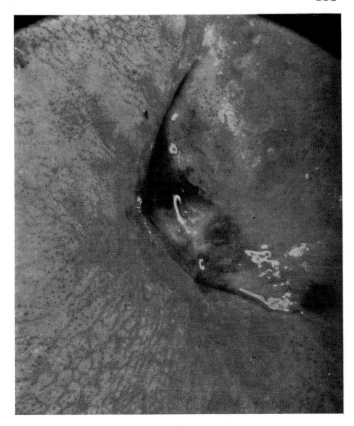

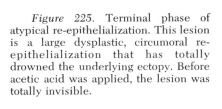

Figure 225. Terminal phase of atypical re-epithelialization. This lesion is a large dysplastic, circumoral re-epithelialization that has totally drowned the underlying ectopy. Before acetic acid was applied, the lesion was totally invisible.

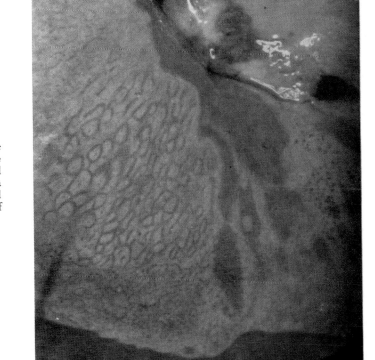

Figure 226. Thanks to the acetic acid, it is even possible to observe some superimposed images (mosaic and ground structure). This is obviously a benign lesion, but it should be destroyed because of its location at the junction of the exocervix with the endocervix.

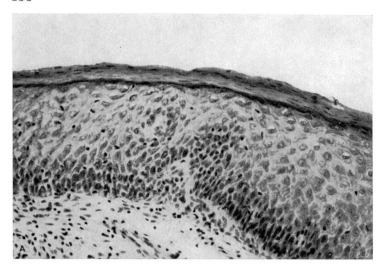
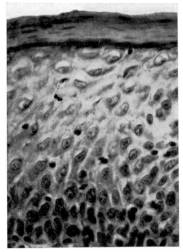

Figure 227. Histologic section at low and high power of an atypical re-epithelialization. The diagnosis was mild dysplasia.

"Mild" dysplasia is, in our conception, the most benign degree of atypical histologic alteration. There is as yet no disturbance in epithelial differentiation, and discreet alterations in maturation are the only ones recognized (Fig. 227). This definition makes mild dysplasia analogous to the grade I dysplasia of the FIGO classification (1961) and to the "regular" or "benign" dysplasia of other authors (de Brux).

Its principal characteristics are as follows:

(1) Squamous metaplastic epithelium, lacking in glycogen, in which all the layers of normoplastic epithelium may be recognized, but whose overall architecture is discreetly disturbed by maturational anomalies, including papillomatosis of the stroma, presenting as edema with leukocytic infiltration and phenomena of vascular neoformation; hyperacanthosis, implying inward growth of the crests with the connective-vascular papillae becoming very evident; excessive maturation of the surface, with phenomena of keratosis and parakeratosis; and moderate thickening of the parabasal layer, with an increase in the number of mitoses (Richart). For all these reasons, the epithelium takes on an undulated or festooned appearance.

(2) Beneath the basement membranes glandular elements are observed, with metaplastic phenomena.

(3) In the periphery of a mild dysplasia it is possible to find the columnar epithelium of the ectopy and the normal stratified squamous mucosa.

The first characteristic defines the dysplasia; the other two define its metaplastic origin.

CYTOLOGY OF ATYPICAL RE-EPITHELIALIZATION

The major portion of cytologic smears from zones of atypical re-epithelialization (97.9 per cent in our series) are catalogued in Papanicolaou's Classes I and II, which gives an idea of the small amount of cytologic transformation found in dysplastic re-epithelialization. Minor cellular alterations lead to a suspicious cytologic diagnosis in only 2 per cent of cases, most of them generally falling into Class II-III. Following these lesions by cytology will demonstrate their progressive normalization. In our series only 0.9 per cent of smears taken in the course of a year presented dysplastic signs (Table 37).

We base an assignment to Class II-III on the presence of dyskaryotic cells, which imply alterations that are quite different from neoplasia and that are attributable to inflammatory or local reparative phenomena (Dexeus and Rawyler, 1962;

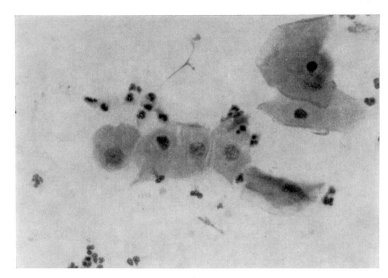

A

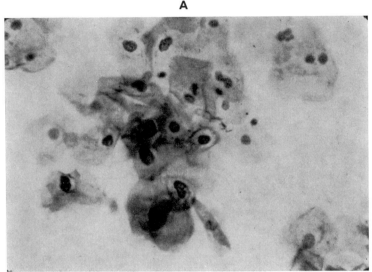

B

Figure 228. Cytologic smear suggestive of an atypical re-epithelialization. *A*, Small maturation anomalies, especially evident in elements of the stratum spinosum. *B*, Group of cells with nuclear anomalies (reinforcement of nuclear membrane, moderate anisonucleosis and perinuclear halos).

Dexeus and Carrera, 1968; Carrera et al., 1969).

To the expert in cervical pathology, the absence of cytologic abnormalities in the presence of lesions which are colposcopically apparent, is not surprising (Table 38). In the majority of cases, regular dysplasia is the substrate, and the histologic lesion is associated with disturbances in maturation but not in cellular differentiation. It is logical that smears will be practically normal.

Cells from all the layers of the cervicovaginal mucosa are seen, and because there are alterations in maturation, it is possible to find at all levels: (a) deep

Table 37. Cytologic Correlation of Active and Residual Atypical Re-epithelialization

Class I	23.93%
Class II	73.99%
Class II-III	1.35%
Class III	0.58%
Class IV and V	0.12%

cells with cytoplasm precociously matured (large normal nucleus and eosinophilic cytoplasm); (b) deep cells with basophilic cytoplasm and precociously matured nucleus (pyknotic or prepyknotic); (c) deep cells with minor nuclear alterations of the retraction or opacification

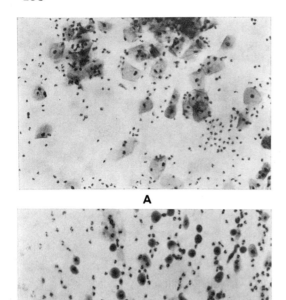

Figure 229. Cytologic smears of atypical re-epithelialization. *A,* Smear with totally normal superficial and intermediate cells, which was interpreted as Class I. Colposcopy showed a striking zone of atypical re-epithelialization. *B,* Atrophic smear, whose only alteration was the presence of parabasal cells with precociously pyknotic nuclei. Even with all this, the smear was simply read as Class II.

type; (d) intermediate cells with basophilic cytoplasm, but a pyknotic nucleus; (e) intermediate cells with normal vesicular nucleus, but eosinophilic cytoplasm like that of the superficial cells; (f) intermediate cells with a voluminous and hyperchromatic nucleus, reinforced or retracted nuclear membrane, and a degree of anisonucleosis; (g) anucleated superficial cells, acidophilic or basophilic; and (h) superficial cells with a pyknotic, hyperchromatic, or slightly dyskaryotic nucleus, adopting tadpole or fiber-like shapes.

The percentages of each of these cellular types and of the aggregate vary greatly, and there will be smears on the one hand in which it is not possible to distinguish any alteration (Fig. 229), and on the other hand smears containing nu-merous atypical cells of the described type. When the predominating element is the parabasal cell, the preparations will be especially suggestive of dysplasia.

CLINICAL COURSE

There are three possible evolutionary routes for a zone of atypical re-epithelialization: (1) disappearance, absorbed by the normal surrounding re-epithelialization process; (2) permanence in the form of a "stable atypical scar"; and (3) evolution toward a "zone of atypical transformation."

Disappearance. A large number of zones of atypical re-epithelialization disappear before forming scars. They vanish within the epithelium that originates after a strictly physiologic metaplastic process. Some zones are rapidly erased, as habitually occurs with those that appear during pregnancy, while in the others regularization is much slower. Finally, it should be said that generally when disappearance is fast, the lesion was not especially dense and showed only minor keratinization, even though it may have had clearly superimposed images (especially mosaics), which were the ones that gave rise to the diagnosis.

The progressive regularization of the lesion until it becomes totally absorbed by the normal surrounding epithelium does not occur in a uniform manner, but rather by areas. Frequently, the edges of the atypical zone remain visible until the last moment (keratinization at the margins is more accented), with the normal maturation of the epithelium initiated in the center of the lesion.

The first indication that the atypical zone is going to be regularized is the difficulty in observing it after the application of acetic acid (Fig. 230). It is visua-

Table 38. Analysis of Class II Smears in Atypical Re-epithelialization

Suggestive of mild dysplasia	40.73%
Totally inexpressive (inflammatory, reparative, etc.)	59.26%

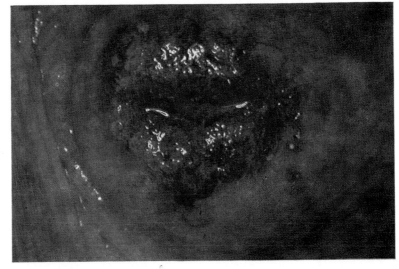

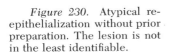*Figure 230.* Atypical re-epithelialization without prior preparation. The lesion is not in the least identifiable.

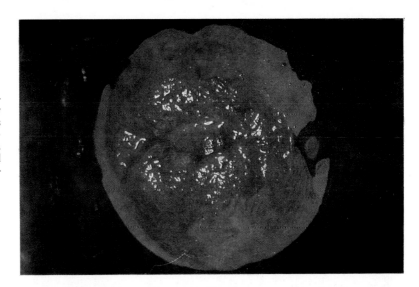

Figure 231. Atypical re-epithelialization visible only after the application of Lugol's solution. The chromatic uniformity of the lesion is evident. Its boundaries with the normal exocervical mucosa are definite.

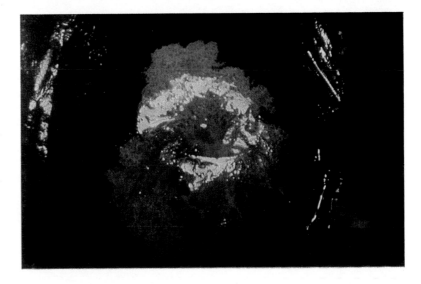

Figure 232. Zone of atypical re-epithelialization in danger of disappearing. The lesion is not visible on direct examination, nor after the application of acetic acid. Only Schiller's test makes it evident. Observe how much of the lesion takes up iodine. Color depends on the degree of maturation. At the 4 and 5 o'clock positions, the limit of the dysplastic zone is no longer visible.

lized only after Schiller's test (Fig. 231). Iodine is taken up unevenly by the atypical plaque, indicating that at some places the epithelium contains glycogen. Progressively, the areas that affix iodine become more extensive, producing a mottled appearance where formerly a uniform iodine-negative plaque was found (Fig. 232). Finally, the whole zone takes up iodine, eliminating the possibility of locating the boundaries of the lesion because the maroon color is uniform throughout the cervix. This process of regularization may take between 2 months and several years.

Lugol's solution very seldom provides clear differentiation between atypical re-epithelialization and atypical transformation, because both lesions are made up of newly formed epithelium, lacking in glycogen in its initial phases.

Permanence. A stable atypical scar is formed when, the ectopy having totally disappeared, the atypical images of the

Table 39. Histologic Correlation of the "Stable Atypical Scar"

Physiologic metaplasia	13.86%
Regular dysplasia	85.34%
Irregular dysplasia	0.86%
In situ carcinoma	0.43%
Invasive carcinoma	0%

dysplastic re-epithelialization persist. These should not be regarded with suspicion, because the limits of the plaque are perfectly clear and stable. In our opinion it is not possible to consider that an evolving atypical zone has been converted into a scar if the internal edge of the zone is within the endocervical canal, because we cannot say that the atypical re-epithelialization has ceased its evolution if we do not see the entire extent of the plaque. It is therefore clear that we label as an atypical scar only a sharply limited lesion, with precise and neat edges that do not touch the cervical os

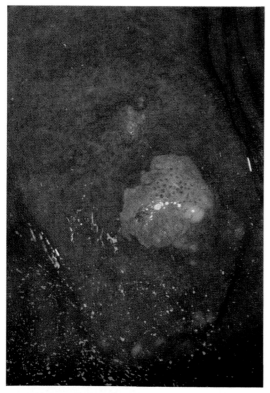

Figure 233. Stable atypical scar, of small size, visualized thanks to the application of acetic acid. It was invisible at direct examination.

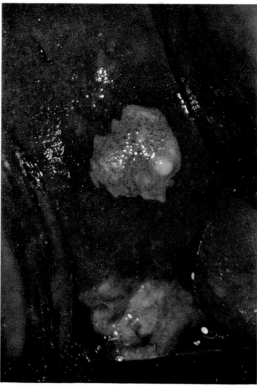

Figure 234. Lugol's solution applied to the same lesion brings out the sharpness of its edges.

once repair of the ectopy has ceased (Figs. 233 and 234).

From a histologic viewpoint, the differences between an evolving zone of atypical re-epithelialization and a stable atypical scar are minimal. Perhaps the most obvious change is an increase in superficial keratosis, which is identified colposcopically by an increase in the visual density. But the differences between the stable scar and the normal surrounding tissue are notable (Bret and Coupez): scarce or absent glycogen content; clear separation between both epithelia at the border of the lesion; and modification of the cellular stratification by keratosis or parakeratosis of the surface, and sometimes due to hyperplasia of basal cells.

The histologic differences lead to the colposcopic findings. The first of these is an iodine-negative zone, of a uniform whitish color. There are also neat and definite limits, which isolate the lesion within the normal cervical tissue (Figs. 235 and 236). It is possible simultaneously to observe several scars of different sizes and shapes, but always sharply limited and isolated. Like evolving re-epithelialization zones, they are usually preferentially located at the 12 and 6 o'clock positions. Finally, the visual intensity of a lesion depends not only on the degree of superficial keratosis or parakeratosis (simple disturbance of maturation), but also on the abnormal density (cellular and nuclear) of the epithelium. However, in the case of the stable atypical scar, the second possibility is rare, and usually it is the keratosis which is responsible for the high visibility.

This superficial alteration, occurring conjointly with stromal papillomatosis, is responsible for the appearance of the lesion: white spots (of variable density) on which are superimposed images of mosaic and ground structure. Generally, when the white spot is nacreous, dense, of a homogeneous color, and visible without much preparation, it is usually not accompanied by superimposed images. However, white spots of poor and irregular visual density usually do exhibit them, even though in the stable scar it is rare to see mixtures of ground and mosaic structure. Instead the usual picture shows both types independently and even isolated. What is seen frequently is the cervix with various plaques of stable scar, some in the shape of mosaic structure and others simply leukoplakic.

The scar that follows atypical re-epithelialization may regress (which is common in menopause), may worsen (if it is subjected to repeated and persistent irritative inflammatory or hormonal stimuli), or may simply persist unchanged. In our experience, the latter course is the most frequent.

In the scar that tends to regress, Schiller's test becomes progressively negative (the tissue acquires glycogen): the scar loses visual density and its borders, formerly sharp, lose stability and vanish. On the contrary, aggravation is marked by an increase in the visibility of the scar and by the development in its midst of an atypical vascularization, with congestive or erosive zones.

Evolution of a Zone of Atypical Transformation. This is the most serious possibility and the one that has to occupy our attention. A small number of zones of atypical re-epithelialization and stable atypical scars (too small to evaluate statistically at present) may evolve toward malignancy, by way of a zone of atypical transformation. In spite of the very low incidence of malignant change, the simple fact that atypical re-epithelialization can lead to cancer requires that we utilize in each case all the possibilities of colposcopy, in attempting to define which lesion may be a candidate for that unfavorable change. In the preceding pages we have discussed the morphologic details that permit us to arrive at a prognosis.

MANAGEMENT

In the initial phase, unless the atypical re-epithelialization is circumferential, an expectant attitude may be adopted. A cytologic examination and an effort to avoid any stimulus that might tend to extend the lesion constitute adequate management. A good ancillary measure is the application of a vaginal sulfonamide

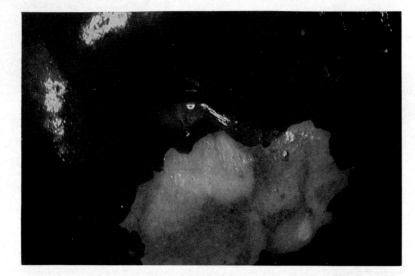

Figure 235. Stable atypical scar after the application of Lugol's solution. The large residual lesion, with precise edges, is revealed only by Schiller's test. A strip of squamous epithelium, already matured, originated by a parallel typical re-epithelialization, is interposed between the scar and the endocervical mucosa, assuring that the lesion is benign.

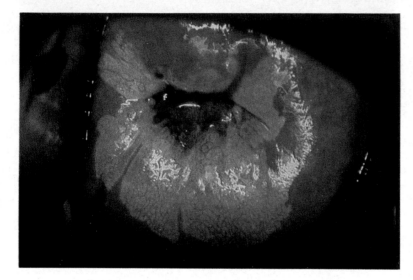

Figure 236. Extensive stable atypical scar, which exhibits a regular mosaic appearance. The prognosis cannot be as optimistic as in the previous case for two reasons: the lesion is already visible after acetic acid is applied, and it is in contact with the endocervical canal. It is advisable to destroy this scar once histologic study has shown that it is not malignant.

cream, which sterilizes the mucosa and tends to stimulate normoplastic re-epithelialization with consequent regularization of the incipient atypical process. On the other hand, when the atypical plaque is extensive from the start, we are advocates of its destruction, but only after cytologic and histologic verification of the absence of malignancy (Lagrutta, Di Paola, Richart). Destruction may be accomplished by diathermic electrocoagulation (Chanen and Hollyock, Richart and Sciarra) or cryosurgery (Ostergard, Chiladze, and others). Some authors (Gambotto) have insisted that diathermy-coagulation has a role in the

pathogenesis of cervical cancer, and that a treated lesion still can become malignant.

In advanced phases of atypical re-epithelialization, measures to be taken will depend on the completed colposcopic data, with a histologic or cytologic study, if necessary. If the lesion is extensive with notable visual density and, above all, if it is in the proximity of the anatomic os, or disappears within its interior, histologic study is imperative. If its results are negative, and if cytologic samples at intervals of 3 months are also negative, one may proceed to destruction of the lesion by electrocoagulation (Figs.

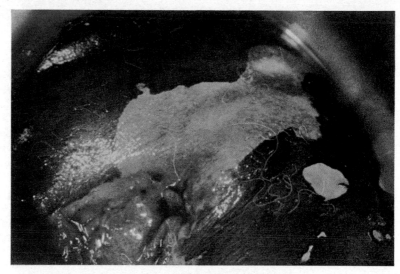

Figure 237. Atypical re-epithelialization at the scar stage. Destruction by coagulation was carried out once histologic study demonstrated that it was benign.

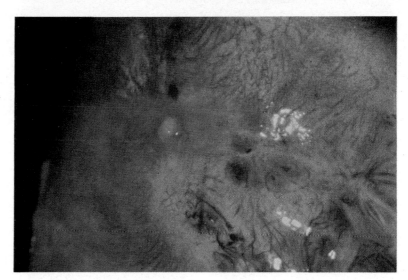

Figure 238. Patterns of vascular hyperplasia over a zone of slight leukokeratosis, both sequelae of coagulation of the anterior cervical lesion three months earlier.

237 and 238), but if they suggest a certain degree of suspicion, surgical conization of the cervix assures adequate histologic study and simultaneous destruction of the lesion. This course of action is especially recommended in multiparous patients near the menopause.

If an inflammatory process adds suspicious images to the atypical plaque and could be an aggravating influence, it is logical to initiate antibiotic therapy. In these cases Aguado prescribes prednisolone, 15 mg. per day for 3 to 6 days. Thereafter, the lesions appear sharper and more apparent, making a correct diagnosis possible. Our opinion of this test is very favorable.

The problem with the stable atypical scar is different. By definition this is a residual and stable lesion. Unless it is large or the variegation of its surface is very accented (mixture of superimposed images, heterogeneous visual density, etc.), there are no indications for either its destruction or a histologic examination. However, electrocoagulation is recommended to eliminate any cervical area that appears to have dysplastic potential. Periodic colposcopic and cytologic examinations are useful.

ATYPICAL TRANSFORMATION

DEFINITION

The "zone of atypical transformation" is the colposcopic expression of the histologic aggravation which the re-epithelialization process may suffer, both typical and atypical, due to disturbances in its maturation and differentiation. It has little to do with repair of ectopy, once this has taken place, but it never appears on a strictly normal cervix (Fig. 239).

SYNONYMS

Atypical Transformation. Zone of colposcopic undifferentiation. Class IV colposcopic image. Zone of high risk of carcinogenesis. *Remaniement atypique.* Suspicious transformation. Zone of uncommon transformation. Zone of undifferentiated abnormal transformation. Zone of grade III transformation. Zone of high degree of proliferation. Suspicious colposcopic atypia.

Following Glatthaar we have accepted the expression "zone of atypical transformation," but not without some hesitation. Our doubts stem from the possibility of confusion with the preceding lesion ("zone of atypical re-epithelialization"), since there are many colposcopists who consider "re-epithelialization" and "transformation" to be synonymous. In some recent publications, "atypical re-epithelialization" is unfortunately grouped with "atypical transformation," creating considerable confusion, not only terminologically, but also conceptually. For this reason, some time ago we used the alternating term "zone of colposcopic undifferentiation" (Carrera), which alluded to the histologic characteristics while attempting to avoid confusion.

Busch et al. grouped the potentially malignant colposcopic lesions (leukokeratosis with differences in levels, vascular atypia, hyperkeratosis, erosions, etc.) under the qualification of Class IV. For the same reasons adduced when speaking about the synonymy between atypical re-epithelialization and Class III (p. 146), we believe that classifications of this type offer more inconveniences than advantages. Martin-Laval and Dajoux speak about "zones of high degree of carcinogenesis" and in a similar manner to that of Busch, establish a numerical ordering of these lesions.

Bret and Coupez coined different terms to define this lesion. The best known is *remaniement atypique,* whose translation (readjustment, reordering, or restructuring) is not distinct. They have also used the expression "zone of metaplastic transformation" to refer to the most frequent colposcopic appearance of in situ carcinoma. This term seems to us correct, but it is evident that the nomenclature proposed by the Zurich school has been more generally accepted.

Unanimity on the word "transformation" even if accompanied by diverse qualifying terms, is virtually total. Hence, Ganse speaks about a "zone of uncommon transformation," Coppleson of a "zone of undifferentiated abnormal transformation," and Coppleson and Reid of a "zone of grade III transformation," differentiating it from that of grade I (typical re-epithelialization) and grade II (equivalent in certain respects to our atypical re-epithelialization). Only a few colposcopists continue using outmoded terminology. Rubinstein, for example, in spite of a perfectly correct description, speaks about a "zone of high degree of proliferation," and Stoltz uses the term "suspicious colposcopic atypia."

Nevertheless, differences exist, because even if all these expressions imply a colposcopic lesion with a high degree of malignant potential, the colposcopic descriptions of the lesions themselves present notable differences.

ORIGIN

To clarify the origin of the "zone of atypical transformation," or of severe dysplasia and in situ carcinoma, requires the solution of two underlying problems:

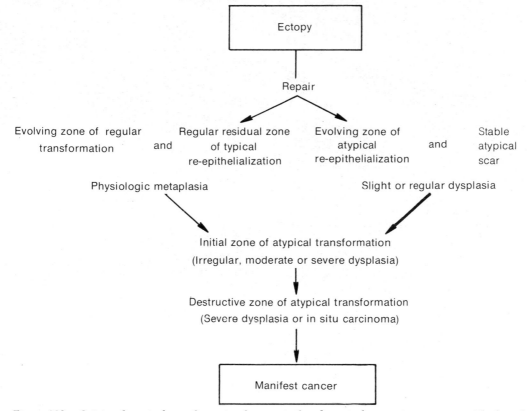

Figure 239. Origin of atypical transformation from typical and atypical reparative processes. The histologic substrate of these lesions is also included.

the place where the suspicious transformation begins and the causes which induce the change. Colposcopy can reply to the first question, but answers to the second are still hypothetical.

At present we believe it is safe to state that atypical transformation may initially appear in (a) the junction between an altered metaplastic tissue (atypical re-epithelialization) and the normal columnar epithelium, or (b) the interior of the ectopic glands that in the course of typical re-epithelialization have suffered an intense metaplastic change with a disturbance in maturation. At either of these locations there is prolonged conflict between the squamous and columnar epithelia. It is extremely unusual to observe atypical transformation in the normal exocervix, the original mucosa, or the mucosa that covers the vagina, even though these are morphologically similar epithelia.

Origin in the Squamo-Columnar Junction. Many investigators have insisted that intraepithelial carcinoma is initiated at this point (Mestwerdt, Richart, Hertig and Mansell, Wielenga, and others), but the conditions under which that event took place were not clear. We do not know of the existence of any proof that severe dysplasia and ultimately in situ carcinoma can be initiated at a strictly normal squamo-columnar border (that is, normal endocervical mucosa and squamous exocervical original mucosa), nor (probably) at a junction between normal columnar epithelium and physiologic squamous metaplastic epithelium. The latter possibility would certainly be the exception and not the rule. On the other hand, colposcopic observations demonstrate without a doubt that at this junction serious colposcopic atypia may appear where previously a zone of atypical re-epithelialization had existed and

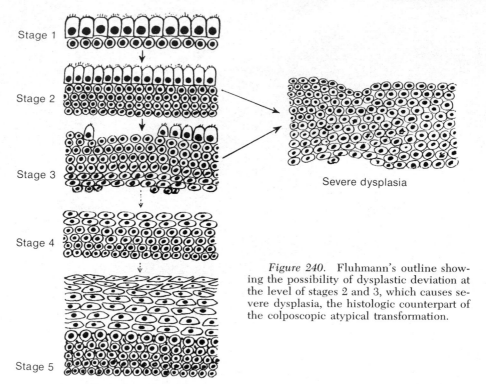

Stage 1

Stage 2

Stage 3

Severe dysplasia

Stage 4

Figure 240. Fluhmann's outline showing the possibility of dysplastic deviation at
the level of stages 2 and 3, which causes severe dysplasia, the histologic counterpart of
the colposcopic atypical transformation.

Stage 5

reached up to the external anatomic os of
the cervix, with persistence of the in-
teraction between the epithelia.

For unknown reasons, in a small
number of cases, the metaplastic process
that initiated the atypical re-epithelialization, when it reaches this
level, and especially in the interior of the
endocervical canal, is interrupted between stages 2 and 3 of Fluhmann's
scheme (Fig. 240). As a consequence,
proliferation of the reserve cells continues, and the squamous differentiation
that would impede the process and lead
to a benign outcome does not take place.
It is as if nature committed a dramatic
error: by trying to retard the metaplastic
re-epithelialization (which at this moment is at its most active), judging by the
fact that it has arrived at the physiologic
limit between the two epithelia, it partially inhibits the metaplastic mechanism
precisely when the squamous differentiation should be initiated. The consequence is obvious: instead of physiologic metaplasia with normal epidermoid
differentiation and with normal or only
slightly disturbed maturation, there appears a metaplastic multiplication of a

hyperplastic variety, which is the matrix
of a severe dysplasia.

According to this, dysplasia and
cancer derive by way of a previous stage
of metaplasia not really from the squamous epithelium, but rather from the
cellular population of columnar origin
(the reserve cells) near the squamo-
columnar border.

Undoubtedly, future research will
demonstrate the existence of some organelles which have as their mission the regulation of epithelial growth by neuroen-
docrine or humoral means, ensuring that
a certain number of epithelial borders
remain stable in the organism. Their
messages initiate or block cellular proliferation, restoring the normal limits lost
by virtue of trauma, inflammation, or
other insult. However, such organelles
may be themselves interfered with totally or partially by a hostile environment
which alters the intracellular metabolism
(lack of oxygen, lack of equilibrium in the
enzymatic balance, necrotic phenomena,
etc.) with the consequence that their
messages are poorly transmitted to the
vanguard of the growing epithelium.

In the present case, detention of the

metaplastic process suffers a partial block which inhibits only the last stages of the reparative mechanism. In this manner, what ordinarily constitutes only one transient stage of the metaplastic process is converted into a permanent and definitive condition. This applies particularly to the disorderly hyperplasia of the reserve cells.

We have never observed a histologically suspicious zone of atypical transformation in the periphery of an ectopy; it always originates near the cervical os. Many reasons can be invoked to explain this fact, such as prolonged epithelial reaction in this area or maximal environmental interference, but the most convincing argument is that metaplastic re-epithelialization is blocked when the reparative process reaches this point.

Origin of Atypical Transformation in an Ectopic Gland. When the atypical transformation process takes place at the level of an ectopic gland that forms part of a typical re-epithelialization zone, the sequence of events usually is (1) partial squamous metaplasia of the epithelial covering of the gland, (2) repeated attempts to block the metaplasia which are themselves prevented by the exaggerated secretion of the intact glandular cells, (3) a permanent struggle between the two types of epithelium, (4) disturbances first in maturation and then in differentiation, (5) extension of the metaplasia to neighboring zones, and (6) possibly carcinogenesis over short or long term.

In these "microepithelial junctions," as they are defined by Coupez, the disturbance in squamous differentiation has as its origin the same organization error that caused the dysplasia at the level of the squamo-columnar junction.

It becomes evident that the atypical transformation zone and consequently the severe dysplasia and neoplastic pathology of the cervix has its origin in the reparative metaplastic epithelium, especially in the one that has suffered a maturation disturbance. By this explanation apparently antagonistic attitudes are harmonized. Carmichael, Fluhmann and Jeaffreson held that epidermoid metaplasia is a "normal" finding in the cervix, whereas the group following Hinselmann believed that such metaplasia is an "obligate stage" in the appearance and development of carcinoma. Both are correct. What occurs is that only a small percentage of cervical metaplasias will continue on the dysplastic route that leads to cancer. The rest will follow a normoplastic route which has as its end an epithelium practically identical to the original mucosa.

Based on our colposcopic observations, we believe in the almost exclusive origin of cancer of the cervix in a previous metaplastic process. This view agrees with the results of histopathologic studies by many authorities (Barcellos, Duarte, Johnson et al., Von Haam, and others). In any event, the rare cancer originating in the germinal layer of the normal stratified epithelium would be invasive so early (Nogales) and have such a rapidly infiltrating growth that there would not be enough time to observe it by colposcopy in its preinvasive phase, which has as its most representative picture that of the zone of atypical transformation.

Table 40. Frequency of Atypical Transformation

	Per Cent of Atypical Images	Per Cent of Total Colposcopies
Mossetti and Russo (1962)	–	0.20
Hernández Alcántara et al. (1971)	11.8	0.80
Youssef (1971)	–	0.90
Zamarriego et al. (1966)	14.2	1.80
González-Merlo (1966)	12.4	2.36
Mateu-Aragonés (1971)	38.59	3.08
Stoltz (1955)	–	3.30
Our Series (1971)	3.7	0.49

As listed by Beato and Barcellos, there are many arguments to justify this stance: (1) the existence of multicentric lesions (the "cancer field" theory of Willis) is always accompanied by metaplasia at different levels (Takeuchi and McKay), as is clearly seen in the initial zone of atypical transformation; (2) the discovery of squamous cell carcinomas which invade the endocervical canal while leaving the exocervical mucosa almost undamaged, (and which arise from secondary zones of atypical transformation that appear in the "collision" site between a zone of atypical re-epithelialization and the columnar endocervical epithelium; (3) the finding of in situ carcinomas limited to the glands (in which a zone of atypical transformation has developed from the glandular sequelae of a zone of typical re-epithelialization); and (4) the existence of endocervical polyps with malignant epidermoid metaplasias.

Summarizing, we know the circumstances of the terrain and place in which a specific normal metaplastic area or a disturbed one may be converted into a zone of atypical transformation, and we have formulated an hypothesis to explain the localization of the phenomenon. Remaining to be explained are the causes of the transformation (p. 211).

FREQUENCY

The zone of atypical transformation is an infrequent colposcopic lesion, at least when the restricted criteria that we maintain are used. This name was used years ago for those atypical lesions of irregular surface, altered vascularization, and uncharacteristic appearance that were not otherwise classifiable. Used in this manner, the percentage of "atypical transformations" was rather high (2 to 3 per cent). At present our figures are much lower: atypical transformation is seen in 0.49 per cent of all colposcopic examinations and 3.7 per cent of the total of atypical lesions. These figures are close to those of Mossetti and Russo (0.2 per cent of all their colposcopies), but are different from those offered by other Spanish authors: González-Merlo 2.36 per

Table 41. Malignant Potential of Atypical Transformation

Limburg (1956)	7.80%
Cramer (1961)	11.80%
Arenas et al. (1961)	12.30%
Bajardi et al. (1959)	17.00%
Wyss (1961)	17.90%
Gil Vernet et al. (1969)	18.25%
Mateu-Aragonés (1971)	19.47%
González-Merlo (1966)	21.50%
Zamarriego et al. (1966)	22.20%
Burghardt and Bajardi (1954)	35.10%
Our Series (1972)	54.09%

cent, Mateu-Aragonés 3.08 per cent (Table 40).

These divergent figures are due chiefly to the difficulty in correctly identifying a zone of atypical transformation, and clearly separating it from some re-epithelializations, typical or atypical, of irregular appearance and with erosion, bleeding and maceration, caused by superimposed inflammatory process. As we have mentioned (p. 154), the principal cause of doubt or diagnostic error is a zone of atypical re-epithelialization subject to infection, because the resulting colposcopic pictures may easily arouse suspicions of malignancy. This fact has led some colposcopists to point to infection as the cause of certain zones of atypical transformation. We believe, however, that apart from the apparent similarity of the colposcopic images, these are two lesions with very different histologic substrates, which we should endeavor to recognize and differentiate by all the means available. Certainly, as colposcopic experience is acquired, the possibility of error is lessened.

COLPOSCOPIC APPEARANCES

There are two stages in the evolution of an "atypical transformation zone:" the initial phase and the destructive phase. The latter, in most cases, is not merely dysplastic but is already a neoplastic lesion (Table 41).

The diagnosis of a zone of atypical

transformation in either stage causes considerable difficulty to the inexperienced colposcopist. The lesion can take many diverse forms, and moreover there exists the possibility of interpreting as atypical transformations other lesions lacking any malignant potential, but subject to inflammatory disturbances which give them a false appearance of seriousness. For example, re-epithelialization processes, typical or atypical, may be subjected to alternating superficial infection and maceration. The fragile metaplastic epithelium, damaged in many places, may offer images so bizarre as to be suspicious.

1. Zone of Initial Atypical Transformation. At the outset, if the dysplastic lesion has not greatly altered the epithelium, it is possible to observe the process at the level of the squamo-columnar junction of the cervical os or in an ectopic gland. We call the former a zone of secondary transformation (secondary to atypical re-epithelialization) and the latter a primary zone of transformation, because it does not derive from a pathologic lesion, but rather from a physiologic metaplasia. Although such a lesion may be located in any part of the cervix, these atypical transformation zones are predisposed to appear at the anterior lip (12 o'clock) and to a lesser extent at 6 o'clock (Richart). This is especially true of secondary transformation; the primary form has a less precise distribution.

ZONE OF PRIMARY INITIAL ATYPICAL TRANSFORMATION. This occurs in cervices subjected to typical re-epi thelialization, but having a considerable number of glandular sequelae in the form of opened and secreting orifices which tend to macerate the circumoral epithelium. Eventually, the secretion diminishes or ceases, because the metaplastic product has converted the primitive "red ring" into a "wax drop" or into a "white ring." These images are distinguished from the strictly normal ones of typical re-epithelialization (p. 118) by their dimensions, (always larger) and by their visual intensity, which reflects extreme cellular and nuclear density (Holtorff). Starting from these elements the dysplastic process advances centrifugally, progressively modifying the

healthy surrounding metaplastic epithelium. In this manner a series of round plaques, interlaced with one another, are formed.

If the cervix is examined through the colposcope without any preparation, some uncharacteristic red zones are observed, which correspond to the aforementioned dysplastic plaques (Fig. 241). After the application of acetic acid, the red zones are transformed into white spots, of higher intensity than those of atypical re-epithelialization, but of imprecise limits, because the optical density is higher near the glands from which they started than in their periphery (Fig. 242). The surface of these leukokeratotic zones is irregular, embossed, with depressions or breaks, and elevations or mounds of a vitreous appearance. Others have emphasized the importance of superimposed images, but in reality they are not consistently found. When they do exist, they are apparent, forming high points above the surface of the cervix and mixing in a bizarre manner one with the other. Bolten insists, and we share his opinion, that when these images are regular and smooth, stromal invasion has not occurred, something which, to the contrary, is very possible when they stand out strongly above the cervical surface. Also, congested and easily eroded zones are observed (Fig. 243). Many of the "red zones" of other authors are included among these cervical pictures. These zones are iodine-negative in Schiller's test.

Agreeing with the Zurich school and also with Palmer and Mateu-Aragonés, we have found the appearance of the blood vessels to be very irregular (Fig. 244), increasing the gravity of the picture (Table 42).

(Text continued on page 172)

Table 42. Malignant Potential of "Vascular Irregularities"

Zamarriego (1966)	10.00%
González-Merlo (1966)	12.35%
Gil Vernet et al. (1969)	20.64%
Mateu-Aragonés (1969) (vessels of types IV and V)	36.90%
Our Series (1972)	29.8%

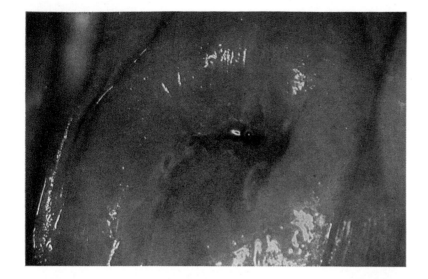

Figure 241. Primary atypical transformation in a very early stage, before the application of acetic acid. A slight reddening of the circumoral region is observed. At this moment an accurate diagnosis is practically impossible.

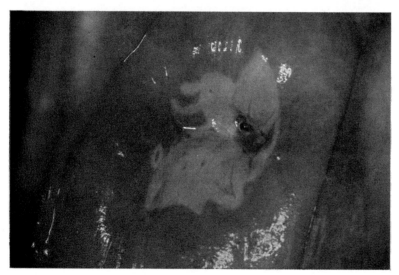

Figure 242. After application of acetic acid, primary atypical transformation is made evident by the presence of a leukoplakiform zone with diffuse edges and glandular orifices. The latter detail permits its differentiation from a zone of atypical re-epithelialization. Undoubtedly this lesion is being observed in an incipient stage.

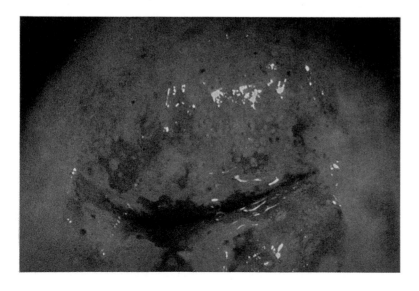

Figure 243. Advanced primary atypical transformation. After acetic acid is applied, a colposcopic complex appears, formed by white zones and red congested and erosive zones, with imprecise and diffuse borders. Numerous glandular orifices suggest the origin of this atypical transformation over the glandular residua of an old typical re-epithelialization. Biopsy discovered an intraepithelial carcinoma.

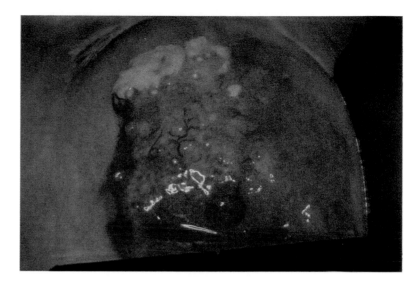

Figure 244. Vascular irregularities forming part of an atypical transformation. A striking leukokeratotic zone is observed.

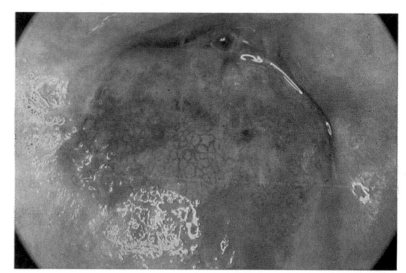

Figure 245. Atypical transformation, secondary to atypical re-epithelialization. In addition to mosaic structure there are congestive, hemorrhagic and erosive zones. No remnants of ectopy are seen. The certification of "secondary" is suggested by the localization (near the anatomic cervical os) and by the characteristics of the residual mosaic structure. Biopsy revealed in situ carcinoma.

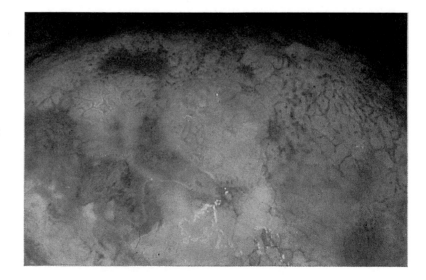

Figure 246. Extensive secondary atypical transformation. This diagnosis is made, aside from the topographical characeristics of the lesion and its constituent images, by the absence of ectopic glandular orifices. In this colpophotograph may be seen a mosaic pattern interrupted by congested and erosive zones.

Table 43. Frequency of "Vascular Irregularities"

	PER CENT OF ATYPICAL IMAGES	PER CENT OF TOTAL COLPOSCOPIES
Hernández Alcántara et al. (1971)	8.17	0.6
Zamarriego et al. (1966)	22.2	2.8
González-Merlo (1966)	22.3	4.2
Our Series (1972)	24.3	3.8

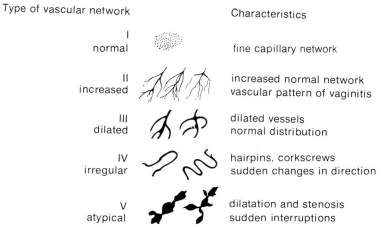

Type of vascular network	Characteristics
I normal	fine capillary network
II increased	increased normal network / vascular pattern of vaginitis
III dilated	dilated vessels / normal distribution
IV irregular	hairpins, corkscrews / sudden changes in direction
V atypical	dilatation and stenosis / sudden interruptions

Figure 247.   Outline of vascular patterns, according to Mateu-Aragónes.

According to Dzioba, if suspicious blood vessels are added to the classic images of mosaic, ground structure, and leukoplakia, there is a 66.6 per cent incidence of severe dysplasia or in situ carcinoma. And if to that colposcopic complex one adds exophytic images, necrosis and irregular vascularization, the percentage of malignancy is 96.6.

Ganse distinguished no less than 12 different types of vessels, attempting to correlate their morphology and the histologic seriousness of the lesion. We consider the classification of Mateu-Aragonés more sensible because it seems especially useful for the inexperienced colposcopist (Fig. 247).

Type I: normal vascular network.

Type II: normal vascular network, but increased.

Type III: dilated, thick vessels, but of normal distribution.

Type IV: dilated and irregular vessels with corkscrew shapes or forked, and with sudden changes in direction.

Type V: markedly atypical vessels with dilatations and strictures in their course, and with sudden interruptions.

True vascular irregularities begin with type III, although the probability of malignancy is low (0.61 per cent). In type IV the incidence of cancer is 15 per cent and in type V, 86 per cent (Table 43).

Kolstad reported an evident correlation between the intercapillary distance and the degree of epithelial atypia and

Table 44. Frequency of Vascular Irregularities According to the Seriousness of the Histology of the Lesion[*]

HISTOLOGIC DIAGNOSIS	PER CENT OF ATYPICAL VESSELS
Benign	0.6
Dysplasia	0.7
In situ carcinoma	16.7
Microinvasive carcinoma	76.9
Invasive carcinoma	96.6

[*]From Kolstad, P.: Acta Obstétrica et Gynecologica Scandinavica, *43*:105–108, 1964.

claimed to see a parallel between the seriousness of the histologic diagnosis and the extent of atypical vessels (Table 44). Koller insisted that a perpendicular orientation of the vessels to the epithelial surface and the absence of a clear circulatory insufficiency were characteristics of preinvasive lesions.

Around these atypical zones of leukokeratosis is a wide congestive zone which separates them from healthy tissue and which Lugol's solution identifies very well if acetic acid has not done so. This colposcopic detail is restricted to this type of lesion; hence it is a detail to consider in the differential diagnosis with atypical re-epithelialization (Holtorff, Kern, Coupez). Nevertheless, some infected zones of atypical re-epithelialization present difficult problems of differential diagnosis.

ZONE OF SECONDARY INITIAL ATYPICAL TRANSFORMATION. These are characterized by two morphologic observations: the initially suspicious zones are very near the anatomic cervical os, and they are occupied by one or several zones of atypical re-epithelialization (Figs. 245 and 246), which may even develop intracervically. On the other hand, their characteristics are remarkably similar to those of the primary initial atypical transformation, except that ectopic glandular orifices are not seen (at least not in the atypical re-epithelialization which is worsening) (Fig. 246).

The fact that re-epithelialization and transformation zones are contiguous can create interesting diagnostic problems, but these tend to resolve by observation of the boundaries of the lesions, their visual density, the existence or absence of vascular irregularities and congestive zones, and the embossment of the surface (Table 46).

With Lugol's solution, it is generally observed that the transformation zone rejects iodine more completely than the re-epithelialization zone; the latter may even stain totally or partially in some sectors (Figs. 252 and 253).

Despite all this, the colposcopic diagnosis of secondary initial atypical transformation is not easy (Kern and Bötzelen). The criteria are based on simple changes of color or transparency of a metaplastic epithelium that has been previously altered (Rieper). Unless there are striking vascular anomalies, the secondary initial transformation may remain undetected in its first stages.

Zone of Destructive Atypical Transformation. In this stage, epithelial damage is very noteworthy in that the mucosal covering breaks up at various points of the exocervix, such breaks becoming more numerous at each examination. For this reason, in addition to the classical superimposed images, numerous congested, erosive, and even ulcerated zones are seen, with bleeding produced upon minimal contact (Fig. 248).

These erosions (Table 45) should lead the colposcopist to think immediately about a possible malignant process (Figs. 249 and 250), if they fulfill some of the following characteristics (Mossetti and Russo): (1) location near the anatomic os of the cervix, especially if they disappear within the interior of the en-

(*Text continued on page 176*)

Table 45. Frequency of True Erosion

	PER CENT OF ATYPICAL IMAGES	PER CENT OF TOTAL COLPOSCOPIES
Hernández Alcántara et al. (1971)	3.56	0.27
Mateu-Aragonés (1971)	4.63	0.37
Guzmán Llovet et al. (1967)	–	0.95
Zamarriego (1966)	8.70	1.10
González-Merlo (1966)	8.60	1.65
Mossetti and Russo (1962)	–	5.50
Bonilla (1965)	–	10.00
Our Series (1972)	6.7	1.05

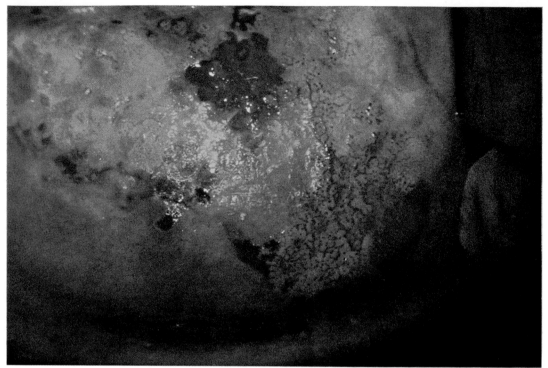

Figure 248.   Destructive atypical transformation. Large plaque of leukokeratosis, which exhibits superimposed images of ground and mosaic structure and which is associated with congested, hemorrhagic and erosive zones. The lesion lacks sharp edges.

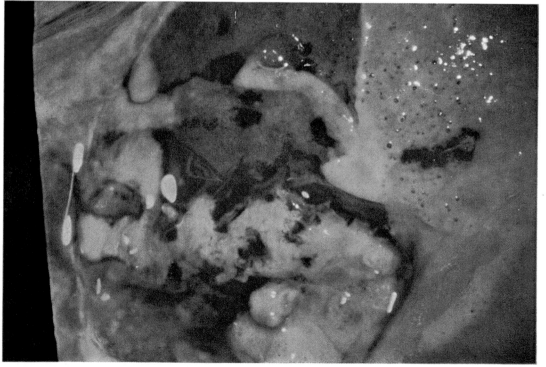

Figure 249.   Extensive and irregular erosion, encircled by a dense plaque of leukokeratosis which shows a papillary ground structure in one sector.

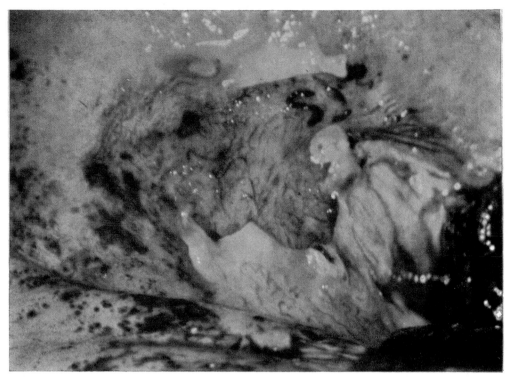

Figure 250. Erosion in the midst of a destructive atypical transformation. Notable vascular irregularities, hemorrhagic zones, and sectors of superficial necrosis are seen.

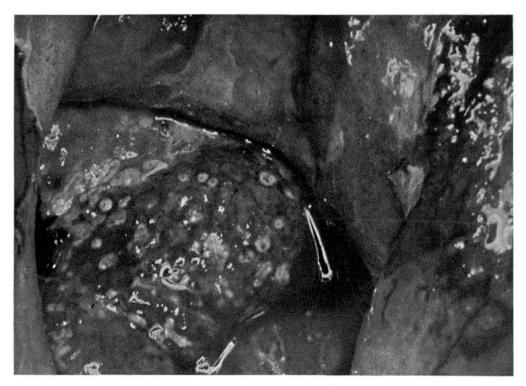

Figure 251. Atypical transformation in a destructive phase. The images of leukokeratosis have been almost totally replaced by ulcerative ones. The last epithelial elements that persist are the zones adjoining the ectopic glandular orifices.

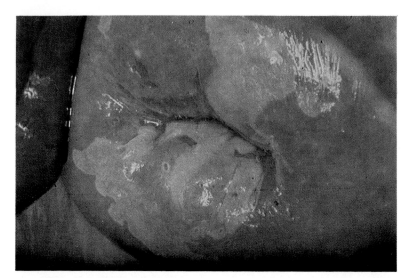

Figure 252. Differential diagnosis between atypical re-epithelialization and atypical transformation. After application of acetic acid, three white zones appear. Between 10 and 12 o'clock is seen a lesion with atypical transformation (poorly defined borders and recognizable glandular orifices in a lesion that disappears into the cervical canal). The other white zone has developed to the periphery of the posterior cervix, covering it lightly; its contours are sharp, its density is minor and it is devoid of glandular orifices, so that it can be called a zone of atypical re-epithelialization. The same can be said about the lesion at 5 o'clock.

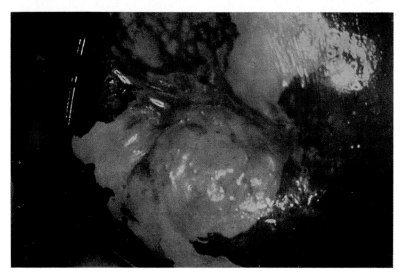

Figure 253. With Lugol's solution, the perfect delineation of an atypical re-epithelialization is confirmed in contrast to the sector with an atypical transformation.

docervical canal; (2) irregular surface, due to the existence of atypical vascularization in the stroma, or due to reactive modifications of the same, which give it a brittle aspect; and (3) atypias in the surrounding epithelium, which exhibit images of leukokeratosis and an irregular vascularization (Fig. 249). The increased probability of malignancy of this lesion is seen (Table 47).

The distinction between a carcinomatous lesion and inflammatory granulation tissue, for example, is not always easy. The general appearance of the lesion many times will orient the observer.

The vessels that remain are highly irregular, dilated, outlined, have atypical pathways and unequal caliber (types IV and V of Mateu-Aragonés). The nu-

merous interruptions and changes in level are especially notable (Fig. 250).

The colposcopic appearance may be truly impressive when, as is very frequent, added trichomonal infection exists. The epithelium then tears with great ease. Further erosions and bleeding can be caused if, prior to the colposcopic exploration, multiple digital examinations have taken place, along with biopsies and instrumentation.

At the end of this destructive process, the leukokeratotic images have practically disappeared, drowned by the erosions and ulcerations. The last epithelial remnants to be shed are the zones adjacent to the ectopic glandular orifices, because here the cellular density is very intense (Fig. 251).

Table 46. Colposcopic Differential Diagnosis between Zone of Atypical
Re-epithelialization and Zone of Atypical Transformation

ZONE OF ATYPICAL RE-EPITHELIALIZATION	ZONE OF ATYPICAL TRANSFORMATION
Barely visible without preparation	Generally visible without preparation
External contours well marked	Ill-defined external contours
Regular, smooth surface	Irregular, embossed surface
Generally situated in the periphery of an ectopy	Rarely associated with ectopy
Without perilesional reaction	Circled by a red congestive zone
Congested or erosive zones are not seen	Frequently associated with congested or erosive and ulcerated zones
Visual density generally weak, more accentuated in the periphery	Marked visual density, especially in the center of the lesion and after acetic acid
Without vascular irregularities	Increased vascularization, frequently irregular
Flat superimposed patterns, barely apparent	Well marked superimposed patterns, sometimes elevated
No glandular orifices are seen in the re-epithelializing zone	Frequent and striking glandular orifices.

Remember that infection may give a zone of atypical re-epithelialization characteristics very similar to those of atypical transformation.

HISTOLOGIC CORRELATIONS

The obligatory biopsy that should follow the colposcopic diagnosis of atypical transformation of either form will be interpreted in 39.3 per cent of cases as irregular dysplasia (6.6 per cent moderate dysplasia, 32.7 per cent severe dysplasia), in 40.9 per cent as in situ carcinoma, in 13.1 per cent as invasive carcinoma, and in only 6.5 per cent as benign (Table 49).

Various authors offer figures similar to ours, and they insist that identification of atypical transformation is more important than the diagnosis of the "matrix areas" of Hinselmann (Glatthaar and Funck Brentano, Palmer, Russo and Macchioni, Wagner and Fettig, Mateu-Aragonés, Coppleson and Reid, Kern and Rissmann). It is clear that zones of atypical transformation include more than half of the severe dysplastic lesions and intraepithelial carcinomas (see Table 49).

In our scheme the irregular dysplasias include grades II and III of the FIGO classification (1961) and the "moderate" and "severe" dysplasias of the system proposed by the WHO (1971). When we speak of moderate dysplasia we refer to a tissue which has suffered a tardy epidermoid differentiation and has seen its maturation highly disturbed. On the contrary, the severe dysplasia signifies a total absence of maturation and differentiation of the covering epithelium.

According to this system, the differences between the slight or regular dysplasia (atypical re-epithelialization) and moderate or severe dysplasia (characteristic of atypical transformation) are striking: The first includes only anomalies of maturation, while the second com-

Table 47. Malignant Potential of
True Erosion

Burghardt and Bajardi (1954)	2.5%
Gil Vernet et al. (1969)	9.31%
Limburg (1956)	9.9%
Bajardi et al. (1959)	10%
Mateu-Aragonés (1971)	12.2%
González-Merlo (1966)	12.72%
Guzman Llovet et al. (1967)	18%
Zamarriego (1966)	18.1%
Our Series (1972)	11.3%

Table 48. Histologic Correlation of Atypical Transformation

	Initial Phase	Destructive Phase	Total
Physiologic metaplasia	0%	0%	0%
Regular dysplasia	12.50%	0%	6.55%
Irregular dysplasia	56.25%	20.61%	39.34%
In situ carcinoma	28.12%	55.18%	40.98%
Invasive carcinoma	3.12%	24.14%	13.11%

prises disordered maturation and differentiation. Which process is found depends on when the disturbing element appears in the metaplastic process (Table 50). If the blockage has taken place in phase 4 of Fluhmann, the epithelium is differentiated but does not adequately mature (slight or regular dysplasia), but if it acts between stages 2 and 3, epidermoid maturation does not occur and proliferation continues (irregular, moderate, or severe dysplasia, according to the degree of failure of differentiation). In Table 30 (p. 131) all these concepts are expressed, using as a basis the reserve cell, and the correspondence between the different classifications is established.

Very succinctly we will describe the three basic histologic pictures seen with atypical transformation.

Moderate Dysplasia (Grade II). The epithelium presents disturbances in differentiation and maturation (Fig. 254).

The major portion of the thickness of the epithelium is occupied by parabasal cells. When they ascend, these cells do not increase in size, but rather remain small and possess a hypertrophic nucleus (voluminous and hyperchromatic), even though retracted. The inversion in the nuclear-cytoplasmic relationship is evident. In some areas it is seen that the cytoplasm changes suddenly to eosinophilic and the nucleus acquires an angulated shape and an intensely black color.

Stratification is doubtful, with the cells arranged in simple heaps perpendicular to the basement membrane. Nevertheless, in some areas, despite its immaturity and slight differentiation, the epithelium resembles epidermoid mucosa.

In the upper part of the epithelium, there is an accented cytoplasmic and nuclear maturation. Stratification is more nearly normal, but nuclei are still atypical, with irregular contour and opacification of the chromatin. Mitoses are more abundant.

Glandular sequelae of the metaplastic reparation persist in the chorion.

Severe Dysplasia (Grade III). (Fig. 255.) There is a complete absence of differentiation, and it is not possible to identify the epithelium as being epidermoid or another type. Stratification in regular columns is absent or sparse. Cellular density is marked, due to the increase of the nuclear volume and the decrease of the cytoplasmic volume. Immaturity is evident, for the germinative cells have lost polarity. There are frequent mitoses, some of them abnormal, and the nuclei are voluminous and irregular.

Table 49. Histologic Correlation of Colposcopic Dysplasia

	Mild	Moderate	Severe	In situ Carcinoma	Invasive Carcinoma
Evolutional atypical re-epithelialization	78.78%	1.14%	0.75%	1.43%	0%
Residual atypical re-epithelialization	85.34%	0.43%	0.43%	0.43%	0%
Atypical transformation	6.55%	6.60%	32.70%	40.98%	13.1%

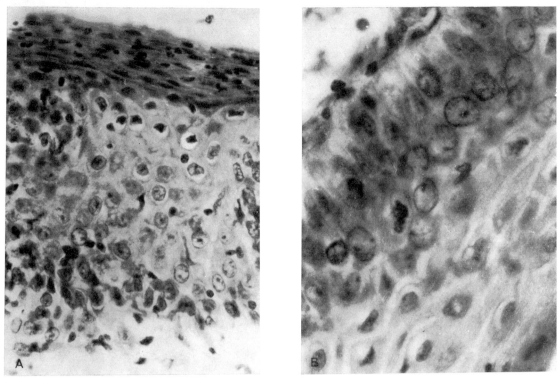

Figure 254. Histologic section showing moderate dysplasia. Colposcopy revealed a zone of very early atypical transformation. *A*, At low magnification; *B*, at higher magnification.

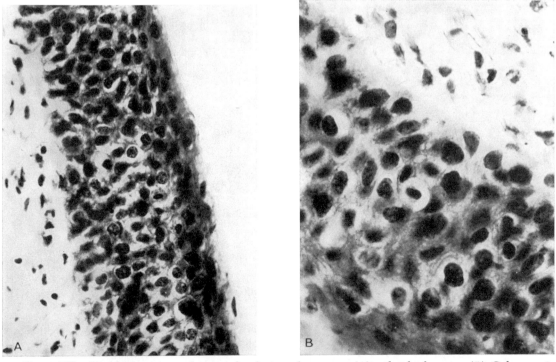

Figure 255. Histologic picture of severe dysplasia, at low power (*A*) and at high power (*B*). Colposcopic examination had revealed a primary atypical transformation.

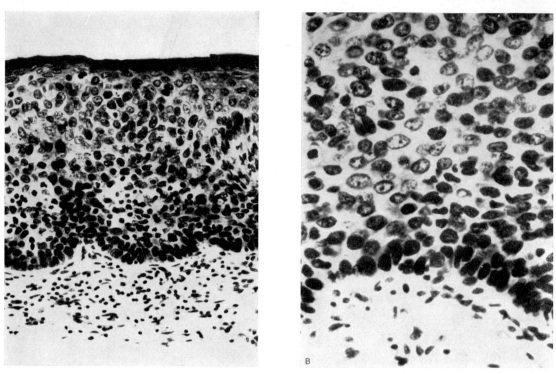

Figure 256. Histology of intraepithelial carcinoma at low (*A*) and high power. (*B*)

Distinguishing between these dysplasias and in situ carcinoma is not easy. de Brux considered cytologic confirmation essential.

In Situ Carcinoma. The histologic alterations are similar to those of irregular dysplasia, but the diagnosis may be established by attention to the nucleus (Fig. 256).

Stratification is again absent or slow, initiated only at the epithelial surface. The cellular density is greater than in severe dysplasia. Differentiation may be normal or not, depending on whether the lesion is a differentiated or undifferentiated in situ carcinoma. There are several notable cellular anomalies, including an increase in the nuclear-cytoplasmic ratio, disappearance of the glycogen content, and a variety of cellular shapes and sizes, except in the undifferentiated form in which all cells are very much alike. Nuclear changes are an increase and an irregular distribution of chromatin, anisonucleosis, and multinucleation. Mitoses are abundant and atypical, with a possibility of polyploidy.

The basement membrane is intact, even though in situ carcinoma may spread to the glandular elements (around 80 to 90 per cent of cases according to Fluhmann, Friedell, and others).

Terminologic confusion has resulted from the attempt to classify intraepithelial carcinomas according to their maturation or differentiation.

CYTOLOGIC CORRELATIONS

From the viewpoint of Papanicolaou's classification, the majority of the smears in atypical transformation should be classified as suspicious (60.6 per cent) and an appreciable number of them should be included within Class IV (29.5 per cent). The lesion is totally benign cytologically in only 9.83 per cent of cases. These figures very eloquently demonstrate the great malignant potential of atypical transformation (Tables 51 and 52). There are considerable differences between the cytologic correla-

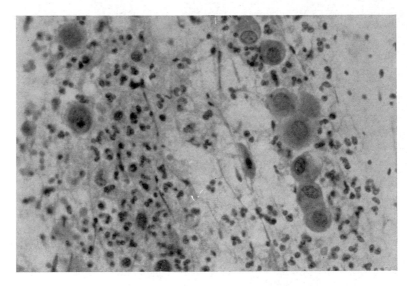

Figure 257. Cytologic smear of moderate dysplasia. Abundant nuclear alterations are observed at the level of the deep cells. However, there are no signs suggesting malignancy.

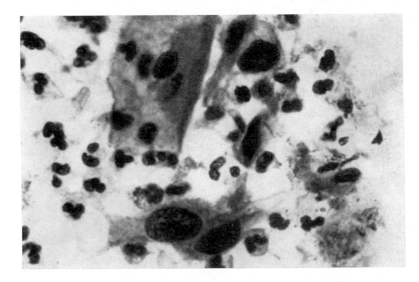

Figure 258. Cytologic smear showing severe dysplasia. Besides the overall cellular morphology, the irregular distribution of the nuclear chromatin and the hyperchromasia exhibited by some nuclei arouse suspicion.

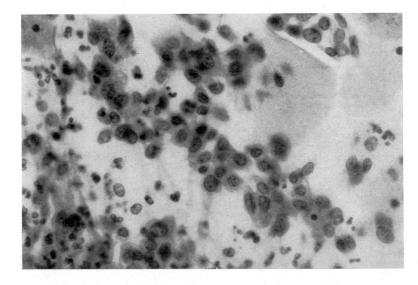

Figure 259. Cytologic smear of intraepithelial carcinoma. Cells of undifferentiated appearance are desquamated in groups. The colposcopic lesion was a "zone of destructive atypical transformation."

Table 50. Cytologic-Histologic Correlation of the Zone of Atypical Transformation

	REGULAR OR MILD DYSPLASIA	IRREGULAR OR MODERATE DYSPLASIA	SEVERE IRREGULAR DYSPLASIA	IN SITU CARCINOMA	INVASIVE CARCINOMA
Class I	0%	0%	0%	0%	0%
Class II	75%	18.75%	0%	0%	0%
Class II-III	25%	75%	37.50%	0%	0%
Class III	0%	0.25%	62.50%	56%	12.50%
Class IV and V	0%	0%	0%	44%	87.50%

tion of initial zone of atypical transformation and that of the destructive phase. The latter carries almost three times the frequency of malignant cytologic findings as the former.

At present there is a gradual abandonment of Papanicolaou's classification, and substitution of a nomenclature comparable to the histologic. In addition to a suspicious diagnosis, the cytologist is now required to determine the histologic lesion which probably caused it. As Meisels pointed out, assigning a case to Papanicolaou's Class III is extremely comfortable. If severe dysplasia or even carcinoma is confirmed, the cytologist's opinion was correct, but if the histologic examination is negative he still cannot be faulted because his diagnosis was only one of suspicion.

The majority of smears from zones of atypical transformation have some common characteristics which cause them to be defined in the present nomenclature as "dysplastic." The number of abnormal cells and the extent of nuclear and cytoplasmic modification permit the establishment of a grading system that encompasses dysplasia (moderate or severe) and in situ carcinoma (Figs. 257 to 259).

General Characteristics

1. An important number of cells present atypical alterations. The percentage of these may provide the first differentiation between severe dysplasia and in situ carcinoma. In the latter, almost all of the cells are dysplastic.

2. The alterations affect cells of all layers. However, in the case of severe dysplasia or in situ carcinoma, basal and parabasal cells predominate.

3. The suspicious cells are grouped in small clumps, of a pseudosyncytial appearance. In the in situ carcinoma they have a certain tendency toward isolated desquamation.

4. The smears appear "dirty," with abundant mucus and inflammatory signs.

Nuclear Characteristics

1. Chromatin is distributed in heavy clusters, irregularly disposed, and the normal uniform chromatinic background disappears. These alterations are especially notable in intraepithelial carcinoma. Anisonucleosis is frequent.

2. The nuclear membrane is irregu-

Table 51. Cytologic Correlation of the Zone of Atypical Transformation

	INITIAL PHASE	DESTRUCTIVE PHASE	TOTAL
Class I	0%	0%	0%
Class II	18.75%	0%	9.83%
Class II-III	34.37%	17.24%	26.22%
Class III	31.25%	37.93%	36.42%
Class IV and V	15.62%	44.82%	29.50%

lar and jagged, and some differences in width may be observed.

3. The nucleoli are prominent.

4. Multinucleation and other phenomena are frequent.

Cytoplasmic Characteristics

1. Modification of the nuclear-cytoplasmic ratio, slightly in severe dysplasia and notably in the in situ carcinoma.

2. The cytoplasm shows an eosinophilic tendency.

3. There is vacuolization and abnormal distribution of the cytoplasm, generally due to retraction of the nucleus.

4. The cell is round in moderate dysplasia, but in severe dysplasia and in situ carcinoma it may be fiber-like or teardrop-shaped.

CLINICAL COURSE

In a considerable number of cases atypical transformation is actually cancer. Naturally, incidence is different for the initial as opposed to the destructive phase. In the first it is 31.2 per cent and in the second 54.1 per cent, according to our series (Table 49).

When histologic study, based on multiple tissue biopsies, reveals a dysplasia of irregular type (moderate or severe), which occurs in the 39 per cent of atypical transformations diagnosed by us, it is difficult to ascertain the potential of this lesion (Fig. 260).

Fox stated that 30 per cent of dysplasias regress, 9 per cent persist and 60 per cent progress to in situ carcinoma. Hall and Walton confirmed that of severe dysplasias, 19 per cent regress, 48 per cent persist, and 33 per cent progress, converting into carcinoma in 29 per cent. Similar figures are given by Coppleson and Reid and by many others, who support Fluhmann's thesis that dysplasia maintains a relation with in situ carcinoma, similar to the one that the latter maintains with invasive carcinoma. Naturally, the progression figures are much lower when all dysplasias are considered (Table 53). Burghardt asserted that any supposed dysplasias that regressed were nothing more than simple epithelial hyperproliferations.

De Brux, who in another era had defended the idea that so-called "precancerous dysplasias" were cancers "masked," now believes that it is necessary to distinguish between two types of dysplasia, which differ in both origin and potentiality. Those whose architecture is regular and with very little dyskaryosis usually are only the atypical metaplastic epidermization of an ectopy. On the contrary, dysplasias whose architecture is very irregular are derived from hyperplasia of the reserve cells, which suffer delayed or inconstant differentiation, with abnormal maturation. Statistically, these are transformed into in situ carcinoma in 50 per cent of cases, while in 20 per cent they regress without total healing.

In our opinion, somewhat less than half of the zones of atypical transformation that are histologically severe dysplasias develop toward carcinoma. It is difficult to determine what percentage of

Table 52.   Evolution of Dysplasia According to Several Authors

	REGRESSION	PERSISTENCE	PROGRESSION
Green (1955)	37%	—	10%
Peckham and Green (1957)	40.5%	—	10.7%
Figge et al. (1957)	26%	65%	4%
Simon and Sheehan (1961)	47%	49%	4.6%
Dougherty et al. (1961)	51%	25%	3%
Scott (1962)	48.9%	43.9%	4.1%
Stern (1963)	40%	49%	12%
Reagan (1964)	54%	30.7%	5.8%
Lagrutta et al. (1966)	46.2%	44%	9.8%
Tortora (1970)	12.5%	—	12.5%

lesions regress and which remain relatively stable, because we do a conization or amputation on all cervices bearing one of these lesions for a long time. The explanation is obvious: it presents a high probability of malignancy and the possibility that jointly with severe dysplasia there exists a true in situ carcinoma, not discovered by biopsy (36 per cent of cases, according to our series).

MANAGEMENT

Simple or multiple biopsy is required in all cases once the possibility of infectious origin is eliminated. If the biopsy gives evidence of an invasive carcinoma, which is not infrequent in a destructive atypical transformation, adequate management may consist of physiotherapy, surgical or combined therapy, according to individual preference and experience. Further elaboration is completely beyond the scope of this book.

Tissue biopsy under colposcopic control (the "selective biopsy" of Limburg) offers trustworthy information 90 per cent of the time in experienced hands (Silver and Woodruf, Christopherson and Gray, Lienhard, Vasquez Ferro, and others). On the contrary, blind biopsy ("simple biopsy" of Schiller) has better than a 30 per cent chance of error which is only partially avoided with the system of four-quadrant biopsy of Foote and Stewart. The so-called ring biopsy of Ayre, which seeks the excision of the transitional zone, has not been widely used. Simple in concept, it is notably complex in execution.

Bolten stated that if biopsy is done under colposcopic control, there never will be more than a grade of difference between the histologic information obtained from the biopsy and that which would be available by conization. In other words, if the biopsy shows severe dysplasia, a cone might reveal an intraepithelial carcinoma but nothing worse. Beller and Khatamee are of the same opinion.

Antoine, and recently Balagueró, advised the abandonment of the single biopsy, even if under colposcopic control, and recommended the practice of conization in all suspicious cases (by cytology or colposcopy), pointing to the multicentric origin of cervical cancer and the frequent extension toward the cervical canal, which may be found in some in situ carcinomas. Our histopathology laboratories are not prepared to receive the avalanche of work which would result from putting into practice this recommendation. Moreover, conization is always a bloody operation, not without risks and sequelae (González-Merlo, Nogales). Unless there is a reason to think about an endocervical origin of the neoplasm, we continue to practice directed biopsies. These must meet the demands listed by Ferrier et al.: adequate site, sufficient material, good orientation (or perpendicular to the surface), and diagnosable (performed on tissue that is not traumatized or necrotized).

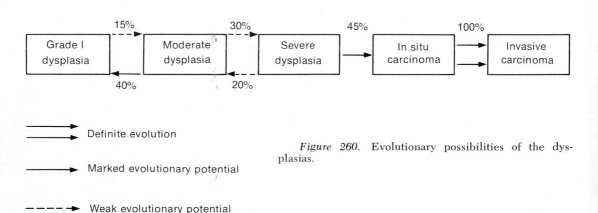

Figure 260. Evolutionary possibilities of the dysplasias.

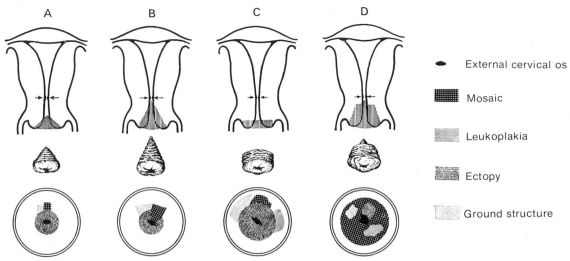

Figure 261. Scheme of the type of conization or amputation advised according to the localization of the lesions observed through the colposcope (according to Lagrutta, Laguens and Quijano). Colposcopy is fundamental to decide on the type of intervention. When the lesion is small and distant from the cervical canal, a minimal conization may be enough (*A*). On the contrary, if it enters the canal, conization excision should go up to the internal cervical os (*B*). If the suspicious image is extensive, but peripheral, the surgical solution will be a minimal amputation (*C*). However, if the lesion is within the cervical canal, the most logical course is ample amputation, with an apical conization (*D*).

If the histologic diagnosis is severe dysplasia or intraepithelial carcinoma, the proper approach is cold conization or amputation, according to the location of the lesions (Fig. 261), with the double objective of obtaining a precise diagnosis and destroying a zone of increased cellular atypia.

To be really effective, conization must include the lower two thirds of the endocervical canal. Curettage of the uterine cavity and the rest of the canal should always be performed in order to avoid missing a neoplasm situated beyond the visible zone of colposcopy, and perhaps not totally eradicated by conization.

If study of numerous serial sections confirms that the lesion is not worse than a severe dysplasia, expectant management should consist of periodic colposcopic and cytologic examination (every 6 months for the first 4 or 5 years, then annually). The same practice may be followed when in situ carcinoma is found, if it is known to be limited to the excised specimen. Some authors believe that even in the case of intraepithelial carcinoma limited to the conization specimen,

it is worthwhile to sacrifice the uterus (TeLinde, Galvin, Way, and others), while others modify this decision depending on age of patient (Hohlbein and Ganse, Held, and others), recommending excision after the menopause. Still, others withhold hysterectomy unless adequate later control is not possible (Kasdon, Stoltz, and others).

On the other hand, if an invasive carcinoma appears at conization or an in situ carcinoma with reasonable doubts about its extension beyond the area of expiration, the unanimous recommendation is extended hysterectomy.* It should include in this case an adequate vaginal cuff, because relapses are frequent (Te Linde, Bret and Coupez, Way et al.), probably due to the existence of multicentric lesions at the moment of intervention, bearing in mind that the exocervix

---

*Invasive cervical carcinomas, more extensive than microinvasive yet still limited to the cervix (that is, Stage I), are generally treated today either by radical hysterectomy or aggressive cancericidal radiotherapy; extended hysterectomy, or modified radical hysterectomy, as recommended here is reserved for those that are superficially invasive at worst. — Ed.

and the upper third of the vagina have a common embryogenesis.

Some authors, such as Scott and Kummert, have emphasized the operative difficulties and the increase of morbidity when hysterectomy is performed within 3 or 4 weeks after diagnostic conization. We have not had any problems in this area, and we continue to think that it is better not to lose much time.

In the less frequent event that the selective biopsy shows only slight or moderate dysplasia, the decision should depend upon the cytologic findings. If the latter confirm the impression of a benign lesion, we pursue a conservative course of quarterly cytologic and colposcopic examinations in the first year, semiannual during the second, and then annual, and the treatment of concomitant pathologic phenomena (infection, endocrine alteration, dystrophic process, etc.). On the other hand, if the cytologic diagnosis is one of suspicion (Class II-III or III) a punch biopsy including the whole of the squamo-columnar junction is imperative (conization, amputation, etc.).

Chanen and Hollyock proposed destruction of these lesions by diathermic electrocoagulation when they are confined to the exocervix. They have obtained a 90 per cent rate of success, with failures (persistence of residual lesions post coagulation) attributed to a deficient technique or to an inadequate selection of patients. They use this technique even if previous biopsy has discovered an in situ carcinoma (19.2 per cent of their cases). Naturally, we cannot recommend this approach, believing that it may be justified only if the study reveals a slight to moderate dysplasia. However, when the pathologist finds severe dysplasia or in situ carcinoma, immediate conization is indicated.

REFERENCES

Aguado Matorras, J.: La cortisona en el diagnóstico diferencial de las lesiones cervicales. Toko-Ginec. Práct., 22:54, 1963.

Antoine, T.: Carcinoma of the cervix. J. Internat. Coll. Surg., 37:277, 1962.

Antoine, T., and Grunberger, V.: Atlas der Kolpomikroskopie. Stuttgart, Georg Thieme Verlag, 1956.

Ayre, J. E.: The vaginal smear: "Precancer" cell studies using a modified technique. Am. J. Obstet. Gynec., 58:1205, 1949.

Ayre, J. E.: What is the pre-cancer cell complex as compared with dyskaryosis? Acta Cytol., 1:50, 1957.

Bajardi, F.: Nomenclature of the atypical epithelium. Acta Cytol., 5:344, 1961.

Balagueró Lladó, L.: El Carcinoma In Situ del Cuello Uterino. Barcelona, Editorial Espaxs, 1971.

Barcellos, J. M., and Nahoum, J. C.: Cuello uterino: Notas de nomenclatura: Concepto de cuello normal y de tercera mucosa. Acta Ginec., 16:315, 1965.

Beato, M., and Barcellos, J. M.: La histogenesis del carcinoma epidermoide del cuello uterino. Arch. Fac. Med. Madrid, 8:367, 1965.

Beller, F. K., and Khatamee, M.: Evaluation of punch biopsy of the cervix under direct colposcopic observation (Target punch biopsy). Obstet. Gynec., 28:622, 1966.

Bolten, K. A.: Colposcopy. In Official Lectures, Part III. IV World Congress of Gynec. and Obstet., Buenos Aires, 1964, p. 228.

Bolten, K. A.: Practical colposcopy in early cervical and vaginal cancer. Clin. Obstet. Gynec., 10:808, 1967.

Bret, J., and Coupez, F.: Colposcopie. Paris, Masson et Cie., 1960.

Bret, J., and Coupez, F.: Colposcopy of leukoplakia. Acta Cytol., 5:117, 1961.

Bret, J., and Coupez, F.: Reserve cell hyperplasia, basal cell hyperplasia and dysplasia. Acta Cytol., 5:259, 1961.

Bret, J., and Coupez, F.: L'épidermisation atypique du col utérin. Rev. Franç Gynéc. Obstét., 59:605, 1964.

Bret, J., and Coupez, F.: Colposcopie. In Encyclopédie Médico-Chirurgicale, Paris, 1969.

Burghardt, E.: Uber die atypische Umwandlungszone. Geburtsh. u. Frauenheilk., 19:676, 1959.

Burghardt, E., and Bacai, T.: L'associazone sistematica della colposcopia e della colpocariologia sulla diagnosi precoce del cancro della portio. Minerva Ginec., 8:738, 1956.

Bur Grato, E., and Lloret, A. P.: El papel de las células de reserva en la génesis de los carcinomas del cuello uterino. Soc. Arg. Pat. Cerv. Ut. y Colposc., Act. Cong. Buenos Aires, 1965.

Busch, W., Hirt, J., Fritsches, W., and Lobenstein, A.: Indice de malignidad de las imágenes colposcópicas, y ensayo de clasificación. Soc. Arg. Pat. Cerv. Ut. y Colposc., Act. Cong. Buenos Aires, 1:190, 1965.

Carrera, J. M.: Estudio citológico de la fisiopatología cervical reparativa. Acta Ginecol., 22:10, 507, 1971.

Carrera, J. M., and Dexeus, S., Jr.: Estudio colposcopico de los cambios cervicales inducidos por anovulatorios orales. Progr. Obstet. Ginec., 14:1, 1971.

Carrera, J. M., Casanelles, R., Dexeus, S., Jr., and Russell, C.: Citologia de las displasias cervicales. Acta Ginec., 20:91, 1969.

Castadot, R. G.: Intérêt du frottis localisé dans les lésions cervicales délimitées par la colposcopie ou le test de Schiller. Bull. Soc. Roy. Belge Gynéc. Obstét., 37:427, 1967.

Chanen, W., and Hollyock, V. E.: Colposcopy and electrocoagulation-diathermy for cervical dysplasia and carcinoma in situ. Obstet. Gynec., 37: 623, 1971.

Chiladze, Z. A., and Bibileishvili, Z. V.: Sixth World Congr. Int. Fed. Gynaec. Obstet., New York, 1970.

Coppleson, M.: The value of colposcopy in the detection of preclinical carcinoma of the cervix. J. Obstet. Gynaec. Brit. Comm., 67:11, 1960.

Coppleson, M.: Colposcopy, cervical carcinoma in situ and the gynaecologist: Based on experience with the method in 200 cases of carcinoma in situ. J. Obstet. Gynaec. Brit. Comm., 71:854, 1964.

Coppleson, M., and Reid, B. L.: Preclinical Carcinoma of the Cervix Uteri: Its Origin, Nature and Management. Oxford, Pergamon Press, 1967.

Coupez, F.: Les dysplasies du col utérin. Rev. Franç. Gynéc. Obstét., 60:579, 1965.

Coupez, F.: Origen, desarrollo y evolución clínica de las displasias del cuello uterino. Progr. Obstet. Ginec., 11:398, 1968.

Coupez, F.: La place de la colposcopie dans l'examen gynécologique actuel. Rev. Franç. Gynéc. Obstét., 65:209, 1970.

Cramer, H.: Die Kolposkopie in der Praxis. Stuttgart, Georg Thieme Verlag, 1956.

Cramer, H.: Kritisches zum Begriff der sogenannten atypischen Umwandlungszone. Geburtsh. u. Frauenheilk., 21:706, 1961.

D'Alessandro, P., and Bernardini, G.: Aspetti istologici di alcune lesioni colposcopiche. Quad. Clin. Obstet. Ginec., 18(Suppl.):1511, 1963.

de Alvarez, R. R., Figge, D. C., and Brown, D. V.: Long-range studies of the biologic behavior of the human uterine cervix: II. Histology, cytology, and clinical course of cervical disease. Am. J. Obstet. Gynec., 74:769, 1957.

de Brux, J.: Morfología histológica y diagnóstico de las displasias y de los carcinomas "in situ" del cuello uterino. Progr. Obstet. Ginec., 7:19, 1964.

de Brux, J., and Dupré-Froment, J.: Le carcinoma intra-épithélial du col utérin doit-il être démembré? Gynéc. Obstét., 59:457, 1960.

de Brux, J., and Dupre-Froment, J.: Papel de la citología en el diagnóstico diferencial de las displasias, del epitelio áctivo de regeneración y del carcinoma "in situ" del cuello uterino. Acta Ginec., 14:1, 1963.

Dexeus, S., Jr.: Imágenes colposcópicas atípicas. Acta Ginec., 16:661, 1965.

Dexeus, S., Jr., and Carrera, J. M.: El frotis displásico. Rev. Cub. Cirug., 7:129, 1968.

Dexeus, S., Jr., and Rawyler, V.: Estudio comparativo de la citología, colposcopia y anatomía pathológica en el diagnóstico precoz del cáncer uterino. Progr. Obstet. Ginec., 5:9, 1962.

Dexeus, S., Jr., and Undabeitia, C.: Un signo colposcópico importante. Progr. Obstet. Ginec., 6: 243, 1963.

Di Paola, G., Vásquez Ferro, E., and Tatti, M. A.: Profilaxis del carcinoma cervical uterino y electrocoagulación. XII. Reunión Nac. Fed. Arg. Soc. Ginec. Obstet., Rosario, 195, 1963.

Dougherty, C. M., Torres, J., and Cotton, N.: The fate of atypical hyperplasia of the uterine cervical epithelium. Proc. First Internat. Congr. Exfol.

Cytol., Vienna, 1961. Philadelphia, J. B. Lippincott Co., 1962.

Duarte, E.: Histogénese e localização do carcinoma epidermoide do colo do utero. Riv. Ginec. Obstet., 107:141, 1960.

Dzioba, A.: Kolposkopische Bilder der Portio vaginalis uteri, die für die beginnende Krebsbildung charakteristisch sind. Zbl. Gynäk., 82: 1464, 1960.

Elsner, H.: Zur kolposkopisch atypischen Umwandlungszone. Zbl. Gynäk., 85:1357, 1963.

Ferrier, Y., Baux, R., and Moreau, G.: Quelques remarques à propos de la biopsie du col dans le diagnostic des épithéliomas malpighiens. Bull. Féd. Soc. Gynéc. Obstét., 9:245, 1957.

Fluhmann, C. F.: Carcinoma in situ and the transitional zone of the cervix uteri. Obstet. Gynec., 16:424, 1960.

Fluhmann, C. F.: The Cervix Uteri and Its Diseases. Philadelphia, W. B. Saunders Co., 1961.

Fox, C. H.: Time necessary for conversion of normal to dysplastic cervical epithelium. Obstet. Gynec., 31:749, 1968.

Friedell, G. H., Hertig, A. T., and Younge, P. A.: Carcinoma In Situ of the Uterine Cervix. Springfield, Ill., Charles C Thomas, 1960.

Galvin, G. A., and TeLinde, R. W.: The present-day status of noninvasive cervical carcinoma. Am. J. Obstet. Gynec., 57:15, 1949.

Gambotto, C.: La diatermocoagulazione nella patogenesi del cancro del collo dell'utero. Minerva Ginec., 14:963, 1962.

Ganse, R.: Zur Frage des atypischen Epithels der Portio. Zbl. Gynäk., 71:217, 1949.

Ganse, R.: Kolpofotogramme zur Einfuhrung in die Kolposkopie. Vol. I and II. Berlin, Akademie Verlag, 1953.

Ganse, R.: Über die Gefässdarstellung kolposkopischer Befunde mit der Quecksilberdampflampe und dem Kolpophot., 76:81, 1954.

Glatthaar, E.: Die Regenerationsvorgänge an der Portio und ihre Bedeutung für die Entstehung des Kollumkarzinoms. Gynaec., 128:25, 1949.

Glatthaar, E.: Epithélium atypique et cancer du col: Leurs rapports à la lumière de l'étude colposcopique répétée. Rev. Franç. Gynéc. Obstét., 49:320, 1954.

Glatthaar, E.: Kolposkopie. In Seitz-Amreich: Biologie und Pathologie des Weibes. Vienna, Urban und Schwarzenberg, 1955.

González Merlo, J., Montalvo, L., Vilar, E., and Botella, J.: Cinco años de experiencia en el diagnóstico precoz del cáncer cervical uterino. Prog. Obstet. Ginec., 7:441, 1964.

González Merlo, J., and Tarancón, A.: Displasias del cuello uterino. Gine. Dips., 11:13, 1971.

Grismondi, G. L.: Analisi di 1559 casi di leucoplachia colposcopica. Riv. Ital. di Ginec., 51:821, 1967.

Guin, G. H.: The incidence and anatomical distribution of basal-cell hyperactivity and its relationship to carcinoma of the cervix uteri. Am. J. Obstet. Gynec., 65:1081, 1953.

Guzmán Llovet, P., Cudemus León, J., de Cudemus, M., and Zambrano, O.: Evaluacion de las exploraciones del cuello uterino. Rev. Obstet. Ginec. Venez., 27:29, 1967.

Hall, J. E., and Rosen, I. H.: Significance of the

Class III cervical smear. Am. J. Obstet. Gynec., 79:709, 1960.

Hamperl, H., and Kaufmann, C.: The cervix uteri at different ages. Obstet. Gynec., 14:621, 1959.

Held, E.: Therapie des nicht invasiven atypischen Plattenepithels. In Früherkennung des Collumcarcinoms: Leistungen und Grenzen der Kolposkopie, Zytologie und Histologie. Berlin, Springer-Verlag, 1957.

Henderson, P. H., Jr., and Buck, C. E.: Cervical leukoplakia. Am. J. Obstet. Gynec., 82:887, 1961.

Hernández Alcántara, A., Calvo de Mora, S., Escalonilla, F., Tubio, J., and Marcos, C.: Estudio citológico y colposcópico de las displasias de cuello uterino. Toko-Ginec. Práct., 30:385, 1971.

Hill, E. C.: Preclinical cervical carcinoma, colposcopy, and the "negative" smear. Am. J. Obstet. Gynec., 95:308, 1966.

Hinselmann, H.: Einfuhrung in die Kolposkopie. Hamburg, Paul Hartung, 1933.

Hinselmann, H.: Approximative Frequenz des atypischen Portioepithels. Zbl. Gynäk., 60:1750, 1936.

Hinselmann, H.: Zur Theorie der kolposkopischen Frühdiagnose und der Verhütung des Karzinoms am Muttermund. Schweiz. Med. Wschr., 70:320, 1940.

Hohlbein, R., and Ganse, R.: Die Therapie des gesteigert atypischen Epithels am Collum uteri und ihre Ergebnisse. Z. Geburtsh. Gynäk., 155:182, 1960.

Holtorff, J.: Kolposkopische Kriterien der "atypischen" Umwandlungszone. Geburtsh. u. Frauenheilk., 20:931, 1960.

Howard, L., Jr., Erickson, C. C., and Stoddard, L. D.: A study of the incidence and histogenesis of endocervical metaplasia and intraepithelial carcinoma: Observations on 400 uteri removed for noncervical disease. Cancer, 4:1210, 1951.

Israel, S.: Colposcopic and cytological studies in leukoplakia of the cervix. J. Obstet. Gynaec., India, 11:45, 1960.

Jakob, A., and Escalante, D.: El Cáncer Pre-invasor del Cuello Uterino. Edit. Bibliog. Arg., Buenos Aires, 1958.

Johnson, L. D., Easterday, C. L., Gore, H., and Hertig, A. T.: The histogenesis of carcinoma in situ of the uterine cervix: A preliminary report of the origin of carcinoma in situ in subcylindrical cell anaplasia. Cancer, 17:213, 1964.

Kaiser, R. F., and Gilliam, A. G.: Some epidemiological aspects of cervical cancer. Public Health Reports, 73:359, 1958.

Kasdon, S. C.: The laboratory, the surgeon and in situ cancer of the cervix: Part I. The laboratory. Obstet. Gynec., 13:576, 1959.

Kasdon, S. C., and Bamford, S. B.: Atlas of In Situ Cytology. Boston, Little, Brown and Co., 1962.

Kern, G.: Colposcopic findings in carcinoma in situ. Am. J. Obstet. Gynec., 82:1409, 1961.

Kern, G.: Preinvasive Carcinoma of the Cervix. Berlin, Springer-Verlag, 1968.

Kern, G., and Bötzelen, H.-P.: Kolposkopischer Befund und Lokalisation des Carcinoma in situ. Arch. Gynäk., 194:564, 1961.

Kern, G., Rissmann, E., and Hund, G.: Die Leistungsfähigkeit der Kolposkopie bei der Frühdiagnostik des Collumcarcinoms. Arch. Gynäk., 199:526, 1964.

Koller, O.: The vascular patterns of cervical cancer. Acta Unio Internat. Contra Cancrum, 15:375, 1959.

Kolstad, P.: The colposcopical diagnosis of dysplasia, carcinoma in situ, and early invasive cancer of the cervix. Acta Obstet. Gynec. Scand., 43(Suppl. 7):105, 1965.

Kos, D., Mikoláš, VI., and Laně, V.: Das Bild des terminalen Blutgefässnetzes auf der karzinomatösen Cervix Uteri. Zbl. Gynäk., 82:1487, 1960.

Kraatz, H.: Earbfiltervorschaltung zur leichteren Erlernung der Kolposkopie. Zbl. Gynäk., 63:2307, 1939.

Kraussold, E.: Untersuchungen über die Bedeutung der Umwelteinflüsse und der sozialen Verhältnisse bei der Entstehung des Kollumkarzinom am Krankengut der Universitäts-Frauenklinik Greifswald von 1938 bis 1957. Zbl. Gynäk., 83:360, 1961.

Krüger, E. H.: Über die Topographie kolposkopischer Befunde und histologischer Epithelveränderungen an der Portio uteri. Zbl. Gynäk., 79:789, 1957.

Kummert, W.: Die Morbidität der Portiokonisation mit nachfolgender Uterusexstirpation. Geburtsh. u. Frauenheilk., 28:1019, 1968.

Lagrutta, J.: Displasias del epitelio cervical uterino: Primer Congreso Español de la World Association for Gynaecological Cancer Prevention. Gine. Dips., 11:13, 1971.

Lagrutta, J., Laguens, R., and Quijano, F.: Histogénesis del carcinoma intraepitelial. Primer Congr. Parag. Obstet. Ginec., Asunción, 1968.

Lagrutta, J., Laguens, R. P., and Quijano, F.: Cáncer de Cuello Uterino: Estados Primarios. Buenos Aires, Editorial Intermedica, 1966.

Lagrutta, J., Laguens, R., Quijano, F., Fernández, C. G. del V. de, and Crego, H.: Tratamiento de las lesiones benignas como profilaxis del cáncer de cuello uterino. XII. Reunión Nac. Fed. Arg. Soc. Ginec. Obstet., Rosario, 1963, p. 189.

Lang, W. R., and Rakoff, A. E.: Colposcopy and cytology: Comparative values in the diagnosis of cervical atypism and malignancy. Obstet. Gynec., 8:312, 1956.

Lienhard, C. P.: Biopsia del cuello uterino biopsia selectiva conización (Indicaciones y técnica). Obstet. Ginec. Lat. Amer., 18:343, 1960.

Limburg, H.: Die Frahdiagnose des Uteruskarzinoms, Histologie, Kolposkopie, Cytologie, Biochemische Methoden. 3rd ed. Stuttgart, Georg Thieme Verlag, 1956.

Margitay-Becht, D.: Kunstgriff zur Vermehrung des mittels Kolposkopie gewonnenen und observierbaren pathologischen Plattenepithel (der sog. Talkum-Test). Zbl. Gynäk., 83:1408, 1961.

Martin-Laval, J., and Dajoux, R.: Clasification des images colposcopiques. Communicat. to Soc. Nat. Gynéc. Obstet. de France, Marseille, 1970.

Masciotta, A.: La Colposcopia Nella Lotta Contro Il Cancro e Nella Diagnosi Ginecologica. Bologna, Licinio Cappelli, 1954.

Mateu Aragonés, J. M.: Importancia del cuadro vascular en la exploración colposcópica: Clasificación de las imágenes vasculares. Acta Gynaec. Obstet. Hisp. Lusit., 13:231, 1964.

Mateu Aragonés, J. M.: Lesiones atípicos del epitelio cervical: Estudio clínico e histológico. Acta Gynaec. Obstet. Hisp. Lusit., 18:1, 1969.

Mateu Aragonés, J. M.: Significación de las atipias colposcópicas: Consideraciones acerca de la importancia de la colposcopia en el estudio de las imágenes vasculares. Rev. Esp. Obstet. Ginec., 28:473, 1969.

Mateu Aragonés, J. M., Trilla Sánchez, V., and Abades, C.: Estudio comparativo entre los hallazgos colposcópicos, citológicos y las alteraciones histopatológicas en las displasias cervicales. Toko-Ginec. Práct., 27:857, 1968.

Mateu Aragonés, J. M., and Trilla Sánchez, V.: Estudio colposcópico de las displasias del cuello uterino. Gine. Dips., 11:91, 1971.

Mateu Aragonés, J. M., Trilla, V., and Bernabé, M.: Lesiones displasicas cervicales. Toko-Pract., 27:872, 1968.

McLaren, H. C.: Conservative management of cervical pre-cancer. J. Obstet. Gynaec. Brit. Comm., 74:487, 1967.

Mestwerdt, G.: Eine neuartige Aufhängevorrichtung für das Kolposkop. Geburtsh. u. Frauenheilk., 10:758, 1950.

Mestwerdt, G.: Atlas der Kolposkopie. Jena, Gustav Fischer, 1953.

Mestwerdt, G.: Valoración clinica de los límites epiteliales a nivel del orificio externo del cuello uterino. Communicat. to Soc. Arg. Pat. Cerv. Ut. y Colposc., Buenos Aires, 1965.

Mestwerdt, G.: Las displasias del cuello uterino: Límites entre la benignidad y la malignidad. Rev. Esp. Obstet. Ginec., 29:331, 1970.

Mestwerdt, G., and Mönckeberg, A.: Über die Beziehungen zwischen Karzinomentwicklung und dem kolposkopisch gefundenen atypischen Epithel an der Portio. Geburtsch. u. Frauenheilk., 7:156, 1947.

Mestwerdt, G., and Wespi, H. J.: Atlas der Kolposkopie. 3rd ed. Stuttgart, Fischer, 1961.

Mikaelian, S., and Haour, P.: Importance de la base de leucoplasie dans le dépistage colposcopique. Bull. Féd. Soc. Gynéc. Obstét., 16:156, 1964.

Misonou, Y., and Sato, T.: Clinical observation on the metaplastic epithelia in uterine cervix and portio vaginalis uteri. Clin. Gynec. Obstet. (Tokyo), 16:707, 1962.

Mossetti, C.: Valutazione delle lesioni precancerosa e cancerosa preinvasiva ed inizialmente invasiva (microcarcinoma): Esame speculare e colposcopico: Tecniche da seguire fino all'indagine bioptica ed istologica. Minerva Ginec., 6:318, 1954.

Mossetti, C., and Russo, A.: La Colposcopia nella Diagnostica Ginecologica. Torino, Ediz. Minerva Medica, 1963.

Navratil, E.: Colposcopy. In Gray, L. A. (ed.): Dysplasia, Carcinoma In Situ and Micro-invasive Carcinoma of the Cervix Uteri. Springfield, Ill., Charles C Thomas, 1964.

Nieburgs, H. E.: What is the pre-cancer cell complex as compared with dyskaryosis (Discussion). Acta Cytol., 1:54, 1957.

Nieburgs, H. E.: Exfoliative cytology of carcinoma in situ during pregnancy. Acta Cytol., 3:96, 1959.

Nogales, F.: Diagnóstico histológico precoz del cancer de cuello uterino, Toko-Gine. Pract., 161:183, 1958.

Nogales, F., Martínez, H., and Parache, I.: Carcinoma in situ: Técnicas para su diagnóstico histopatológico. I. Reiunión de la sección Española de la Asociación Mundial de Prevención del Cáncer Ginecológico, Málaga-Torremolinos, 1966.

Ober, K. G.: Variations topographiques de la jonction de l'épithélium cylindrique et pavimenteux cervical en fonction de l'âge. Rev. Franç. Gynéc. Obstét., 56:593, 1961.

Ober, K. G., Kaufmann, C., and Hamperl, H.: Carcinoma in situ, beginnendes Karzinom und klinischer Krebs der Cervix uteri. Geburtsh. u. Frauenheilk., 21:259, 1961.

Olson, A. W., and Nichols, E. E.: Leukoplakia of the cervix—the mosaic and papillary pattern. Am. J. Obstet. Gynec., 82:895, 1961.

Ostergard, D. R., Townsend, D. E., and Hirose, F. M.: Treatment of chronic cervicitis by cryotherapy. Am. J. Obstet. Gynec., 102:426, 1968.

Palmer, R.: Sur la colposcopie et les biopsies dans le diagnostic des cancers du col uterin. Acta Gynaec. Obstet. Hisp. Lusit., 8:315, 1959.

Pereyra, A. J.: The relationship of sexual activity to cervical cancer: Cancer of the cervix in a prison population. Obstet. Gynec., 17:154, 1961.

Pineda, et al. Displasias. Gine. Dips., 11:245, 1971.

Pratas, A., and Roriz, M. L.: Límite de benignidad en las alteraciones diplásticas del cuello uterino. X. Congr. Hisp. Portug. de Obst. y Ginec., Palma de Mallorca, 1970.

Rawson, A. J., and Knoblich, R.: A clinicopathologic study of 56 cases showing atypical epithelial changes of the cervix uteri. Am. J. Obstet. Gynec., 73:120, 1957.

Reagan, J. W.: Dysplasia of the uterine cervix. In Gray, L. A. (ed.): Dysplasia, Carcinoma In Situ and Micro-invasive Carcinoma of the Cervix Uteri. Springfield, Ill., Charles C Thomas, 1964.

Reagan, J. W., and Patten, S. F., Jr.: Dysplasia: A basic reaction to injury in the uterine cervix. Ann. N. Y. Acad. Sci., 97:662, 1962.

Richart, R. M.: Colpomicroscopic studies of the distribution of dysplasia and carcinoma in situ on the exposed portion of the human uterine cervix. Cancer, 18:950, 1965.

Richart, R. M.: Colpomicroscopic studies of cervical intraepithelial neoplasia. Cancer, 19:395, 1966.

Richart, R. M.: Natural history of cervical intraepithelial neoplasia. Clin. Obstet. Gynec., 10:748, 1967.

Richart, R. M., and Sciarra, J. J.: Treatment of cervical dysplasia by outpatient electrocauterization. Am. J. Obstet. Gynec., 101:200, 1968.

Rieper, J. P.: Colposcopia ne gravidez (consideracoes etiopatogeneticas sobre o carcinoma do colo uterino). Anais Brasil. Ginec., 18:25, 1953.

Rodrigues, F. V.: Um estudo histotopográfico das mucosas do colo uterino. Thesis, University of Brazil, 1964.

Rodríguez-Soriano, J. A.: Personal communication, 1965.

Rodríguez-Soriano, J. A.: Las displasias del cérvix uterino en la lucha contra el cáncer. A través de la exploración de 6000 pacientes. Gine. Dips., 11: 67, 1971.

Rodríguez-Soriano, J. A., and Benasco Naval, C.: La citología tipo III y su correlación colposcópica. Acta Ginec., 19:823, 1968.

Rodríguez-Soriano, J. A., Serradel Terreres, E., and Márquez, M.: La colposcopia en el diagnóstico precoz del cancer cervical uterino. Toko-Ginec. Práct., 17:584, 1958.

Rubinstein, E.: On the proliferation of the squamous epithelium on the portio vaginalis uteri: A colposcopic, histologic and cytologic study. Acta Obstet. Gynec. Scand., 45(Suppl. 6):7, 1966.

Russo, A., and Macchioni, B.: La posizione dell'indagine colposcopica nel dépistage del carcinoma cervicale preclinico: Considerazioni su 120 casi di carcinoma preinvasivo e microcarcinoma. Minerva Ginec., 14:351, 1962.

Sammartino, R.: Relaciones de las modificaciones fisiológicas y patológicas del cuello uterino con el carcinoma. Communicat. to Soc. Arg. Pat. Cerv. Ut. y Colposc., Buenos Aires, 1965.

Schiller, W.: Leukoplakia, leucokeratosis, and carcinoma of the cervix. Am. J. Obstet. Gynec., 35:17, 1938.

Scott, R. B.: Clinical treatment of dysplasia and carcinoma in situ of the cervix. In Gray, L. A. (ed.): Dysplasia, Carcinoma In Situ and Micro-invasive Carcinoma of the Cervix Uteri. Springfield, Ill., Charles C Thomas, 1964.

Song, J.: The Human Uterus: Morphogenesis and Embryological Basis for Cancer. Springfield, Ill., Charles C Thomas, 1964.

Štafl, A., Linhartová, A., and Dohnal, V.: Das kolposkopische Bild der Felderung und seine Pathogenese. Arch. Gynäk., 199:223, 1963.

Stern, E., and Neely, P. M.: Carcinoma and dysplasia of the cervix: A comparison of rates for new and returning populations. Acta Cytol., 7:357, 1963.

Stern, E., and Neely, P. M.: Dysplasia of the uterine cervix: Incidence of regression, recurrence, and cancer. Cancer, 17:508, 1964.

Stoltz, H.: Aspectos colposcópicos do carcinoma grao o. Anais Brasileiros Ginec., 40:213, 1955.

Stoltz, H.: Prática atual do diagnóstico precoce e tratamento do carcinoma estádio "o" do colo do útero no instituto de ginecologia da universidade do Brasil. Anais Brasil. Ginec., 46:69, 1958.

Takeuchi, A., and McKay, D. G.: The area of the cervix involved by carcinoma in situ and anaplasia (atypical hyperplasia). Obstet. Gynec., 15:134, 1960.

Te Linde, R. W.: Hysterectomy for carcinoma in situ. In Meigs, J. V. (ed.): Surgical Treatment of Cancer of the Cervix. New York, Grune and Stratton, 1954.

Terentieva, L. S.: The assessment of diagnostic methods of investigation in hyperplastic processes of the uterine cervix. Akush. Ginek., 40:113, 1964.

Tortora, M.: Les dysplasies du col utérin: Aspects cliniques et diagnostiques. Gine. Dips., 11:101, 1971.

Uyttenbroeck, F.: Lésions exocervicales prémalignes. Bull. Féd. Soc. Gynéc. Obstét., 16:120, 1964.

Varga, A.: The relationship of cervical dysplasia to in situ and invasive carcinoma of the cervix. Am. J. Obstet. Gynec., 95:759, 1966.

Vasquez, E., Di Paola, G. R., and Tatti, M. A.: Epitelios atípicos del cuello uterino: Su localización colposcópica. Reunión Nac. F.A.S.G.O., Mar del Plata, 1962.

Vasquez Ferro, E. C.: La biopsia selectiva del cuello uterino. Semana Médica, 115:741, 1959.

Villalba, R., Anzola, C., and Erminy, A.: Lesiones precancerosas del cervix en la pesquisa del cancer. Rev. Obstet. Ginec. Venez., 28:389, 1968.

von Haam, E., and Old, J. W.: Reserve cell hyperplasia, squamous metaplasia and epidermization. In Gray, L. A. (ed.): Dysplasia, Carcinoma In Situ and Micro-invasive Carcinoma of the Cervix Uteri. Springfield, Ill., Charles C Thomas, 1964.

Wagner, D., and Fettig, O.: Zytologische und histologische Untersuchungen zur atypischen Um wandlungszone. Geburtsh. u. Frauenheilk., 21:156, 1961.

Way, S., Hennigan, M., and Wright, V. C.: Some experiences with pre-invasive and micro-invasive carcinoma of the cervix. J. Obstet. Gynaec. Brit. Comm., 75:593, 1968.

Wespi, H.: Progresión y regresión de las atipias cervicales. Communicat. to Soc. Arg. Pat. Cerv. Ut. y Colposc., Buenos Aires, 1965.

Wespi, H. J.: Early Carcinoma of the Uterine Cervix: Pathogenesis and Detection. New York, Grune and Stratton, 1949.

Wielenga, G., Old, J. W., and von Haam, E.: Squamous carcinoma in situ of the uterine cervix: II. Topography and clinical correlations. Cancer, 18:1612, 1965.

Willis, R. A.: Pathology of Tumours. 3rd ed. Washington, Butterworths, 1960.

Chapter Eight

NEOPLASTIC CERVIX

The uterine cervix may be the seat of innumerable neoplasms of diverse origin and clinical significance. Colposcopy, though not indispensable to their diagnosis, constitutes a technique capable of contributing toward their differentiation, especially when the tumors are so small that they could be missed by the usual methods of exploration.

Furthermore, even when cancer is clinically evident and colposcopy seems useless, there are still some indications for its use, namely to secure information about the origin of the neoplasm.

CLASSIFICATION

The classification of neoplasms is especially difficult if, like the cervix, the organ has two different types of epithelium, a connective tissue rich in vessels, and the possibility of containing embryonic rests. A histogenetic classification may have scientific value, but it lacks practical utility. This chapter deals not only with the true neoplasms (tumors of autonomous and indefinite growth), but also with other types of proliferation which clinically appear as "tumors." To this end it would be futile to adopt a complex histologic classification.

The traditional classification of tumors into benign and malignant categories has undisputed clinical value. Histology tends to support this distinction, and colposcopy can assist in evaluating the morphologic signs that distinguish the two types of tumors (Table 53).

We restrict our attention to the more frequently encountered tumors, avoiding the exceptional ones, such as tumors of the vascular or nervous systems and the mesonephric cysts. Besides being rare, these are poorly defined colposcopically. However, we have chosen to include brief mentions of uterine tumors which may project through the cervical os and become accessible to colposcopic study.

Table 53. Classification of Tumors of the Cervix

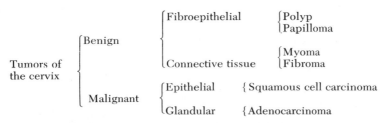

191

BENIGN NEOPLASMS

In this category are some true neoplasms (fibromyomas) and some dystrophies (polyps and papillomas). The fact that in all cases a tumor or mass is observed, justifies this grouping.

ORIGIN

Polyps. Diverse theories have been invoked to explain the presence of a cervical polyp.

1. It is accepted that in the majority of cases a chronic infectious process accompanies the polyp (Israel), and it is suggested that this could cause the hyperplasia of the endocervical mucosa that in turn leads to formation of the tumor. In our experience, 70 per cent of endocervical polypoid formations are accompanied by intensely inflammatory cytologic smears and by colposcopic images of similar implication (such as congestive and hyperemic exocervical mucosa).

2. The endocrine origin of many of these neoplasms seems evident. Khakimova and Gustowski affirm that in 50 per cent of cases these polyps are accompanied by a uterine disorder such as endometrial hyperplasia or polyposis, which points to an endocrine origin. The immediate cause is probably an excess of estrogens. The fact that pregnancy can bring about the appearance of cervical polyps also argues for this origin. We have observed the appearance of new polyps in 1.6 per cent of pregnant women during the second and third trimesters.

Rodriguez–Soriano and Márquez pointed out that most cervical polyps appear between the ages of 35 and 55 years, when anovulatory cycles are frequent. This would also suggest a hyperestrogenic stimulus.

3. Considering cervical polyps as vascular formations, resulting from congestion of the cervical vessels (Fluhmann), may be valid for some (the angiomatous polyps), but not for the majority.

Papillomas. For a long time the papilloma was considered to be of venereal origin regardless of its topography. At present, and realizing that in some diseases of this type (gonorrhea especially), papillomas are habitually observed, other etiologic possibilities are postulated.

1. Potential irritative factors include poor hygiene, neglected infectious leukorrhea (trichomonal, for example), endocervicitis, and introduction of foreign bodies into the vagina. These factors would help to explain the frequent appearance of polyps with venereal diseases.

2. In many cases hormonal factors may be involved and even when they cannot be called responsible for the papilloma, they may constitute an important stimulus to its growth. This is why papillomas undergo considerable growth during pregnancy, forming large vegetating masses which may even constitute an obstacle to vaginal delivery. In almost all cases observed by us, both factors coincide: gestation and infectious vaginitis.

3. The possibility has been suggested that in some cases papillomas originate from viral infection. This seems to be the likely origin of a special type of papilloma called "condyloma acuminata," but not for the rest of these lesions.

Fibromyomas. Numerous hypotheses have been conceived to explain the origin of fibromyomas of the uterus in general, invoking factors such as heredity, race, sterility, and uterine hypoplasia, which we will not discuss here. Recently, hyperestrogenism has come to be regarded as the most important stimulus (Moench). The hormonal imbalance presumably acts on those areas of the organ with circulatory difficulties. Fibromyomas are seldom seen at the level of the cervix, probably because muscular tissue in this zone is scanty and the cervix does not participate in the menstrual cycle.

Cervical fibroma rarely appears alone as a uterine tumor. On the majority of occasions it coexists with nodules of the corpus.

FREQUENCY

The overall frequency of benign neoplasms is notable (6.1 per cent of all of our colposcopic observations), because of the large number of endocervical polyps which are diagnosed (98.3 per cent of all benign tumors of the cervix).

The incidence of endocervical polyp as an isolated or associated colposcopic image is 6 per cent in our material. On the contrary, papillomas are found in only 0.095 per cent of cases (1 per cent of all benign tumors of the cervix), and there are even fewer cervical fibromas evident at colposcopy (0.035 per cent).

Our figures on cervical polyps fully coincide with those given by others: González-Merlo, 5.8 per cent; Mateu-Aragonés, 5.05 per cent; Arenas et al., 6.6 per cent (Table 54).

Table 54. Frequency of Endocervical Polyps

Moreno (1971)	1.31%
Figuero et al. (1971)	1.40%
Guzmán Llovet et al. (1967)	1.75%
Guerrero et al. (1957)	2.70%
Bory, De Brux and Curt (1959)	3.00%
Bonilla (1965)	4.20%
Mateu-Aragonés (1971)	5.05%
González-Merlo (1966)	5.80%
Arenas et al. (1961)	6.60%
Our Series (1972)	6%

COLPOSCOPIC APPEARANCE AND HISTOLOGIC AND CYTOLOGIC CORRELATION

Polyps

These are the most frequent neoplasms of the cervix. They arise in the endocervix. Among those that appear in the colposcope, some have long pedicles, but others may be sessile if their site of implantation is near the external os.

From a colposcopic viewpoint, it is possible to describe diverse types, which project various histologic structures (Table 55).

Mucous Polyps. These are the most frequent, constituting 77.5 per cent of our material. They are small tumors of pink color and relatively smooth surface, upon which it is possible to observe the fissures (primary and secondary) of the normal endocervical tissue (Fig. 262). In some cases the fissures are relatively scarce, and there may be papillary prominences resembling those of ectopy. The details are especially observed after the acetic acid test, with which they become paler. Schiller's test, on the contrary, stains them in a dark pink tone, unless there are metaplasic phenomena on the surface.

The existence of squamous metaplasia at the level of the surface of the polyp may modify its colposcopic appearance in a significant manner. After application of acetic acid, some whitish zones are seen, similar to those of an initial zone of typical re-epithelialization, which on occasion tend to alternate with nonepithelialized glandular crypts and small retention cysts (Figs. 263 and 264). These retention cysts are often hemorrhagic, because they are easily traumatized.

Epidermization of the polyp is almost never complete, with persistence of some zones of endocervical epithelium. Abundant vessels often accompany the squamous epithelium and give a peculiar

Table 55. Frequency of Polyps According to Colposcopic-Histologic Type

AUTHOR	MUCOUS	ADENO-MATOUS	FIBROUS	DECIDUAL	ANGIO-MATOUS	GRANULO-MATOUS
Aaro et al.	—	90	4	—	0.7	—
Jimi	—	44	—	—	—	—
Moreno		88	3.8	—	1.5	—
Usandizaga et al.	75.77	—	4.26	1.26	1.69	—
Winter	79.29	—	20.71	—	—	—
Our Series	77.5	15.4	3.6	2.2	0.9	0.3

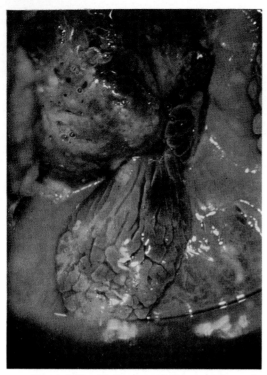

Figure 262. Endocervical mucous polyp. The most peculiar colposcopic detail is the existence of fissures in its surface.

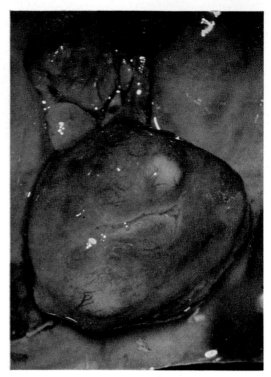

Figure 263. Mucous polyp, almost totally epidermized.

appearance to the surface of the polyp (Figs. 265 and 266). Necrosis imparts a characteristic whitish color, especially striking when tissue death is total (Fig. 267). Similarly, the presence of infection can create problems in identification (Khakimova). The polyp may have reddish spots caused by an inflammatory vascular hypertrophy.

The differential diagnosis includes endometrial polyps which, due to the length of their pedicle, reach the external cervical os. Commonly these are larger and more reddish in color; although they are clearly glandular, their surface presents fewer fissures and their papillae are smaller. Their content is serous and not mucous (Fig. 268). Later reference will be made to the characteristics of the sarcoma which adopts a polypoid disposition (see p. 224).

The histologic structure of a cervical polyp recalls the mucosa from which it originates. The polyp is covered by a mucous columnar epithelium, whose cytoplasm is intensely PAS-positive (Fig.

269). This epithelium with its glandular formations continues toward the interior; the glands may be distended by mucus which has not been able to drain out because the glandular orifices are occluded by areas of squamous epithelium on the surface of the polyp (Fig. 270). The absence of contact between this squamous epithelium and that of the exocervix clearly demonstrates its metaplastic origin. Study of the squamous epithelium reveals a substantial proportion of dysplasias (32 per cent of cases according to Berrios).

On some occasions the surface epithelium is separated, and the appearance of erosion exists. The stroma is rich in blood vessels, which explains the easy production of hemorrhages and the intense pink color of the polyp. Frequently edema and inflammatory phenomena with polymorphonuclear leukocytes, lymphocytes, and macrophages.

Adenomatous Polyps. Here the colposcopic picture is quite similar to that of ectopy. An adenomatous polyp is much

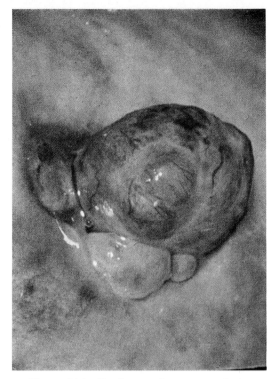

Figure 264. Epidermized mucous polyp, exhibiting notable vascularization and some retention cysts.

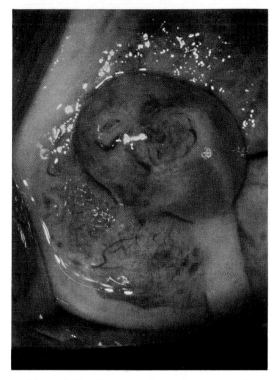

Figure 265. Very vascularized mucous polyp. Its surface, partially epidermized, presents a vessel which crosses from one extreme to the other.

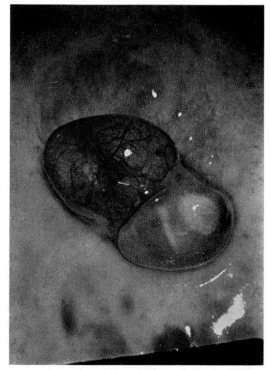

Figure 266. Mucous polyps, totally epidermized. One of them presents a voluminous retention cyst, covered by vessels.

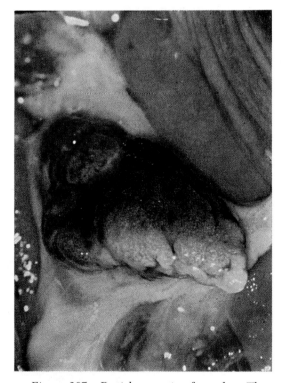

Figure 267. Partial necrosis of a polyp. The whitish apical color is a sign of necrobiosis.

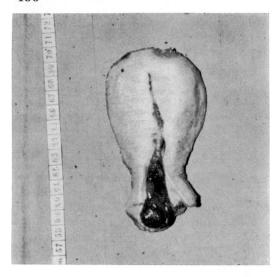

Figure 268. Benign endometrial polyp with a long pedicle making it visible outside the cervix (hysterectomy specimen).

panied by erosions, vascular hypertrophy and hemorrhagic infarcts which are seen at colposcopy as blue-black spots most numerous in the apical portion of the neoplasm. Adenomatous polyps are seen with some frequency in menopausal women. In many cases, they have evolved from mucous polyps.

Some authors (Aaro et al., Moreno) have listed adenomatous polyps as the most frequent form of polyp but have included the mucous type within this division. In our statistics 15.4 per cent of all polyps are adenomatous.

Histologic findings also resemble those of cervical ectopy, consisting of papillae with a core of connective tissue and blood vessels and a columnar epithelial covering. But in the polyp the glands are much more branched, and there is a notable glandular hyperplasia. On occasions true cystic, mucoid dilatations are seen (Fig. 271). The vessels are dilated in the apical portion or the so-called "telangiectatic portion" of the polyp.

These two varieties of polyps are the only ones that under certain circum-

redder than a mucous polyp and its consistency and even its size are greater (Fig. 273). Also, total or partial epidermization is possible (Fig. 274). Inflammatory accidents are frequent, often accom-

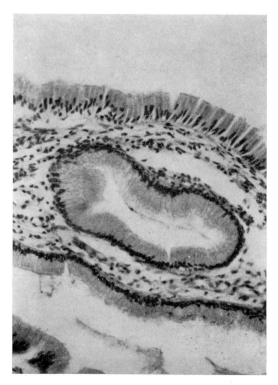

Figure 269. Histologic section of an endocervical mucous polyp, without phenomena of superficial squamous metaplasia.

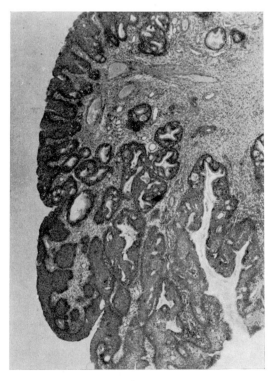

Figure 270. Histologic section of a mucous polyp, epidermized by metaplastic squamous epithelium.

stances may be accompanied by particular cytologic findings. In the case of a large mucous or adenomatous polyp that hangs from the external os, it is possible that in the vaginal vault there will be secretory cells, isolated or in plaques. On the contrary, the direct "scraping" of the polyp itself usually yields scanty columnar cells or none at all.

We have already mentioned (p. 192) that smears of the polyps tend to exhibit nonspecific inflammatory signs (Table 56). However, some ulcerated polyps may show suspicious cytologic signs (Bolten).

Fibrous Polyps. These are larger and have a firmer consistency; their surface is smoother, because it is poor in glandular elements. Fibrous polyps are purple, with frequent petechiae or hemorrhages, due in part to rich vascularization. Many times their identification is difficult due to the bizarre coexistence of necrotic, hyperemic, hemorrhagic and even erosive zones (Fig. 275). They constitute 3.6 per cent of our polyps.

Histologic study reveals that they are practically bare of epithelium, while the

Table 56. Cytologic Correlation of Polyps

Class I	25%
Class II	69%
Class II-III and III	4.8%
Class IV	1.1%

stroma is dense, rich in connective tissue and poor in nuclei. They contain abundant vessels and it is not rare to find smooth muscle fibers in their interior.

Decidual Polyps. Pregnancy may considerably modify the colposcopic appearance of a mucous or adenomatous polyp. On page 240 there is a discussion of the colposcopic and histologic characteristics which these neoplasms may show during pregnancy (Fig. 276).

Angiomatous Polyps. Even though histologically the possibility of different varieties of such polyps may exist (telangiectatic, true angiomatous, etc.), from a colposcopic viewpoint they have a common appearance. They are of a good size, of bluish or purplish color, generally sessile, and have no glandular elements

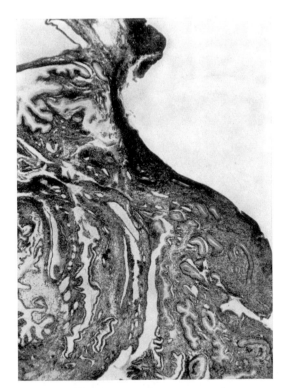

Figure 271. An adenomatous polyp.

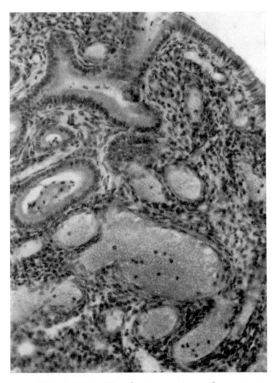

Figure 272. Histologic section of an angiomatous polyp.

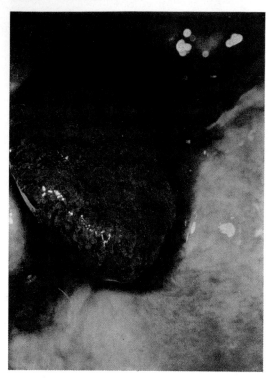

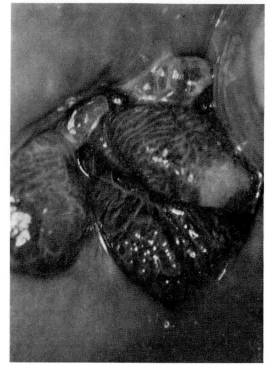

Figure 273. Adenomatous polyp. Its intense reddish color and the similarity of its surface to that of an ectopy attract the attention.

Figure 274. Adenomatous polyps, largely epidermized.

(Fig. 277). They are scarce and constitute only 0.9 per cent of our series of polyps.

Whatever their histologic type, they are all characterized by extensive vascular changes (Fig. 272), including both small vessels and voluminous and dilated ones. The angioblasts are abundant in a true angiomatous polyp, and scarce or nonexistent in the telangiectatic variety. In the latter, the great vascular ectasia is very striking. While true angiomatous polyps commonly relapse, the telangiectatic ones have very little tendency to reappear after excision (Esteba Cabellería et al.).

Granulomatous Polyp. On occasions (0.3 per cent of all polyps) the vaginal granuloma of a hysterectomy scar adopts a polypoid appearance, which makes it resemble a necrotic mucous polyp. Colposcopy reveals a vegetating formation, multilobulated, with a smooth, vascularized and bleeding surface. Its base of implantation is wide. It is red without preparation, turning white after the application of acetic acid (Fig. 278).

Histology reveals nothing more definite than nonspecific granulation tissue (Fig. 279).

Papillomas

These could also be called "exocervical polyps." They can arise at the level of the cervicovaginal mucosa, or in the periphery of an ectopy that undergoes the process of metaplastic cure.

Even though some authors report higher frequencies (Nuñez Montiel et al. gave an incidence of 0.8 per cent), we have a relatively small percentage of 0.095 per cent of colposcopies.

From a colposcopic viewpoint it is possible to distinguish up to five varieties: the arborescent papilloma (cock's-comb polyp of Hertig or pedunculated papilloma); the smooth papilloma (or true exocervical polyp); the condylomatous papilloma (identified commonly as sessile papilloma, verrucous papilloma, or condyloma acuminata); the keratinized

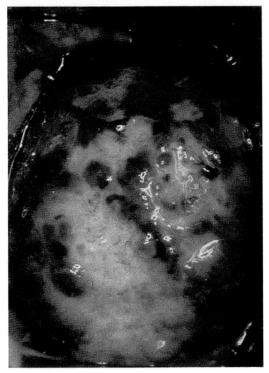

Figure 275. Fibrous polyp, with ulceration and hemorrhagic zones on its surface.

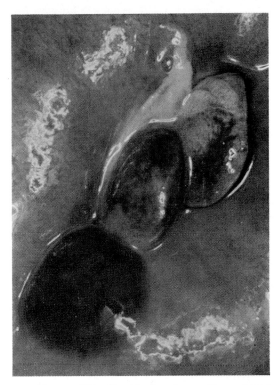

Figure 276. Decidual polyps. The whitish color of part of their surface is characteristic.

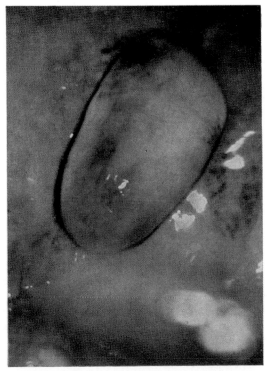

Figure 277. Angiomatous polyp.

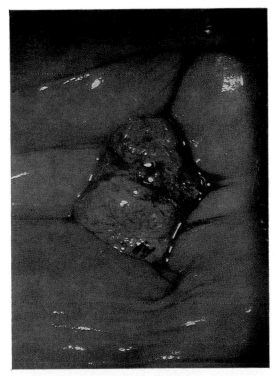

Figure 278. Vaginal granuloma, which adopts a polypoid appearance.

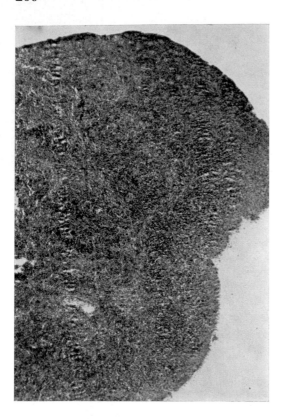

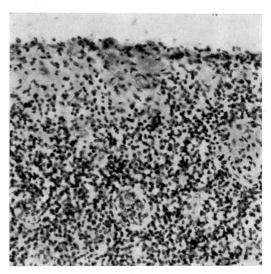

Figure 279. Vaginal granuloma at low and high magnification.

papilloma (also called leukoplastic papilloma); and finally the plaquelike papilloma (which is also given the qualifications of superficial, extensive, etc.).

Arborescent Papilloma. This is the most striking colposcopic form and probably the most frequent. It is most commonly localized to the lateral vaginal fornices and the adjacent area of the cervix. Without preparation of any type, identification is difficult. The arborescent papilloma resembles a suspicious proliferation, especially when vascular irregularities of the "corkscrew" type are seen and when the lesion bleeds easily upon contact. On occasion it is also possible to confuse this papilloma with a polyp having extensive metaplastic phenomena.

With the acetic acid test, the appearance of the arborescent papilloma is completely modified. Something resembling a cluster of papillae is observed, generally similar to the colposcopic appearance of ectopy but of a much whiter and opalescent color (Figs. 280 and 281). This similarity to ectopy is caused by prolifer-

ation of squamous epithelium over the papillae of ectopy in many instances.

During gestation these papillomas increase in size considerably, forming extensive vegetating masses which cover much of the vaginal fornices (Fig. 284).

The whitish color of the granulations of the papillomas ordinarily becomes evident only after the acetic acid test. However, on occasion, because of hyperplasia of the superficial layers, it is already visible to the naked eye. The pedicle of these papillomas is usually very evident.

Smooth Papilloma. This type appears as an isolated neoplasm, with a small or absent pedicle, which emerges from the exocervix near the external os (Figs. 285 and 286). Its appearance is like that of the endocervical polyp, and it may be distinguished by its point of implantation, by the smoothness of its surface (totally lacking the fissures or depressions that characterize endocervical polyps), and by a covering of squamous epithelium identical to that of the rest of the cervix. They are usually small and are only exceptionally observed in groups.

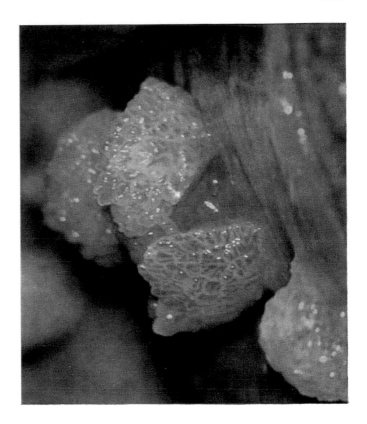

Figure 280. Arborescent papilloma, situated on the lateral wall of the vagina. Observe its papillary structure, which is somewhat like that of ectopy. The vessels are abundant, and each papilla shows several capillaries of somewhat irregular shape.

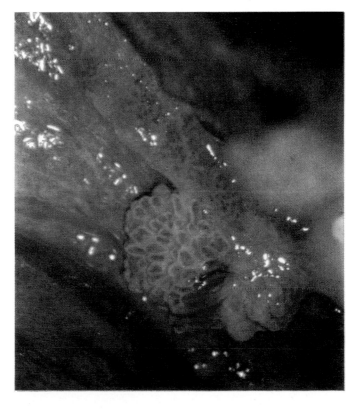

Figure 281. Single arborescent papilloma, with very marked papillae and easy identification of its capillary vessels.

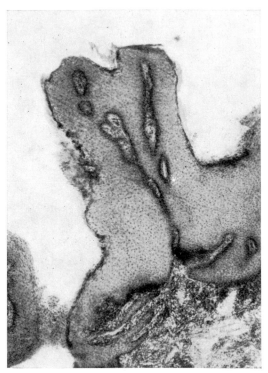

Figure 282. Histologic section of arborescent papilloma.

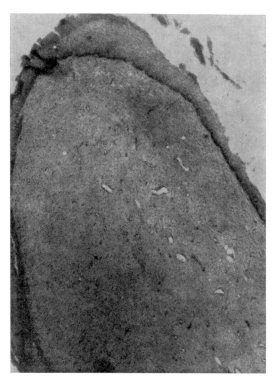

Figure 283. Histologic appearance of smooth vaginal papillomas.

Condylomatous Papilloma. In our experience these are second in frequency to the arborescent variety. We have always seen them in the anterior and posterior vaginal fornices, and most often at the point of the anterior cervicovaginal reflection. When they are established on the exocervix, the anterior lip is the one most commonly affected (Figs. 287 to 289).

They appear as whitish prominences, with sharp contours, and do not bleed even when an attempt is made to dislodge them. This maneuver, incidentally, does not accomplish anything. With the acetic acid test, some of these formations may exhibit a pseudomosaic-like surface, but this is not common. They do not take up iodine, or are stained only in part.

Commonly, several of these neoplasms are seen, and as in the arborescent variety, they may form vegetating masses (Fig. 287).

Keratinized Papilloma. Some forms of papilloma undergo keratinization,

which may be so intense that they resemble leukoplakias. Two varieties are possible. The isolated keratinized papilloma, also called "cotton ball," looks like small concretions of adherent mucus, irregular in shape and size (Fig. 290). The so-called "iceberg" papilloma has the appearance of a thick plaque of verrucous leukoplakia. Its keratinization is so deep that it is perfectly visible on direct examination, and its appearance changes very little with the acetic acid test (Fig. 291).

Plaquelike Papilloma. This is a rare variety, which under certain circumstances may be mistaken for a zone of ectopy. This is because the papilloma is made up of an aggregate of more or less keratinized papillae, individually fixed to the subjacent mucosa. Each papillary element resembles the "gloved finger" of ectopy (Fig. 292).

Although opinions are not unanimous, the tendency is to adopt a common histologic description for all these forms. Accordingly, papillomas are characterized by acanthosis with hyperkeratosis

(*Text continued on page 208*)

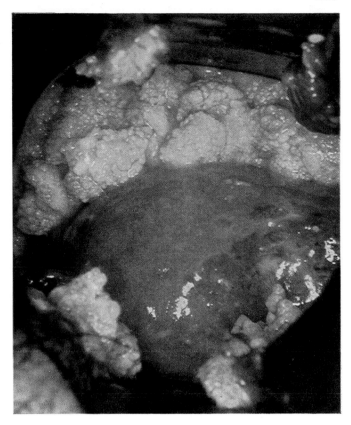

Figure 284. Arborescent papillomas grouped in the form of vegetating masses, which occupy all of the anterior vaginal fornix and part of the posterior. Their intense keratinization is striking.

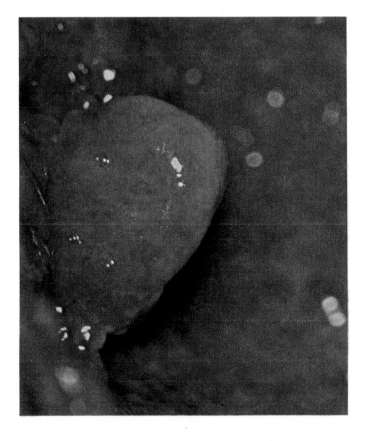

Figure 285. Smooth papilloma, at high magnification, situated on the anterior lip of the cervix. The smoothness of its surface is notable because it is so different from the arborescent variety. In this case white spots are observed, which should be interpreted as a papillary elevation in response to irritation.

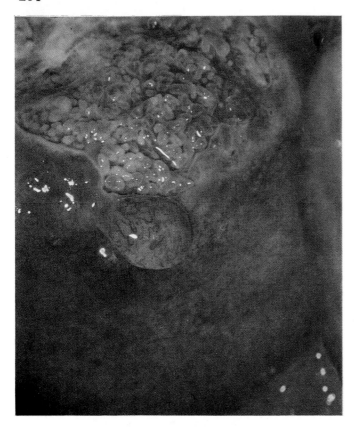

Figure 286. Small smooth papilloma, situated in the periphery of an ectopy. The appearance of its surface is identical to that of the exocervical epithelium which almost surrounds it.

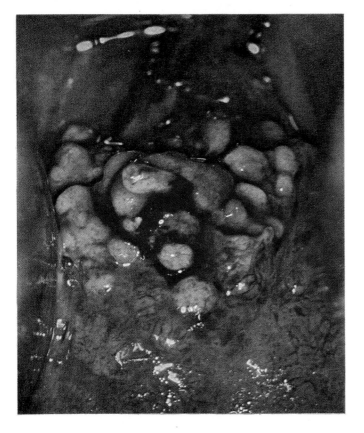

Figure 287. Group of condylomatous papillomas in a vegetating mass. Superimposed infection and the easy bleeding of the interpapillary tissue may induce a suspicious diagnosis, which should be avoided through identification of each element in the total picture.

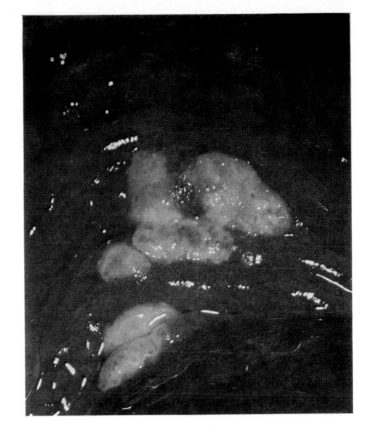

Figure 288. Condylomatous (or verrucous) papillomas at the base of the anterior vaginal fornix. They tend to form plaques.

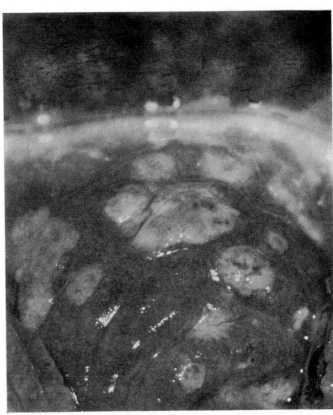

Figure 289. Group of acuminate condylomas (condylomatous papillomas), of diverse sizes. Separation has been attempted but has only caused minute superficial erosions. The interpapillomatous mucosa presents inflammatory signs.

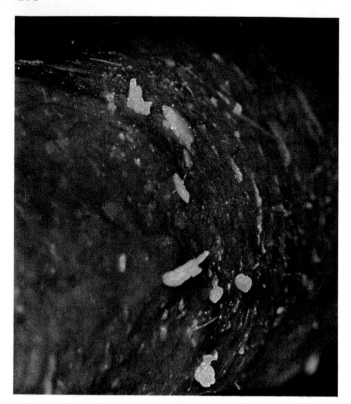

Figure 290. Keratinized papilloma in the form of "cotton balls." It is possible to confuse this picture with particles of mucus adhered to the cervix. Cleaning with acetic acid and careful colposcopic observation will avoid the error.

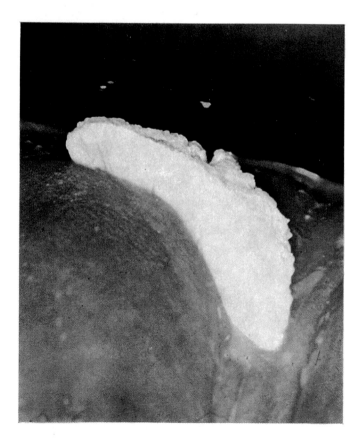

Figure 291. Keratinized papilloma, adopting the form of a large plaque of verrucous leukoplakia. Observe the marked elevation of the lesion.

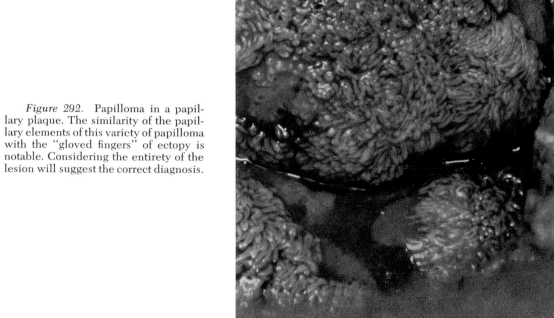

Figure 292. Papilloma in a papillary plaque. The similarity of the papillary elements of this variety of papilloma with the "gloved fingers" of ectopy is notable. Considering the entirety of the lesion will suggest the correct diagnosis.

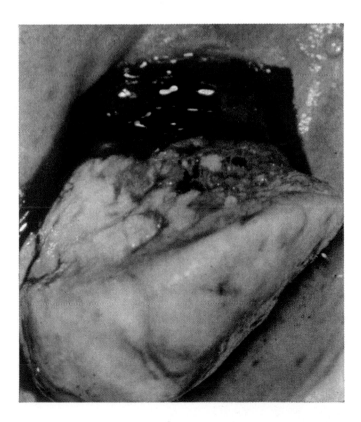

Figure 293. Polypoid mass arising from the uterus. It was not a true polyp, but a suspicious protruding tumor of a pseudopolypoid form.

and parakeratosis of the squamous epithelium which covers them (Figs. 283, 294 and 295), phenomena which explain their peculiar colposcopic appearance. The arborescent pedunculated papilloma especially exhibits a typical branching arrangement, with multiple papillary prolongations of the squamous epithelium. There is practically no connective tissue between these multiple epithelial strips (Fig. 282).

Benign epithelial alterations are frequent, and so are mitoses. The adjacent stroma is well vascularized, and there is often a chronic inflammatory infiltration around the dilated vessels.

Cytology reveals nothing characteristic but does call attention to the great percentage of inflammatory smears (in our experience 100 per cent, mostly indicating a trichomoniasis, with its peculiar cytologic modifications such as perinuclear halos, multinucleation, and presence of basal cells).

Fibromyomas

By colposcopy it is possible to observe three varieties of fibromyomas. The first is the cervicovaginal fibroma, which is found in the vagina. Its base, sessile or pedunculated, is established in the vaginal or exocervical mucosa. The polypoid fibromyoma is in the endocervix, and appears in the vagina thanks to a long pedicle. Rarely, the prolapse of a submucous fibroma from the uterine cavity may be observed.

We have seen only five cases through the colposcope (0.035 per cent of all our observations). Two of these were sessile neoplasms, of the size of a cherry, on the vaginal portion of the cervical os. Before preparation they had a smooth, pink surface. In one of them there were suspicious hemorrhagic and hyperemic sectors. After the application of acetic acid, the appearance became much paler and vitreous.

In two other cases, the colposcopic appearance was that of a fibrous polyp, because they were endocervical. Histology established the true diagnosis. Our remaining case was a uterine myoma that had prolapsed. Colposcopy revealed a reddish, irregular surface, with areas of extensive necrosis, alternating with bleeding, erosive, or frankly ulcerated areas. If the clinical diagnosis had not been clear, colposcopy could have led us astray.

Pathologic study of these lesions reveals characteristics of any fibroma — a bundle of smooth muscle fibers separated by abundant connective tissue. The muscle fibers are longer than those of normal myometrium, accentuating the characteristic whorled morphology. Mitoses are rare.

CLINICAL COURSE

Malignant degeneration of polyps is infrequent (0.2 to 1.5 per cent). It is possible to suspect such degeneration colposcopically if images of leukokeratosis and vascular irregularities are established above the common phenomena of epidermization (metaplasia) (Table 57). Sarcomatous degeneration of a polyp is probably nonexistent, but there are sarcomas which adopt polypoid shapes. For this reason histopathologic study of all excised polypoid formations is recommended including examination of the base of implantation (Fig. 293).

Colposcopy is useful to verify the complete extirpation of the tumor. By opening the speculum widely, it is usually possible to learn where the polyp was implanted in the endocervical canal, thus assuring that its eradication is complete.

Malignant degeneration of a polyp is diagnosed too often (see Table 57). In many cases, repeat examination of cytologic smears reveals that what was considered malignant was nothing more than simple phenomena of squamous metaplasia or areas of glandular hyperplasia. On the other hand, a polypoid carcinoma should be differentiated from a polyp with malignant degeneration and from a botryoid sarcoma, which, as has already been said, may take on a polypoid form. In these obvious cases the recommendation to eradicate the lesion completely is more pressing, because many malig-

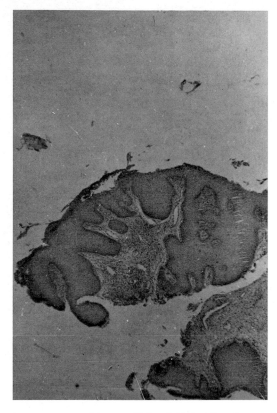 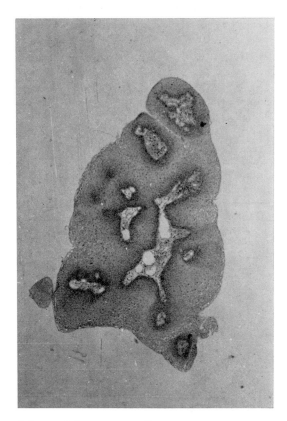

Figures 294 and *295*.   Histologic aspects of the condylomatous papillomas.

nant cells are found in the base of these neoplasms.

Polyps, as benign as they may be, have little tendency to disappear spontaneously, even when they become necrotic. In spite of apparently complete extirpation, recurrence is not exceptional, and in the presence of a recurrent polyp, one must always think about sarcoma. Colposcopically, its characteristics are clearly different from those of a common polyp: erosive surface, vascular irregularities, and proliferating areas without a papillary appearance.

Malignant transformation of papillomas is much more frequent, being estimated to occur in 5 to 10 per cent of cases (Gilbert and Ganse). Because of the peculiar appearance of some of these neoplasms, which is usually suspicious, colposcopy may not be of much help in determining which are undergoing malignant degeneration.

Papillomas may exist unnoticed for years, until pregnancy occurs. Then the papilloma becomes clinically evident, because it increases extraordinarily in volume, occupying the whole of the vagina (causing irritative discomfort, bleeding, and dyspareunia) or even ap-

Table 57.   Frequency of Malignant Degeneration of Polyps

Aaro et al.	0.2%
Farrar and Nedoss	0.2%
Winter	0.26%
Fluhmann	1.0%
Usandizaga et al.	1.26%
Moreno	1.5%
Nogales and Manglano	3.0%
Guzmán Llovet et al.	4.22%
Huber	12.9%
Our Series	1.1%

pearing externally. On many occasions, these regress after delivery, without leaving any trace.

Cervical fibromyomas have no greater a tendency toward malignant change than those in any other part of the uterus. Logically any such degeneration would be in the form of a sarcoma. There are no precise data in the literature, but it seems logical that the best candidates would be those bearing phenomena of superficial necrosis and abnormal vascularization.

The evolution of cervical fibromas observed by colposcopy is usually uneventful. This definitely does not include those fibromas of great volume which cause compression of the adjacent organs. Diagnosis of these neoplasms is made by simple vaginal examination and not by colposcopy.

MANAGEMENT

Extirpation is the only adequate treatment for these benign neoplasms. When colposcopy correctly identifies these small tumors, permitting an accurate prediction of their histologic characteristics, it also facilitates the clinical gynecologist's approach, giving him advanced information needed for correct management.

Extirpation of polyps is usually no problem. If the polyp is small and colposcopy characterizes it as a mucous or adenomatous polyp, without superficial phenomena of epidermization or ulceration, it may be removed by a simple twist (Aaro et al.). On the contrary, if it is a fibrous or angiomatous polyp, or mucoglandular with extensive areas of squamous metaplasia, it is advisable to use wide punch forceps or a small scalpel, which permits complete excision after prior cervical dilatation. These polyps are, at least potentially, the ones that may be the seat of carcinomatous or sarcomatous degeneration. For similar reasons, histologic examination is obligatory in the latter type, while in the former it may be omitted (Fig. 296).

Various instruments have been advocated to completely remove the tumor, including Gavert's forceps, Eve's polypotome, and Palmer's forceps for polyps. Careful curettage of the implantation site remains the only secure procedure.

The correct conduct in the presence of papilloma, solitary or multiple, is extirpation by surgical excision or electrocautery. However, in the pregnant woman it is advisable to postpone treatment until after delivery, because under these circumstances bleeding is produced that may be difficult to control. Moreover, even large papillomatous formations often totally regress after delivery.

Fibromyomas should also be extirpated completely, and as they are usually sessile and the study of the base of implantation is important (because of possible sarcomatous degeneration), the most adequate procedure is surgical.

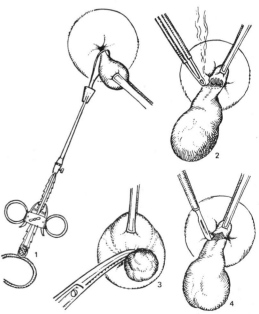

Figure 296. Techniques of enucleation of a polyp, according to its type. A pedunculated polyp, well characterized colposcopically, is extirpated by a polypotome (1) or simple torsion with forceps (3). A sessile polyp without colposcopic atypia is enucleated with a diathermic loop (2). A colposcopically suspicious polyp is extirpated with a scalpel (4), followed by curettage of the implantation site. On occasion it will be necessary to dilate the cervical canal.

MALIGNANT TUMORS

With the colposcope two types of cervical malignant tumors may be observed: squamous cell carcinoma of the exocervix and endocervical adenocarcinoma, once the latter protrudes through the external os. We will also refer to the colposcopic appearance of endometrial neoplasms when, as is not infrequent, these emerge through the cervical os.

ORIGIN

We have already explained (p. 165) the initial mechanism by which a simple process of physiologic metaplasia could lead to a dysplastic lesion or an in situ carcinoma. When we refer to the origin of the "zone of atypical transformation" the place and terrain of carcinogenesis become clear.

At present we agree with those who believe that the appearance of cancer of the uterine cervix is not a sudden phenomenon, but rather the end of a long chain of processes, each more atypical, which is initiated in the squamous metaplasia of a re-epithelialization (Coppleson and Reid). The intermediate stages are represented by the different types of dysplasia.

Except for invasive carcinoma, which is not likely to regress, all the intermediate stages have the ability to do so, and none of them have to evolve inevitably toward cancer. In an important percentage of cases they may remain stable for an indefinite period. It is not possible, therefore, in any one case, to guess the probable evolution, especially when the average duration of each one of these stages is measured in years. Dunn and Martin asserted that the average duration of the dysplastic phase was 3.8 years and that of preinvasive carcinoma 8.1 years. Richart and Barron, in their large series of 557 cases of dysplasia observed that mild dysplasias which evolved to intraepithelial cancer took an average of 7 years, moderate dysplasias almost 5, and the severe, 1 year. The period of transition to carcinoma was 44 months on the average.

It is evident that the likelihood of regression diminishes as the grade of atypia increases, whereas the possibility of progression is each day increased. There is a notable jump in the malignant potential between a moderate dysplasia and a severe one (see Fig. 297). Since the histologic equivalent of "atypical re-epithelialization" is mild dysplasia, and that of "atypical transformation" is severe dysplasia, it is not difficult to make the correct assumptions from the colposcopic pictures.

Remaining to be determined are the factors capable of initiating or accelerating these transformations of increasing atypia. According to the well known outline of Van Potter, there are some "initiating" factors capable of transforming a normal cell into a dysplastic cell; "promoting" factors which convert the latter into a dependent cancerous cell, reactive to the action of certain drugs and hormones; and finally, factors of "progression" which result in a cancerous cell with totally autonomous growth. It is not known whether this sequence can be abbreviated, and whether a cell can be transformed directly from a normal to an autonomous cancerous cell by the action of an unknown virus (see Fig. 298).

Factors capable of accelerating an already established neoplastic process are well understood, but we know very little of those equipped with true inductive capacity (carcinogenetic factors). As has been suggested in connection with the origin of atypical transformation, future research may demonstrate the existence of an error in organization in the cellular intercommunication.

As factors of promotion and progression, the following have been listed.

Maternity. The larger the number of children, the greater the risk.

Sexual Activity. Cervical cancer is rare in the virgin and frequent in prostitutes. There has been a suggestion that Trichomonas vaginalis is implicated (Table 58).

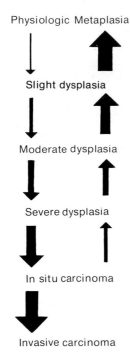

Figure 297. Outline of the relationship between metaplasia, dysplasia and cancer. Possibilities of progression and regression.

Race. Jewish women seem to be refractory to cervical cancer, probably due to circumcision in the male.

Heredity, at least in the experimental field.

Local irritative lesions, which promote atypical cervical re-epithelialization.

Local circulatory deficiencies, as are found in the cervix remaining after subtotal hysterectomy.

Hormonal imbalance (hyperestrogenism).

A given somatic constitution. There is a tendency noted for the disease to occur in large women of endomorphic habitus.

FREQUENCY

The incidence of cervical cancers observed on a gynecologic service, where early diagnoses are obtained by colposcopy and cytology is about 1 per cent. Differences between the figures quoted by different centers depends not only on the quality of the examination, but also on the organization of the particular institution and on the types of patients with whom it deals (Table 59).

Our own figure of 1.07 per cent is similar to that of other centers which function in an analogous manner (Calvo de Mora, 1.21 per cent)—in other words, with simple clinical criteria of selection (gynecologic and obstetric patients who attend a hospital or are referred by gynecologists)—but would be lower for those who undertake a systematic colposcopic and cytologic screening (Zinser, 0.66 per cent) and relatively higher where colposcopy or cytology is done only in the presence of clinical suspicion (Walz, 3.5 per cent).

Evidently, the figures are somewhat lower when screening is done exclusively by cytology (Von Haam 0.38 per cent, Calabresi 0.62 per cent). On the other hand, they perceptibly diminish in the event of "re-screenings." Christopherson gave a 0.69 per cent incidence of cervical cancers detected by initial screening, while after a subsequent examination the figure declined to 0.1 per cent.

Dividing our cases into preclinical

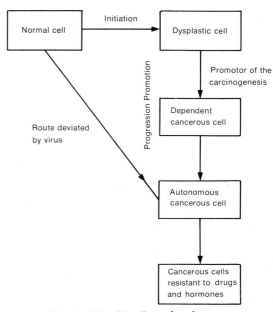

Figure 298. Van Potter's schema.

Table 58. Incidence of Dysplasia and Carcinoma in Patients With and
Without *Trichomonas vaginalis* Infections*

CYTOLOGIC DIAGNOSIS	PATIENTS WITHOUT T. VAGINALIS (TOTAL: 56,986)	PATIENTS WITH T. VAGINALIS (TOTAL: 6,884)	P VALUE
Dysplasia	887 (1.6%)	256 (3.7%)	<0.001
In situ carcinoma	214 (0.4%)	75 (1.1%)	<0.001
Invasive carcinoma	129 (0.2%)	25 (0.4%)	<0.02
Total	356 (5.2%)	1,230 (2.2%)	<0.001

*Meisels (1969)

cancers (discovered by colposcopy, but not evident by ordinary exploration) and clinical cancers (diagnosable without the help of colposcopy), we observe that frequency of the former is 0.46 per cent, while that of the latter is 0.61 per cent (Table 60).

The number of preclinical carcinomas varies widely in different series, from very high figures (Limburg, 1.75 per cent; Battaglia, 1.4 per cent; González-Merlo, 2.04 per cent; Calvo de Mora, 0.92 per cent) to extraordinarily low ones (Zinser, 0.13 per cent; Manelis, 0.1 per cent). The differences undoubtedly relate to the type of patients subjected to the examination. However, in very large series, the percentage usually lies between 0.4 and 0.9 per cent (Table 61).

COLPOSCOPIC APPEARANCE AND HISTOLOGIC CORRELATION

Squamous Cell Carcinoma (Epidermoid Carcinoma). The so-called preclinical stage usually corresponds to the histologic designations of intraepithelial carcinoma and microcarcinoma, and the clinical stage represents frankly invasive carcinoma.

PRECLINICAL STAGE. In this early phase the colposcopic appearance of the lesion is similar to that of "destructive atypical transformation." In 54 per cent of these last mentioned lesions, an inapparent cancer is hidden. This means that from a colposcopic viewpoint, the step from severe dysplasia to in situ carci-

Table 59. Frequency of Cervical Cancer in a Screening Program

AUTHORS	PER CENT In situ CARCINOMA	PER CENT INVASIVE CARCINOMA	TOTAL
Von Haam (1965)	0.22	0.16	0.38
Glatthaar (1954)	0.39	0.13	0.52
Calabresi (1958)	0.32	0.30	0.62
Zinser (1965)	0.24	0.42	0.66
Christopherson (1966)	0.39	0.30	0.69
Mateu-Aragonés (1969)	0.08	0.69	0.77
Berger (1952)	0.20	0.59	0.79
Calvo de Mora and Tubio (1971)	0.25	0.95	1.21
Walz (1958)	0.80	2.70	3.50
Our Series (1972)	0.46	0.61	1.07

Table 60. Results of Colposcopic Examination at the Cancer Center,
Provincial Maternity Hospital, Barcelona

	1964	1965	1966	1967	1968	1969	1970	1971	TOTAL	
Patients observed	536	3352	2902	1850	1573	1237	1772	1862	15,084	
Patients excluded	3	50	82	33	73	27	37	31	336	
Patients diagnosed	533	3302	2820	1817	1500	1210	1735	1831	14,748	
									No.	%
Typical images	403	2779	2418	1480	1259	984	1379	1560	12,262	83.14
Atypical images	120	472	336	288	231	226	356	271	2300	15.61
Unclassified images	10	51	66	49	10	0	0	0	186	1.24
Preclinical carcinomas	4	14	14	6	12	8	3	8	69	0.46
Clinical carcinomas	3	24	14	16	10	12	5	6	90	0.61
Total carcinomas	7	38	28	22	22	20	8	14	159	1.07

Table 61. Diagnosis of Preclinical Carcinoma Colposcopy
(Minimum of 15,000 Observations)

AUTHORS	OBSERVATIONS	PRECLINICAL CARCINOMA	%
Zinser (1951)	32,631	43	0.13
Hohlbein (1957)	95,427	—	0.41
Rieper (1966)	15,000	79	0.52
Wespi and Glatthaar (1955)	16,501	91	0.55
Navratil (1964)	55,000	663	0.82
Calvo de Mora (1971)	23,114	214	0.92
Our Series (1972)	15,084	69	0.46

noma generally is not abrupt (Azocar). However, the appearance of the cervix is considerably altered once the invasion of the stroma has taken place. The topography is also similar, because a notable preference for the median areas of both cervical labia is observed (at the 12 and 6 o'clock positions), while the lateral commissures, at least at first, are only seldom affected (Johnson) (Fig. 299).

Hillemanns and Moog observed that the preference of carcinomatous lesions for the anterior lip increases as there are more children, suggesting a relationship to the trauma of childbirth. However, the areas of the cervix that are most frequently exposed to obstetrical tears (3 and 9 o'clock) are precisely those least involved by the carcinomatous transformation.

The signs which make us consider the destructive zone of atypical transformation as the site of an incipient cancer are as follows.

1. Progressive extension of the atypical transformation encroaching on the erosive or ulcerated red zones, which alternate with congested sectors and remnants of leukokeratotic images in destruction (Figs. 300 to 302). The epithelial elements that usually resist transformation for the longest period are those near the ectopic glandular orifices. Silver nitrate may help to identify the ulcerated zones. Despite this progressive epithelial destruction, in the center of the grade I cancers, clearly visible zones of mosaic, ground structure, or leukoplakia are still seen, especially at the edges of the clearly neoplastic tissue (Fig. 302).

2. Irregular surface, with embossments and accentuated differences of level between the various sectors of the exocervix (Mestwerdt), which suggest invasion of the stroma (Fig. 302). On occasion, regular depressions are seen alternating with small elevations. They usually are due to mosaic segments of mucosa having been completely denuded, leaving geometric impressions upon the stroma (Fig. 303).

3. The more or less undamaged epithelium which has not as yet been shedded has a pale, vitreous appearance, with yellow-white or reddish zones. In some areas it gives an impression resembling fat, and the sensation of a crumbling and breaking epithelium is evident (Fig. 304). The variegation of the epithelium attracts immediate attention, and is one of the signs of malignant change.

4. A slight contact is all that is necessary to produce hemorrhage, which is difficult to control and which complicates further exploration (Figs. 300 and 308).

5. Significant vascular irregularities affect the shape, size, course, and caliber of the vessels. Dilatations and stenoses are clearly visible in the course of twisted vessels, whose distribution is capricious in appearance, but at least in the periphery it is radial (Fig. 307). The green filter may help in identifying these vessels (Fig. 306).

More than 40 years ago Hinselmann referred to the so-called "adaptive vascular hypertrophy," which he classified as "sufficient" and "insufficient." In effect, it is common to observe, along with proliferating, well vascularized areas, others in necrosis due to vascular insufficiency. This observation usually indicates a destructive, infiltrating, neoplastic growth.

When a cervical carcinoma is irradiated, one of the first colposcopic signs of a favorable response is disappearance of the atypical vessels (Ganse, Mannarino, Bajardi, and others).

The importance of these vessels in the identification of a suspicious zone is evident and we owe to Mateu-Aragonés

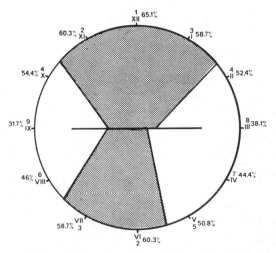

Figure 299.   Circumferential localization of in situ carcinoma, according to Johnson.

the codification of their alterations in a logical and practical scheme. However, on occasion their role has been over-emphasized. Ganse has said that the vascular picture may offer more data about the malignancy of a tumor than its own histologic picture. There is no doubt that on many occasions the vascular pattern is the colposcopic signal for further study of a cervix for carcinoma (Burghardt). Although we do not as yet believe that there are certain pathognomonic vascularization patterns of the precancerous areas or the intraepithelial carcinoma, vessels in corkscrew or forked formations are always suspicious.

6. Around this zone of re-epithelialization and morphologic variegation, a sector of undamaged epithelium may be observed, but this has a whitish appearance after the application of acetic acid, and it does not take up iodine. Many times the significance of this zone is questionable. It may be a remnant of an atypical transformation not as yet affected by the destructive process. On other occasions it is a centrifugal extension of the neoplasm, colonizing previously healthy areas (Fig. 308).

Total absence of vessels in the periphery of a neoplastic lesion is a suspicious finding. The rapid growth of the tumor may lead to avascularized areas.

Many of these signs were described by Mestwerdt as belonging to "microcarcinoma," and Palmer has called them "colposcopic alarm signals." Their occurrence as part of the so-called zone of atypical transformation has given rise to the belief that they are related to the repair of an ectopy, which from a dynamic standpoint is not correct.

After the menopause, a squamous cell carcinoma may be totally hidden in the interior of the endocervical canal because of the frequent inward displacement, at this time, of the squamo-columnar junction (see p. 60). To avoid missing one of these cancers, all patients with major or minor colposcopic alterations in the external os should undergo endocervical histologic study, especially if previous observation has diagnosed ectopy.

Study of the endocervical mucosa may be by meticulous endocervical curettage or by biopsy with the aid of Gusberg's forceps (Fig. 309). We have obtained good results with this ingenious instrument. Endocervicoscopy with the Ganse or the Martin-Laval intracervical specula has not as yet become common practice.

CLINICAL STAGE. Colposcopy is not required to confirm the diagnosis of an established invasive cancer, for there is clinical evidence that does not generally require optical confirmation. The existence of necrosis, edema, and persistent hemorrhage makes careful colposcopic exploration difficult.

As does the clinician, the colposcopist classifies apparent cervical cancer into two categories exophytic and endophytic, with mixed types (Fig. 310). Exophytic cancers (three-fourths of the total) proliferate on the surface, often adopting the form of a cauliflower. They grow from one of the two lips of the cervix, generally the upper one, although by infiltrating the other they form a single lesion.

This variety carries the most favorable prognosis because its growth is slow. Its superficial development, extending toward the vaginal mucosa, indicates that the connective tissue offers effective resistance to its progression. On the other hand, appearance of this form is usually preceded by a long period of dysplastic change, of the atypical transformation type, susceptible to accurate colposcopic diagnosis. This type of cancer is commonly found in young women.

The most striking elements at colposcopy are neoplastic papillae of diverse size, color and shape, grouped in irregular mounds which are visible to the naked eye. Contact with these irregular and exuberant lesions causes easy bleeding (Figs. 311 and 312).

It is curious that although recognition of this stage of cervical cancer does not present any problem clinically, there may be doubts in the mind of a beginning colposcopist. The papillae may be mistaken for those of ectopy, especially an infected ectopy, because they have a similar shape and volume. The differentiating colposcopic signs that suggest cancer are the paler color of the cancerous papillae; their conglutination in blocks; ease

(*Text continued on page 220*)

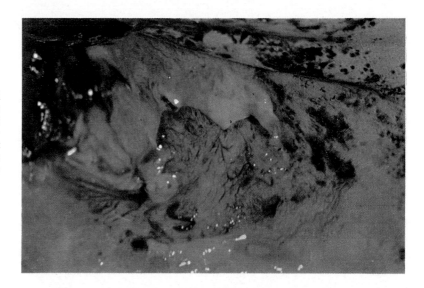

Figure 300. Ulcerated zone which shows the vascular irregularities of the subjacent stroma. Some plaques of leukokeratosis persist without shedding. (The same patient as in Figure 250 with a green filter on the colposcope.)

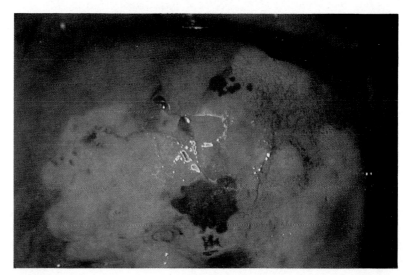

Figure 301. In situ carcinoma observed colposcopically without preparation. The congested and erosive zones alternate with more or less undamaged leukokeratotic plaques.

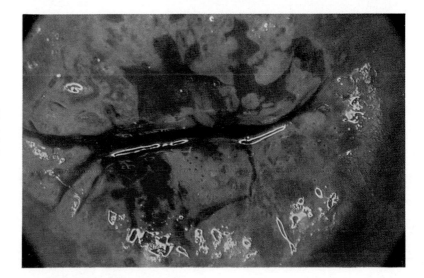

Figure 302. Preclinical cancer with incipient invasion. This is an "atypical transformation" in phase of destruction.

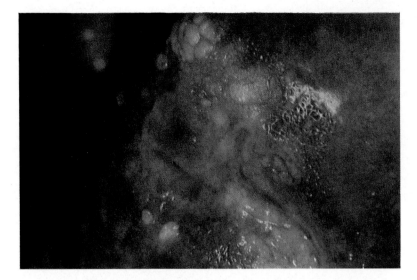

Figure 303. Images of keratinization in mosaic and in leukoplakic plaques, progressively replaced by congested and erosive processes. At the right are some depressions which correspond to blocks of mucosa in mosaic, which have been torn off by drying prior to colposcopic observation. Histopathologic study determined the existence of an intracpithelial carcinoma.

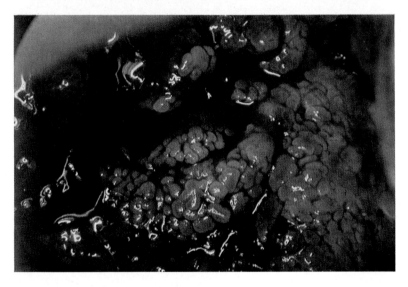

Figure 304. Zones of superficial necrosis and epithelial ulceration coexist with zones of mucosa of a white-yellow color, and of an appearance similar to that of lard, which crumble easily.

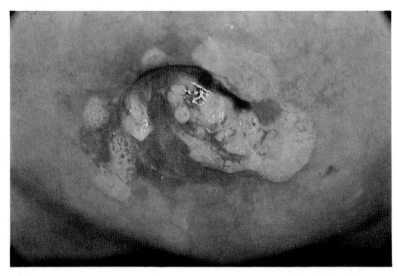

Figure 305. Colposcopic observation of a zone of atypical transformation, containing an intraepithelial carcinoma. Acetic acid makes visible some leukoplakic plaques with diffuse edges, small vascular irregularities and glandular orifices.

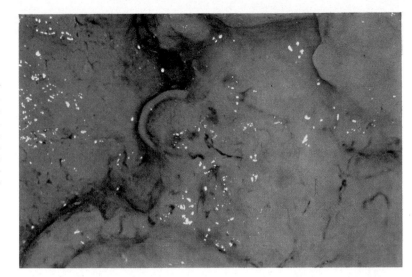

Figure 306. The vascular irregularities of a zone of neoplastic transformation, presenting a variegated surface, seen through a green filter. Vessels in "hairpin" and in "corkscrew" shapes may be observed for only short distances because they constantly change their level.

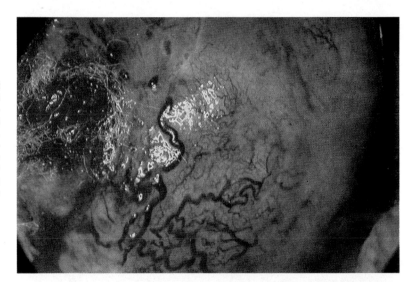

Figure 307. Important vascular irregularities in the periphery of a neoplastic lesion. The typical arborescent distribution has disappeared. Vessels of very unequal caliber are seen, subject to dilatation and sudden stenosis. They may suddenly descend into the stroma and then again become exteriorized.

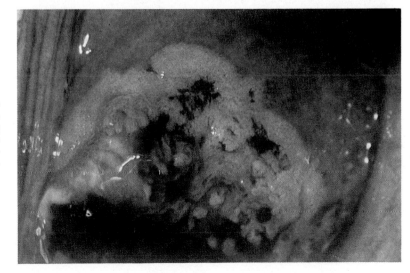

Figure 308. Orificial carcinoma, circled by an extensive white area (appearing after the acetic acid application), which may be interpreted as a superficial extension of a central neoplasia.

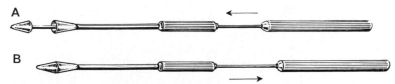

Figure 309. Gusberg's forceps for endocervical biopsy. It is introduced while open (*A*) into the cervical canal. When closed (*B*) it imprisons a fragment of endocervical tissue. Withdrawal must be careful, so as not to lose the material obtained.

of bleeding; fragile, woody consistency, crumbling with slight trauma, and a denuded surface, without epithelium. However, it is the general appearance of the lesion, with its exuberance, its vascular irregularities, and its easy bleeding, that confirms the colposcopic diagnosis (Fig. 312).

Exophytic transformation usually occupies a considerable portion of the cervix. Only in rare cases will the colposcopist observe a limited exophytic neoplasm, clearly malignant, with small zones of central necrosis and areas of ground and mosaic structure in its periphery.

In the endophytic form (one-fourth of cases), the neoplastic growth occurs deep in the tissues. What attracts the colposcopist's attention is the existence of a great ulcerous excavation, with bleeding and irregular walls, which thins the walls of the cervix, providing the sensation of seeing into the uterine corpus. What remains of the cervix is necrotic, to the extent that the colposcopic vision is poor. There is no epithelium, and the connective tissue bleeds or is destroyed when held to obtain a biopsy (Fig. 314).

This variety of cancer has been called a "drama in one act" by Feyrter, due to its extraordinarily rapid evolution, which does not allow an early diagnosis to be made (Ashworth). It is seen especially in women of advanced age.

On rare occasions is it possible to ob-

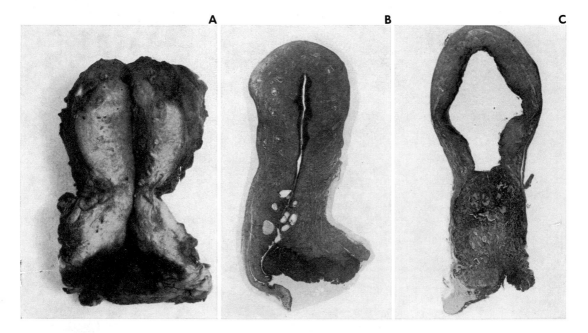

Figure 310. Macroscopic varieties of carcinoma of the cervix. *A* and *C* show endophytic, infiltrating growth, while *B* is an endophytic cancer limited to the anterior lip of the cervix.

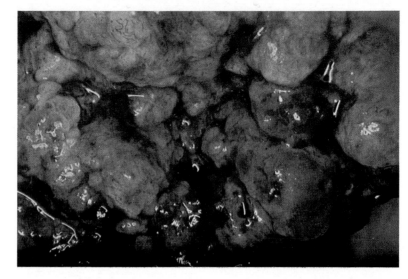

Figure 311. Exophytic excrescent cancer, with papillary mounds of very diverse sizes. Simple placement of a speculum causes bleeding.

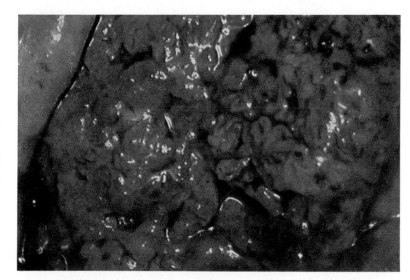

Figure 312. Exophytic carcinoma exhibiting the characteristic neoplastic papillae which permits its distinction from common ectopy. For this differential diagnosis it is useful to observe the paler color of the cancerous papillae and their fragile consistency and easy bleeding.

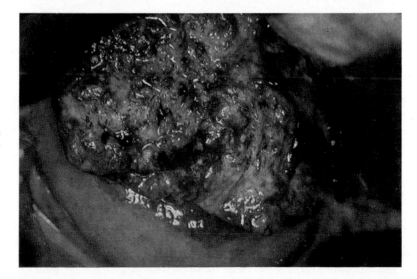

Figure 313. An exophytic cancer with a very bizarre surface.

serve an endophytic carcinoma in its initial stages. At most, it may be possible to observe its ulcerative stage, when it has not yet deepened excessively and has a more or less wide ulceration, always in contact with the anatomic os of the cervix (Figs. 315 and 316), encircled by an ample congestive zone, with additional images of papillary ground structure in some cases. Its growth is so rapid that if a therapeutic decision is not made at this time, in a few weeks the colposcopist will be surprised to find sudden crumbling of the cervix.

An extreme form is the so-called "barrel carcinoma" in which only the exterior covering of the cervix remains. The rest has been destroyed by the neoplastic process. This variety carries the worst prognosis, because vascular and lymphatic invasion occurs very early.

The histologic characteristics that define an invasive squamous cell carcinoma are similar to those of the carcinoma in situ (p. 182). We will only add, in accordance with Hillemanns, that when invasion occurs, the number of mitoses increases significantly, as does the nuclear volume (Fig. 319). The fundamental difference between one and the other lies in the invasion of the stroma by the tumoral growth and the involvement of the lymphatics.

"Microcarcinoma" may be considered as an intermediate stage between the in situ and the frankly invasive carcinoma. At present the concept of invasion is subject to revision, because the structure of the tissues surrounding the tumor is not identical in all cases (Masson, Herovici), nor does the infiltration of the stroma always occur in the same manner (Hamperl).

Extension of a neoplastic focus may occur by assimilation (induction of predisposed neighboring zones) or by exclusion (displacement of adjacent structures). Commonly, a clear division is established between normal and cancerous epithelium (Schiller's pathologic line).

With respect to the grade of cellular differentiation, squamous cell carcinomas have been grouped as immature or undifferentiated and mature or differentiated. Botella and Nogales substituted this classification for that of "müllerian" and "malpighian" carcinoma in the belief that the undifferentiated form originates from an indirect metaplasia, and the mature variety in the germinative layer of the polystratified epithelium of the cervix.

Undifferentiated carcinomas are formed by groups of small cells of great uniformity, which form compact accumulations; nuclear density is due to scarceness of cytoplasm. The nuclei are hyperchromatic. Keratinization is not observed, or if it exists, is very scarce. The direction of cellular maturation is toward the free surface of the tumor strip (Fig. 317).

Differentiated carcinomas are characterized by a high degree of keratinization, including pearl formation. The latter are formed by very atypical cells, including distorted giant ones. Maturation of the cells take place in the direction of the invasive cords (Figs. 318 and 319).

Generally, a histologically undifferentiated carcinoma constitutes the substrate of the exophytic form, whereas the differentiated type represents the endophytic variety. While the former usually is seen in the form of an in situ carcinoma, with the possibility that it may remain latent for a long period, the latter has a very rapid evolution, in such a manner that it is seldom possible to discover it in the intraepithelial phase.

Endocervical Adenocarcinoma (Glandular Epithelioma or Endocervical Cylindrical Epithelioma). In the rare cases in which adenocarcinoma of the endocervix is initiated near the external cervical os, colposcopy may be able to visualize it in the first stages of its growth (D'Allesandro et al.). It may adopt a papillomatous or ulcerated form having a gray color after acetic acid, with no colposcopic signs that permit its differentiation from the exophytic variety of the epidermoid cancer, except that its appearance more closely resembles that of an exuberant cervical ectopy.

Papillae are also observed in the shape of bunches of grapes but having an irregular appearance due to the intense epithelial proliferation. The capillaries present the shape of a comma or cork-

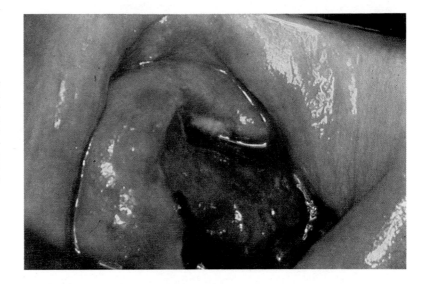

Figure 314. Hemorrhagic ulceration corresponding to an endophytic infiltrating carcinoma. The tissue destruction has already affected a sizable portion of the wall of the cervix. Exploration with a flexible probe discovered a ligneous hardening of the bottom of the ulceration.

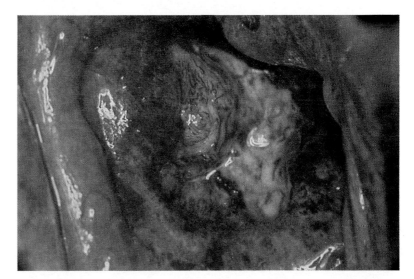

Figure 315. Circumoral ulceration observed without preparation. There is an area of necrobiosis, notable vascular irregularities, and ample zones of neoplastic infiltration. The acetic acid test would demonstrate the existence of an ample atypical transformation over the anterior lip of the cervix.

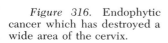

Figure 316. Endophytic cancer which has destroyed a wide area of the cervix.

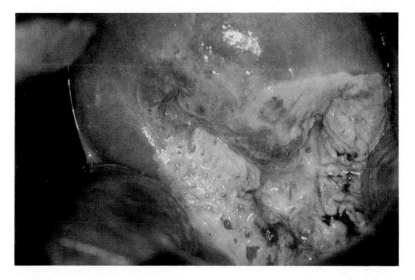

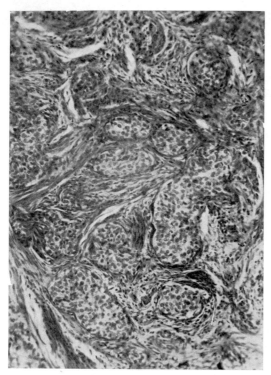

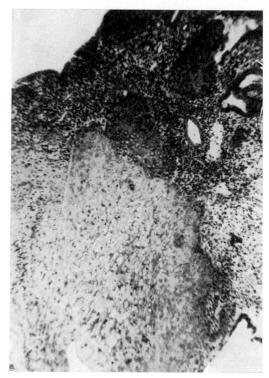

Figure 317. Histologic section of an undifferentiated cervical carcinoma.

Figure 318. Histologic section of a differentiated cervical carcinoma.

screw. They are tortuous and of great caliber, having notable irregularities in their course and overlying the epithelium (Bolten).

From a histologic standpoint, in addition to the erasing of the glandular pattern and the notable architectural pleomorphism, there is an alteration of the cell population characterized by tall, clear columnar cells with an increased content of mucus. Nuclear hyperchromasia, alteration of the nuclear-cytoplasmic ratio, and a profusion of mitoses in all fields are also notable. The stroma is found infiltrated by lymphocytic cells (Fig. 320).

Colposcopic Diagnosis of a Malignant Endometrial Tumor. An endometrial tumor (adenocarcinoma or sarcoma) may adopt a more or less polypoid structure and become visible in the vagina by protruding through the cervical canal. An endometrial adenocarcinoma cannot be distinguished colposcopically from its endocervical homologue. On the contrary, the colposcopic diagnosis of an en-

dometrial sarcoma is perfectly feasible, as long as it is not so large that when it distorts the structure of the cervix its origin cannot be seen. Uterine sarcoma should always be considered in the presence of a neoplasm that is endocervical in appearance, with characteristics of malignancy, but lacking papillary structure.

In our experience, the colposcopic image is that of an exophytic tumor, but not papillary, with an embossed surface and abundant atypical vessels (types III, IV and V). Hemorrhagic zones are observed, as are ulcerations covered by grayish exudate. The appearance is extraordinarily bizarre (Figs. 321 and 322). Instrumental exploration demonstrates the fragility of the neoplasm (Dexeus et al.).

The microscopic characteristics of the endometrial sarcoma include an enormous variety of histologic types. One of the most notable characteristics is the presence of myxomatous tissue, made up of cells with streaming cytoplasmic projections. Immature cartilaginous cells

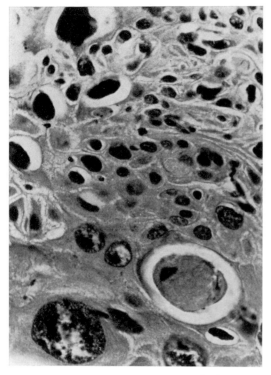

Figure 319. Histologic section at high magnification of a differentiated cervical carcinoma.

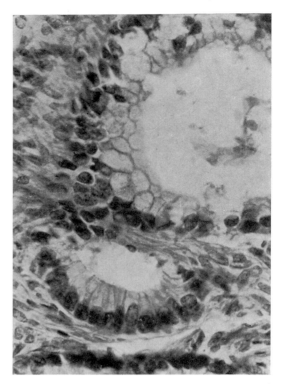

Figure 320. A mucous endocervical adenocarcinoma.

may even be observed, representing the transition between cartilaginous and myxomatous elements. Other elements are striated and smooth muscle fibers and adipose tissue (Fig. 323). These irregular microscopic characteristics explain the bizarre colposcopic appearance.

CYTOLOGIC CORRELATION

In the preclinical cancer diagnosed by colposcopy and confirmed by biopsy, cytologic smears confirm the malignancy (Papanicolaou's Class IV or V) in 82 per cent of cases. In 9.6 per cent of cases, the cytologic diagnosis is suspicious (Class II-III or III of Papanicolaou), and 8.3 per cent fall into Class I or II or are in other words false negatives.

In our series, 5.6 per cent of preclinical cancers (mostly microcarcinomas and endocervical adenocarcinomas) were diagnosed exclusively by cytology and were missed at the first colposcopic ex-

amination (Table 62). In the clinical cancer, agreement between cytology and colposcopy is the rule.

In the light of these results, and of those of a great number of gynecologists who use both methods simultaneously (Navratil, Limberg, Gerli, Zinser and Kern, and others), the combined use of colposcopy and cytology seems to be necessary. Each compensates for the limitations of the other, and the percentage of correct diagnoses can reach 99 per cent (Table 63).

The principal limitations of cytology, besides the inherent difficulty of training personnel, are the existence of carcinomas which do not shed cells (approximately 2 per cent of cervical cancers) and the fact that it is a blind procedure, giving no information about the location of the assumed cancer. Colposcopy, meanwhile, totally ignores intrauterine cancers and most endocervical tumors, because they are outside its area of vision.

According to González-Merlo et al., colposcopy is somewhat superior to cytol-

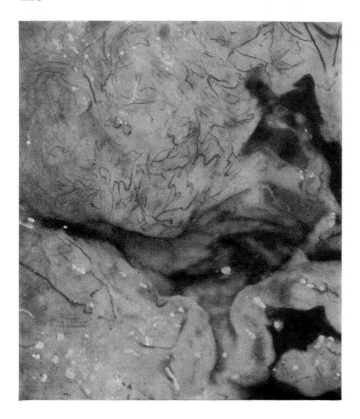

Figure 321. Uterine sarcoma (mixed mesodermal tumor), diagnosed through colposcopy. Observe the existence of an exophytic, but not papillary, neoplastic mass, of irregular surface, crossed by innumerable vessels with diverse irregularities.

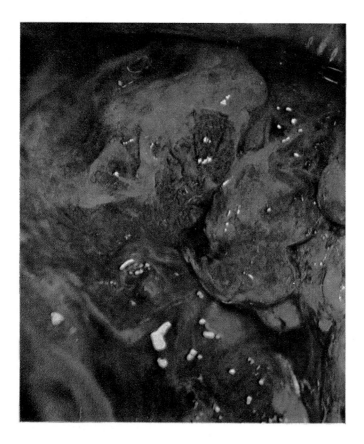

Figure 322. The same image as in Figure 321 observed through a green filter. The existence of large erosive zones is clearly seen.

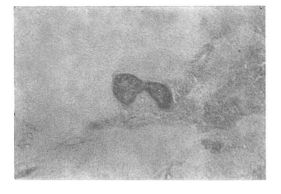

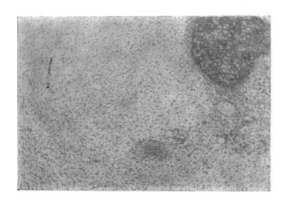
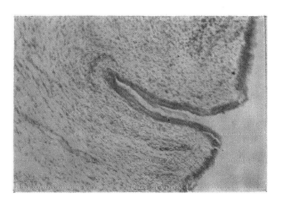

Figure 323. Histopathologic study of the endometrial sarcoma seen in Figures 321 and 322. It was a mixed mesodermal tumor. In these smears, the cartilaginous and myxomatous elements are perfectly distinguishable (alcian blue stain).

ogy in diagnosis of dysplasias, microcarcinomas and intraepithelial carcinomas, but inferior in discovering extensive hidden areas of malignancy, such as endocervical adenocarcinoma.

Characteristics that suggest malignancy in a cytologic smear corresponding to a squamous cell carcinoma are found both in the nucleus and in the cytoplasm (Figs. 324 and 325). The general characteristics are similar to those described for the dysplastic smear (p. 182).

Nuclear Characteristics

1. Increase in the size of the nucleus, which may be gigantic. Inequality of nuclear sizes (anisokaryosis) is especially evident.

2. Alterations in shape. Reniform, elongated, lobulated, and pear-shaped nuclei are seen (poikilokaryosis).

3. Multinucleation.

4. Chromatin clumped in large granules of different sizes, irregularly distributed, but especially disposed along the nuclear membrane.

5. Hyperchromasia, due to an increase in the nucleic acids of the chromatin.

6. Increase in number and size of nucleoli, which alters the nuclear-nucleolar ratio.

7. Increase in the width of the nuclear membrane, which also appears irregular.

8. Abnormal mitoses, with varying degrees of chromosome multiplication.

Characteristics of the Cytoplasm

1. Modification of the nuclear-cytoplasmic ratio in favor of the nucleus, despite the fact that an overall increase in cell volume is observed, and on occasion there are giant cells.

Table 62. False Negatives Obtained by Cytology and Colposcopy
in the Diagnosis of Cancer of the Cervix

	CYTOLOGIC FALSE NEGATIVES	COLPOSCOPIC FALSE NEGATIVES
	%	%
Walz (1952)	10	13.3
Burghardt and Bajardi (1954)	15.6	24
Held et al. (1954)	13	8
Cramer (1956)	8.9	6.7
Antoine (1964)	5	11
González-Merlo et al. (1966)	25.8	9.6
Lagrutta et al. (1966)	14.2	3.1
Our Series (1972)	8.3	5.6

2. Changes in the affinity for stains. Generally, the cytoplasm is eosinophilic in well differentiated carcinomas, while it is basophilic in the undifferentiated ones.

3. Cytoplasmic vacuolization, with inclusions.

4. Modifications of the cellular shape (anisocytosis). Abundant spindle-shaped, tadpole-shaped, and fiberlike cells appear.

Some authors (Graham) feel that it is possible to arrive at the diagnosis of mature or immature carcinoma based on cytology, in the same manner that others (Kasdon and Bamford, Nieburgs and Pund) describe specific cytologic modifications seen with invasion of the stroma. Nevertheless, there is agreement that these distinctions are not always possible (de Watteville, Meigs, Limburg, and others). Wagner has argued that the number of basal atypical cells significantly increases to about 70 per cent if invasion exists, while the percentage of dyskaryotic superficial cells decreases to less than 30 per cent.

In regard to the cytology of endocervical adenocarcinoma, the criteria of malignancy that we have given for the squamous carcinoma are valid in general. The glandular appearance of many of the neoplastic cells and the type of desquamation, in more or less organized plaques or groups, provide the differentiation.

CLINICAL COURSE

The "natural" evolution of the intraepithelial carcinoma is toward invasion of the stroma, at short or long term. But stromal invasion is neither obligatory nor fatal, as demonstrated by a multitude of statistics. Approximately 60 per cent of in situ carcinomas progress to invasive carcinoma within 10 years (Boyes et al.). This is confirmed by the statistical finding that invasive carcinoma is found in

Table 63. Diagnosis of Cancer of the Cervix Through the
Simultaneous Use of Cytology and Colposcopy

	CYTOLOGICALLY CORRECT DIAGNOSES	COLPOSCOPICALLY CORRECT DIAGNOSES	JOINTLY CORRECT DIAGNOSES
Limburg (1958)	89%	97%	99.4%
Navratil (1964)	87%	79.1%	98.8%
Coppleson and Reid (1967)	93%	92%	98%
Cope (1969)	90%	95%	95%
Our Series (1972)	91%	94.1%	98.9%

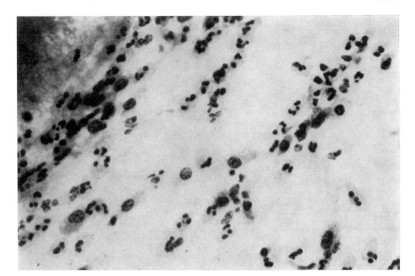

Figure 324. Cytologic smear of an intraepithelial carcinoma.

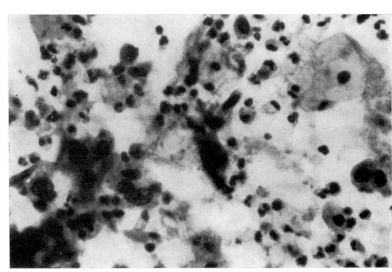

Figure 325. Cytologic smear of an invasive carcinoma.

patients 10 years older on average than those with intraepithelial cancer (Kneer and Hillemanns).

However, the period of time that a given intraepithelial carcinoma needs to become invasive varies from a few months (two, in a case reported by Limburg) to many years (12, according to Smith and Pemberton), depending both on the aggressiveness of the tumor and on the specific resistance of the host.

Generally, the in situ carcinoma which will become invasive most rapidly is the one whose colposcopic expression is an advanced atypical transformation with very striking destructive processes

(erosions and ulcerations) and irregular vascularization.

It is difficult to determine the percentage of intraepithelial carcinomas which regress, but it is somewhere between 10 and 30 per cent. The balance persist without change for an indefinite period, which may be as long as 17 years.

Ayre and Koss, and others, claim to have obtained regression by the use of topical tetracyclines, which seem to be capable of provoking maceration of tissue with shedding of an epithelial strip en bloc. Koss also reported excision of a carcinomatous focus by simple biopsy, relying upon subsequent reparative or inflammatory phenomena to eliminate the possible neoplastic remnants (Fig. 326).

Those intraepithelial carcinomas discovered colposcopically in the midst of secondary atypical transformation with superimposed erosive zones and normally patterned but hypertrophic vessels, are those that are most likely to regress. The changes that can take place in this type of cervix over an interval of a few days are surprising. Hence, what today seems to be an atypical image of benign prognosis may have been called suspicious two weeks earlier. In general, once an atypical lesion is demonstrated as unstable and mutable over a short period of time, one must doubt its true malignant nature.

Most of the assumed in situ carcinomas which apparently regress are diagnosed during pregnancy (McLaren, Campos et al., de Brux and Dupré, Froment, Bret and Coupez). Hence the necessity for prudence and for delaying a therapeutic decision until after delivery. Quite probably as our diagnostic methods improve, the number of these doubtful "on-off" carcinomas will diminish.

Colposcopy makes no contribution to evaluating the evolution of invasive carcinoma or the degree of extension of a neoplasm, which is preferentially evaluated by clinical or surgical procedures instead of colposcopy.

USE OF COLPOSCOPY IN MANAGEMENT

Colposcopy plays a part in three fundamental kinds of characterization of a carcinoma that are important to therapy. The first of these is the differentiation between intraepithelial and invasive carcinoma. Biopsy under colposcopic control will guarantee that the sample does not include a marginal zone of the neoplasm, which might lead to a false diagnosis of in situ carcinoma in the presence of a clearly invasive carcinoma. As stated by Novak, the diagnosis of in situ carcinoma should not be accepted until the complete cervix has been submitted to an orderly histologic examination.

Extension of an in situ carcinoma of the cervix to the vagina may also be diagnosed, or at least suspected, by colposcopy. In the presence of an image suggestive of cervical carcinoma, the colposcopist should not be content to observe the cervix alone, but must include examination of the vaginal walls and especially the fornices. It may be useful, in this respect to use the standard speculum alternately with the lateral retractors.

The vaginal vault is involved in the cervical neoplastic process in 1.5 per cent (Topek) to 6 per cent (Bolten and Jacques) of cases. The vaginal lesions are colposcopically less evident than the cer-

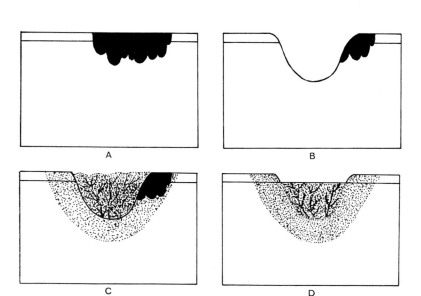

Figure 326. Possibility of eradication by biopsy of a carcinomatous area of small size, according to Koss. See text for explanation.

vical, and biopsy generally reveals a lesser seriousness. Excision of the vaginal lesions is necessary, however, and to omit this step is to risk recurrence of the disease (Bolten and Jacques).

Colposcopy is a vital element in postoperative follow-up, to watch for the appearance of recurrences at the level of the vaginal scar. Taking into account that half of these appear during the first year, it is imperative to be careful with postoperative examinations during this period of time, performing colposcopic and cytologic examinations every two to three months. Later, these may be spaced at six-monthly or yearly intervals. This control is especially necessary in the exophytic variety of squamous cell carcinoma, because of the frequency of its extension to the vaginal mucosa (Fig. 327).

Vaginal recurrence usually is evidenced by a small exophytic formation which to the naked eye may be confused with a common granuloma. However, the colposcopic examination offers definite signs of malignancy: atypical papillary structure and irregular vascular formations. Rarely, there may be an ample zone of atypical transformation which completely occupies the vaginal fornices.

Colposcopy may also be useful to observe the effects of radiation in women subjected to conventional or supervoltage radiotherapy. Therapeutic success is revealed by the rapid disappearance of the vascular anomalies (p. 216), even though a diffuse vascular network may persist for a period in apparently normal tissue.

Rutledge, and also Bolten, held that colposcopy was superior to cytology in the diagnosis of recurrences after radiotherapy because cytologic disturbances of the radiation response type hamper the diagnosis of recurrence for the next three years. By contrast, colposcopy reveals recurrences without difficulty thanks to the reappearance of vascular anomalies.

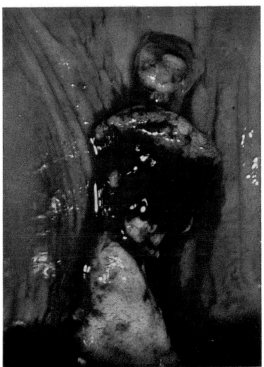

Figure 327.   Recurrence in the vaginal fornix of a cervical carcinoma treated by total hysterectomy five months previously. A partially necrotized granuloma is observed, cerebriform in character, and histologic study revealed that it was made up of neoplastic tissue.

REFERENCES

Aaro, L. A., Jacobson, L. J., and Soule, E. H.: Endocervical polyps. Obstet. Gynec., *21*:659, 1963.

Ashworth, C. T., Luibel, F. J., and Sanders, E.: Epithelium of normal cervix uteri studied with electron microscopy and histochemistry. Am. J. Obstet. Gynec., 79:1149, 1960.

Ayre, J. E.: Regression of cervical carcinoma in situ following aureomycin: A further report. South. Med. J., *45*:915, 1952.

Azócar Espin, B.: Analisis ginecologico de 600 biopsias selectivas del cuello uterino. Rev. Obstet. Ginec. Venez., *26*:599, 1966.

Baçaj, T., and Fioretti, P.: Contributo alla conoscenza dei papillomi squamocellulari della portio. Arch. Ostet. Ginec., 65:723, 1960.

Bajardi, F., Lang, W. R., de Moraes, A., and Rieper, J. P.: Colposcopy of the irradiated uterine cervix. Acta Cytol., 3:369, 1959.

Balagueró Lladó, L.: Diagnóstico precoz del cáncer de cuello uterino en la I Clínica Ginecológica Universitaria de Viena. Rev. Esp. Obstet. Ginec., *26*:244, 1967.

Balagueró Lladó, L.: El Carcinoma In Situ del Cuello Uterino. Editorial Espaxs, Barcelona, 1971.

Battaglia, G. B., and Leoni, R.: Il contributo della colposcopia alla diagnosi precoce del carcinoma della portio: Rilievi Clinico-statistici. Riv. Ostet. Ginec., *19*:78, 1964.

Berríos, G.: Lesiones poliposas de cuello uterino estudio histopatologico. Revista Obstet. Ginec. Venezuela, 26:95, 1966.

Bolten, K. A.: Practical colposcopy in early cervical and vaginal cancer. Clin. Obstet. Gynec., 10:808, 1967.

Bolten, K. A., and Jacques, W. E.: Introduction to Colposcopy. New York, Grune and Stratton, 1960.

Bonilla, F.: Diagnóstico precoz del cáncer genital. Rev. Esp. Obstet. Ginec., 24:327, 1965.

Boyes, D. A., Fidler, H. K., and Lock, D. R.: Significance of in situ carcinoma of the uterine cervix. Brit. Med. J., 1:203, 1962.

Bret, J., and Biojout, G.: Les expulsions de caduque au cours de la grossesse. Rev. Franç. Gynéc. Obstét., 62:413, 1967.

Bret, J., and Coupez, F.: Aspects colposcopiques des éliminations de caduque au cours de la grossesse: Etiologie et pronostic. Bull. Féd. Soc. Gynéc. Obstét., 12:356, 1960.

Bret, J., and Coupez, F.: Colposcopie. Paris, Masson et Cie., 1960.

Bret, J., and Coupez, F.: Four cases of vaginal recurrences of invasive or intra-epithelial carcinoma of the uterine cervix. Acta Cytol., 7:277, 1963.

Calabresi, P., Arvold, N. V., and Stovall, W. D.: Cytology screening for uterine cancer through physicians' offices: Report of 65,163 women examined over a period of ten years (1947–1956). J.A.M.A., 168:243, 1958.

Calvo de Mora, S., and Tubio, J.: Screening colposcópia en veintitrés mil enfermas ginecológicas. Communicat. to VII Cong. Nacional de citologia, Seville, 1971.

Carrera, J. M., and Dexeus Trias de Bes, S.: El cuello uterino durante la gestación: Estudio colposcópico, citológico e histológico. Rev. Esp. Obstet. Ginec., 29:401, 1970.

Cartier, R.: Recherches comparatives colpophotographiques et histopathologiques sur les lésions dystrophiques et cancéreuses du col utérin. Gynéc. Obstét., 63:451, 1964.

Christopherson, W. M., and Parker, J. E.: Control of cervix cancer in women of low income in a community. Cancer, 24:64, 1969.

Coppleson, M.: Colposcopy, cervical carcinoma in situ and the gynaecologist: Based on experience with the method in 200 cases of carcinoma in situ. J. Obstet. Gynaec. Brit. Comm., 71:854, 1964.

Coppleson, M., and Reid, B. L.: Preclinical Carcinoma of the Cervix Uteri: Its Origin, Nature and Management. Oxford, Pergamon Press, 1967.

Coupez, F.: La place de la colposcopie dans l'examen gynécologique actuel. Rev. Franç. Gynéc. Obstét., 65:209, 1970.

D'Alessandro, P., Bettocchi, S., and Garulli, R.: L'Adenocarcinoma primitivo della cervice uterina. Quad. Clin. Ostet. Ginec., 20:439, 1965.

de Brux, J., Dupré-Froment, J., and Dexeus, S.: Histomorphologie des carcinomes "épidermoïdes" du col utérin. Gynéc. Obstét., 62:211, 1963.

De Salvia, P., and Centonze, M.: Aspetti citologici dei polipi cervicali e loro modificazioni gravidiche. Minerva Ginec., 14:410, 1962.

de Watteville, H., Geisendorf, W., and Damon, L.: Le diagnostic précoce du cancer du col et son traitement au stade non invasif. Bull. Féd. Soc. Gynéc. Obstét., 4(Suppl. 1): 37, 1952.

Dexeus, S., Jr., and Rawyler, V.: Estudio comparativo de la citología, colposcopia y anatomía pathológica en el diagnóstico precoz del cáncer uterino. Progr. Obstet. Ginec., 5:9, 1962.

Dexeus, S., Jr., Carrera, J. M., Casanelles, R., and Palacin, A.: Screening ginecológico sistemático: Análisis de los resultados. Acta Oncol., 4:283, 1965.

Dexeus, S., Jr., Carrera, J. M., and Palacin, A.: Carcinoma in situ en la vejez. Bol. Asoc. Obstet. Ginec. Acad. Cienc. Med., 1:303, 1966.

Dexeus, S., Jr., Casanelles, R., Carrera, J. M., and Font, V.: La citología y la colposcopia en el diagnóstico precoz del cáncer uterino. Acta Ginec., 19:881, 1968.

Dexeus, S., Jr., Casanelles, F., Carrera, J. M., and Xiol, G.: La cytologie et la colposcopie dans le diagnostic précoce del cancer de l'uterus. Communicat. to S. P. A., 1968.

Dexeus, S., Jr., Palacín, A., Carrera, J. M., and Casanelles, R.: Tumor mesodérmico mixto del cérvix uterino. Acta Ginec., 17:729, 1966.

Dunn, J. E., Jr., and Martin, P. L.: Morphogenesis of cervical cancer. Cancer, 20:1899, 1967.

Esteba Cabellería, J., Usandizaga, J. A., and Mateu Aragonés, J. M.: Pólipos cervicales de tipo angiomatoso. Toko-Ginec. Práct., 22:24, 1963.

Fanghänel, M.: Über das Verhalten und die Rückbildung der Portio vaginalis uteri post partum im kolposkopischen Bild. Zbl. Gynäk., 88: 409, 1966.

Feyrter, F.: Symposium über "Carcinoma in situ" der Nordwestdeutschen Gesellschaft für Gynäkologie in Hamburg. Geburtsh. u. Frauenheilk., 15:869, 1955.

Fioretti, P., Bonzani, A., and Andriani, A.: Associazione dell'esame colposcopico e colpocitologico nella diagnosi precoce del carcinoma del collo dell'utero in gravidanza e puerperio. Arch. Ostet. Ginec., 68:725, 1963.

Fluhmann, C. F.: Mucous polypi of the cervix uteri. Northwest Med., 26:244, 1927.

Ganse, R.: Die Veränderungen der atypischen Gefässe des Portiokarzinoms unter Telecobaltbestrahlung. Geburtsh. u. Frauenheilk., 27:476, 1967.

Ganse, R., Krimmenau, R., and Brey, J.: Papillomatöse Veränderungen der Portio und deren karzinomatöse Potenz. Geburtsh. u. Frauenheilk., 22:232, 1962.

Gerli, M., and Berlingieri, D.: L'impiego associato della colpocitologia e della colposcopica nella diagnosi precoce del cancro del collo dell'utero. Minerva Ginec., 14:539, 1962.

Gilbert, E. F., and Palladino, A.: Squamous papillomas of the uterine cervix: Review of the literature and report of a giant papillary carcinoma. Am. J. Clin. Path., 46:115, 1966.

Gil-Vernet, E., Gil-Vernet, E., Gil-Vernet, L., and Escasany, P.: Estudio de las lesiones displásicas contiguas al carcinoma in situ e invasivo del cuello uterino. Gine. Dips., 10:91, 1970.

González Merlo, J., Montalvo, L., Vilar, E., and Botella, J.: Experiencia de cinco años en el diagnóstico precoz del carcinoma cervical-uterino. Progr. Obstet Ginec., 8:441, 1964.

González Merlo, J., Vilar, E., Sánchez, J., and Silva, V.: Siete años de campaña colposcópica. Communicat. to Sec. Esp. Asoc. Mund. Prev. del Cáncer Ginec., Málaga-Torremolinos, 1966.

Graham, M. R.: The Cytologic Diagnosis of Cancer. 3rd ed. Philadelphia, W. B. Saunders Co., 1972.

Gustowski, A.: The frequency of cancer of the vaginal portion as a complication of the preexisting polypus of the cervix. Ginek. Polska, 34:255, 1963.

Hamperl, H.: Über das infiltrierende (invasive) Tumorwachstum (Untersuchungen am Carcinom und am sog. Carcinoma in situ). Virchows Arch. Path. Anat., 340:185, 1966.

Herovici, C.: Étude de la réaction du tissu conjonctif dans les tumeurs malignes du col utérin. Bull. Assoc. Franç. du Cancer, 50:519, 1963.

Hillemanns, H. G., and Moog, P.: Epithelgrenze und Geburtstrauma. Geburtsh. u. Frauenheilk., 26:519, 1966.

Hillemanns, H. G., and Prestel, E.: Karyometric mit dem Teilchengrössenanalysator (TGZ) am Beispiel des Cervixcarcinoms und seiner Vorstufen. Z. Krebsforsch., 71:316, 1968.

Hillemanns, H. G., and Rha, K.: Die Cytoplasma-Kernrelation bei der Krebsentstehung am Collum uteri. Z. Krebsforsch., 64:262, 1961.

Hillemanns, H. G., Fröhlich, D., and Prestel, E.: Zellzahl und Mitosefrequenz bei Entstehung des Cervixcarcinoms (zum Carcinoma in situ und Mikrocarcinom der Cervix). Arch. Gynäk., 206:292, 1968.

Hinselmann, H.: Diagnose des Portiocarcinoms nebst Frühdiagnose. In Veit-Stoeckel: Handbuch der Gynäkologie, Vol. 6. Munich, Bergmann, 1930.

Hinselmann, H.: Der Nachweis der aktiven Ausgestaltung der Gefässe beim jungen Portiokarzinom als neues differentialdiagnostisches Hilfsmittel. Zbl. Gynäk., 64:1810, 1940.

Israel, S. L.: A study of cervical polyps. Am. J. Obstet. Gynec., 39:45, 1940.

Johnson, L. D.: The histopathological approach to early cervical neoplasia. Obstet. Gynec. Surv., 24:735, 1969.

Kahan, L.: Communication at Third World Congress. Rio de Janeiro, 1968.

Kasdon, S. C., and Bamford, S. B.: Atlas of In Situ Cytology. Boston, Little, Brown and Co., 1962.

Kern, G., and Bötzelen, H.-P.: Kolposkopischer Befund und Lokalisation des Carcinoma in situ. Arch. Gynäk., 194:564, 1961.

Kern, G., Rissmann, E., and Hund, G.: Die Leistungsfähigkeit der Kolposkopie bei der Frühdiagnostik des Collumcarcinoms. Arch. Gynäk., 199:526, 1964.

Khakimova, S., and Petrushkova, N.: The treatment of polyps in the mucosa of the uterine cervix. Zdravookhr. Tadzh., 39:28, 1961.

Kneer, M., and Hillemanns, H. G.: Das Oberflächenkarzinom der Portio uteri. Münch. Med. Wschr., 99:647, 1957.

Koller, O.: The Vascular Patterns of the Uterine Cervix. Oslo, Universitetsforlaget, 1963.

Kolstad, P.: The colposcopical diagnosis of dysplasia, carcinoma in situ, and early invasive cancer of the cervix. Acta Obstet. Gynec. Scand., 43(Suppl. 7):105, 1965.

Koss, L. G., Stewart, F. W., Foote, F. W., Jordan, M. J., Bader, G. M., and Day, E.: Some histological aspects of behavior of epidermoid carcinoma in situ and related lesions of the uterine cervix:

A long-term prospective study. Cancer, 16:1160, 1963.

Limburg, H.: Comparison between cytology and colposcopy in the diagnosis of early cervical carcinoma. Am. J. Obstet. Gynec., 75:1298, 1958.

Limburg, H.: Die Bedeutung des Vaginalabstrichs für die Erkennung des Uteruscarcinoms. Arch. Gynäk., 178:279, 1950.

Manelis, M. E.: The efficacy of colpocervicoscopy in prophylactic examinations. Vop. Onkol., 15:70, 1969.

Mannarino, T., Garcea, N., Larciprete, F., and Bucci, M.: Quadri colposcopici ed aspetti citoistologici del cancro del collo dell'utero radiumtrattato. Clin. Ostet. Ginec., 69:55, 1967.

Martin-Laval, J., and Dajoux, R.: L'endocervicoscopie. Communicat. to Soc. Nat. Gynéc. Obstét. de France, Marseille, 1970.

Masson, P.: Tumeurs Humaines: Histologie, Diagnostics et Techniques, 2nd ed. Maloine, Paris, 1956.

Mateu Aragonés, J. M.: Importancia del cuadro vascular en la exploración colposcópica: Clasificación de las imágenes vasculares. Acta Gynaec. Obstet. Hisp. Lusit., 13:231, 1964.

Mateu Aragonés, J. M.: Significación de las atipias colposcópicas: Consideraciones acerca de la importancia de la colposcopia en el estudio de las imágenes vasculares. Rev. Esp. Obstet. Ginec., 28:473, 1969.

Mateu Aragonés, J. M.: La exploración colposcópica en la práctica ginecológica: Lesiones benignas. Orbe Ginec. Obstet., 19, 1971.

Meigs, J. V.: The cytologic diagnosis of carcinoma of the cervix. Harper Hosp. Bull., 7:275, 1949.

Mestwerdt, G., and Wespi, H. J.: Atlas der Kolposkopie. 3rd ed. Stuttgart, Gustav Fischer, 1961.

Mestwerdt, G.: Enfermedades del hocico de tenca y del cuello uterino. In Schwalm and Döderlein (Eds.): Clínica Obstétrico-Ginecológica, Vol. 5, 1st Edit. Madrid, Editorial Alhambra, 1966.

Mestwerdt, G.: Las displasias del cuello uterino: Límites entre la benignidad y la malignidad. Rev. Esp. Obstet. Ginec., 29:331, 1970.

Moench, G. L.: A consideration of some of the aspects of sterility. Am. J. Obstet. Gynec., 13:334, 1927.

Morales, J. M., González, R., and Torres, C.: La citología vaginal y la colposcopia: Su valor en el diagnóstico del cáncer preclínico del cuello uterino. Prog. Obstet. Ginec., 11:405, 1968.

Navratil, E., Burghardt, E., Bajardi, F., and Nash, W.: Simultaneous colposcopy and cytology used in screening for carcinoma of the cervix. Am. J. Obstet. Gynec., 75:1292, 1958.

Nemes, J., and Farkas, A.: A kolposzkopia és cytológia együttes alkalmazásával elért újabb eredményeink, a méhnyakrák korai kórismézésénél. Magyar Nöorvosok Lapja, 24:148, 1961.

Nieburgs, H. E., and Pund, E. K.: Specific malignant cells exfoliated from preinvasive cancer of the cervix uteri. Am. J. Obstet. Gynec., 58:532, 1949.

Nogales, F., and Botella, J.: Modalidades histogenéticas, histopatológicas, y biopatológicas del carcinoma cervical uterino. Obstet. Ginec. Lat. Amer., 23:89, 1965.

Núñez Montiel, J. T., García Galvé, H., Molina, R.,

and Wenger, F.: Papilomas del cuello uterino. Rev. Obstet. Ginec. Venez., 30:351, 1970.

Núñez Montiel, J. T., Rodriguez-Barboza, J., Molina, R. A., and Gamero, G.: Colposcopic exploration of the endocervix. Prog. Clin. Cancer, 4:203, 1970.

Pardo Vargas, F.: Cancer del cuello uterino: Su pesquisa en 6.427 mujeres. Rev. Colombiana Obstet. Ginec., 17:107, 1966.

Potter, V. R.: New prospects in cancer biochemistry. Adv. Enzyme Regulation, 1:279, 1963.

Richart, R. M., and Barron, B. A.: A follow-up study of patients with cervical dysplasia. Am. J. Obstet. Gynec., 105:386, 1969.

Rodríguez-Soriano, J. A., and Márquez Ramírez, M.: Contribución al estudio de los pólipos cervicales. Toko-Ginec. Práct., 22:9, 1963.

Rutledge, F.: Cancer of the vagina. Am. J. Obstet. Gynec., 97:635, 1967.

Smith, G. V. S., and Pemberton, F. A.: The picture of very early carcinoma of the uterine cervix. Surg. Gynec. Obstet., 59:1, 1934.

Topek, N. H.: Surgical treatment of carcinoma in situ of the cervix. Clin. Obstet. Gynec., 10:853, 1967.

Usandizaga, J. A., Mateu Aragonés, J. M., and Caballería, J. E.: Pólipos del cuello uterino: Ensayo de clasificación histológica. Acta Gynaec. Obstet. Hisp. Lusit., 12:214, 1963.

Wagner, D.: Differential-zytologische Untersuchungen zum Spontanverhalten von atypischem Portioepithel. Geburtsh. u. Frauenheilk., 28:445, 1968.

Wagner, D., and Schlaich, P.: Zur Frage der Rückbildung von atypischem Plattenepithel an der Cervix uteri. Arch. Gynäk., 199:379, 1964.

Walz, W.: Über die Früherfassung des Portiokarzinoms: Ergebnisse aus einem Zeitraum von 5 Jahren. Geburtsh. u. Frauenheilk., 18:243, 1958.

Zerolo Davidson, J. M., and Recaséns, E.: Cancer del cuello uterino (Cádiz, 1960–1965). Acta Ginec., 17:15, 1966.

Zinser, H. K.: Folgerungen aus den Ergebnissen eines zytologischen Karzinom-Such-Programms. Geburtsh. u. Frauenheilk., 25:781, 1965.

Zinser, H. K., and Kern, G.: Kritische Betrachtungen zur Karzinomfrühdiagnostik. Geburtsh. u. Frauenheilk., 18:105, 1958.

Chapter Nine

COLPOSCOPY DURING
PREGNANCY

A discussion of colposcopic findings during pregnancy is of particular importance because, on the one hand, pregnant women are generally examined in a more systematic and complete manner, and on the other hand, the histologic modifications suffered by the pregnant cervix notably transform the colposcopic appearance. It is absolutely necessary to be aware of these transformations in order to avoid misinterpretation. Rather than adding to each chapter a section dedicated to pregnancy, we have undertaken to deal with this topic separately, trying to avoid dispersion of the descriptions, and to assure better comprehension of this important subject.

TECHNIQUE

Even though colposcopic exploration during pregnancy requires no specific precautions, the colposcopist will encounter some special problems. Proper exposure of the cervix and of the vaginal fornices requires a speculum with wide and long valves, because the edema and softening of the vaginal mucosa markedly increase the capaciousness of the organ. Complementary introduction of a lateral retractor or even of a second speculum to retract the vaginal walls may be necessary.

Preparation of the cervix should be very careful, so that its particularly fragile and hemorrhagic mucosa is not damaged. Before the direct examination, the sur-

face of the cervix should be cleaned only with physiologic saline, a fluid which may help dissolve viscous and adhesive mucus. A cotton swab should be used to apply the saline, because gauze compresses are in this case excessively traumatic.

Once the cytologic sample has been taken, the colposcopic examination proceeds in the same phases as in gynecology: direct examination, acetic acid test, and Schiller's test. It is possible to observe any of the lesions studied in the preceding chapters, but these are generally modified by the pregnancy. The edema, ectropion and inflammation will obscure the recognition of some well-known patterns and the identification of others that arise at this time.

During pregnancy, biopsy requires obtaining adequate material without producing hemorrhage. We are satisfied with the O.R.L. universal biopsy forceps and the Krause forceps, but any punch biopsy instrument that is sufficiently fine and sharp may serve perfectly well.

HISTOLOGIC CHANGES

The colposcopic appearance of the cervix during pregnancy is a consequence of the histologic modifications which the cervix undergoes during this period. Although the first histopathologic studies of the pregnant cervix date from 1885 (Bayer), it was not until after World War II that a systematic classification of

235

its morphologic modifications was prepared. At present, the majority of descriptions follow the criteria espoused by Epperson et al., which characterize the cervical histopathology through the study of its three basic elements: epithelium, stroma and glands (Table 64).

Epithelium

The modifications at this level are, undoubtedly, the most important, because they are responsible for the conflicting colposcopic images. The stratified squamous epithelium reacts to the presence of estrogens with a specific hyperactivity. Since these steroids increase the synthesis of DNA and stimulate the metabolism of the basal layers, while an excess of progesterone inhibits cellular maturation, two consequences in the histologic preparation may be observed. The first is a thickening of the epithelium, due to increases in all its layers; the second is basal hyperactivity, characterized by an increase in the number of mitoses and the presence of poorly differentiated cells at the level of the intermediate and superficial layers of the epithelium (Fig. 328).

Other less characteristic histologic findings are the existence of some erosive zones and the presence of columnar epithelium. Jointly with Fernández-Cid, we studied a type of "decidual reaction" that affects only the epithelium. The stroma does not show any decidual transformation (superficial deciduosis) except for the changes of a normal gestation. The epithelial cells suffer considerable hypertrophy at the expense of a perinuclear edema of the cytoplasm, which is reminiscent of the so-called "ballooning degeneration" (Fig. 329).

Stroma

The most characteristic stromal phenomena during pregnancy are increased vascularization, inflammatory infiltration, edema and, above all, the so-called decidual reaction or "decidualization."

Modifications of vascularization appear as soon as the woman becomes pregnant, but initially they are minor, increasing in intensity nearer to term. The vascular network is much denser and the caliber of the vessels is much greater. Visually, the hyperemia is reflected by the congestion, and at times, especially at term, it is converted into a true angiomatous state.

Table 64.   Histologic Modifications Observed in the Gravid Cervix

| | DURING PREGNANCY | | AFTER DELIVERY | |
	Number	Per cent	Number	Per cent
Epithelium				
Basal hyperactivity	13	10	1	3.8
General hyperplasia	38	29.2	3	11.5
Columnar epithelium	27	20.7	5	19.2
Erosive zones	29	22.3	9	34.6
Stroma				
Increased vascularization	27	20.7	3	11.5
Edema	26	20	2	7.6
Decidual reaction	14	10.7	0	0
Leukocytic infiltration	78	60	15	57.6
Glands				
Glandular hyperplasia	59	45.3	9	34.6
Epithelial hyperplasia	14	10.7	2	7.6
Adenomatous hyperplasia	16	12.3	1	3.8
Epidermization (metaplasia)	19	14.6	3	11.5

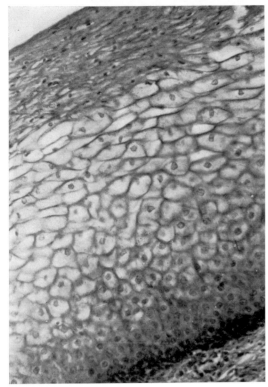

Figure 328. Histologic section of an exocervical mucosa during pregnancy, where increases in the overall width and the basal cell hyperactivity of the epithelium are observed.

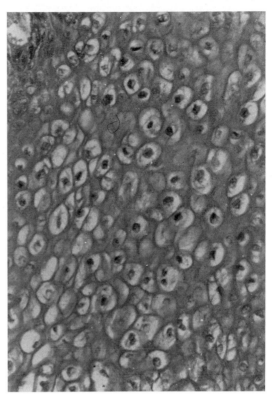

Figure 329. Histology of the so-called superficial or epithelial deciduosis. Observe the hypertrophy of the epithelial cells, due to intracellular edema. The overall appearance notably resembles that of decidua.

Edema of the stroma is persistent and a consequence of the vascular hyperplasia and hypertrophy which are accompanied by an extravascular serous transudation. These phenomena produce a progressive increase in the size of the cervix, which at the time of delivery may have doubled or tripled in volume.

The inflammatory infiltration of a leukocytic type, is also very striking. It is the microscopic equivalent of the frequent infections and dystrophic phenomena which accompany pregnancy.

The decidual reaction or decidualization is the most specific histologic finding of the pregnant cervix, and is of greatest interest to us, because it creates colposcopic images that are totally unknown in gynecology (Fig. 330).

Bayer (1885) was the first to describe the presence of cells similar to those of the decidua in the gravid cervix. Volk, Seitz and Blumberg detailed the histo-

logic appearance of these cells in 1906 and 1907, and after 1945 numerous American papers underlined the frequency of the phenomenon (MacIlrath, Murphy and Herbut, Fluhmann, Epperson, Campos and Soihet, to mention only the better known).

The origin of this "decidualization" has been the subject of various hypotheses and of some experimental papers. It has been deduced that it may be secondary to the transformation of a focus of endometriosis (very rare) or to the evolution of undifferentiated embryonic cells (more frequent).

The incidence of this "deciduosis" is difficult to determine. Bercu-Bardicef, Orr, Russo, Samuel, and others have given figures between 10 and 34 per cent. Colposcopy does not afford any greater precision, because it does not register more than those decidual reactions sufficiently important and close to the sur-

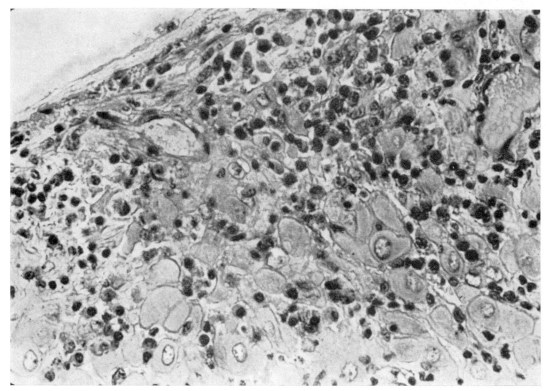

Figure 330. Histologic section of an exocervix bearing an ulcerated deciduosis. An intense decidualization of the stroma is observed, with a practically vanished covering epithelium.

face to modify the appearance of the cervix, something that in our experience occurs in less than 5 per cent of all the cervices examined (Table 14, p. 56).

Glands

Modifications of the glandular component of the cervix are of four types: (1) An increase in the *number* of glands (glandular hyperplasia), which Nesbitt and Hellman observed in 28.7 per cent of cases, Carrow and Gruni in 23 per cent, and we in 45.3 per cent. (2) An increase in the *size* of each gland (glandular hypertrophy), which is usually accompanied by a true adenomatous hyperplasia, whose frequency Nesbitt gives as between 10 and 40 per cent. (3) Hyperplasia of the epithelium that coats the glands. (4) Phenomena of epidermization or squamous metaplasia of the same, from the so-called reserve cells (p. 108).

COLPOSCOPIC APPEARANCES

These will be considered in two categories, according to whether the colposcopic images were nonexistent before the pregnancy and are observed as a consequence of the pregnancy, or whether they are simple modifications of lesions existing before the pregnancy.

New Colposcopic Images in a Previously Normal Cervix. In addition to congestion and general edema, which increase as term approaches, and which give a characteristic red-violet color to the cervix, there are four types of new images that may appear during pregnancy: ectropion (or mechanical ectopy), cystic glandular hypertrophy, deciduosis and polypoid formations.

The *mechanical ectropion* of pregnancy presents some special characteristics. It appears during the first trimester, generally localized to the upper lip.

Its size is moderate and its papillae are relatively regular. However, the most characteristic sign is that its outer edges are ringlike, without any sign of peripheral re-epithelialization or of central metaplastic plaques. The step from squamous to columnar epithelium is abrupt, without a transition zone, and with the limits of the ectropion being especially notable because both epithelia are not at the same level (Fig. 331).

Cystic glandular hyperplasia is also observed during the first months of gestation. It is formed by retention cysts, of mucoid contents and of a translucent or yellowish appearance. Their sizes are variable, even though generally they are not very large. They usually are situated around the cervical os. While in some cases they are not numerous and are localized to a specific part of the cervix, in others they may be seen in considerable numbers and adopt an aspect similar to that of the cystic glandular hypertrophy of the premenopause (Fig. 332).

Deciduosis, in its different types, is the most specific colposcopic lesion of pregnancy. Understanding it is important, because in its ulcerated form it may be the origin of bleeding episodes which can be erroneously attributed to a threatened abortion, or a suspicious cervical lesion.

The appearance of cervical deciduosis depends fundamentally on its histologic base. Hence the lesion will adopt different characteristics according to the depth, density and extent of the underlying lesion and will reflect its influence upon the stratified covering.

Aside from the rare superficial deciduosis, which affects only the covering epithelium (see p. 240), the usual or stromal deciduosis may be classified according to whether the decidual transformation takes place in the normal squamous mucosa, in the columnar mucosa of an ectopy, or in the residua of re-epithelialization (Table 65).

Here we will deal only with the epidermal deciduosis, so called because the decidual cells are situated beneath the stratified epithelium of epidermoid origin. On pages 240 and 245, we will describe the other possibilities. From the colposcopic viewpoint (Bret and Coupez), we distinguish the following varieties:

Flat form. Without preparation, this is manifested by a red congestive zone, poorly demarcated, which turns slightly whitish after the acetic acid test (Fig. 333). Lugol's solution will erase it completely. It is practically level with the undamaged mucosa. When it is associated with a stable atypical scar, problems of differential diagnosis may ensue.

Focal form. This involves a compact and superficial focus of decidual cells that causes a sudden elevation of the epithelium. It does not attract attention because of its size, which is small, but because of its elevation (Fig. 334). Upon direct colposcopic observation it has the

Table 65. Classification of Deciduosis

Deciduosis		Superficial or epithelial	
		Subepidermal	Flat
			Focal
			Ulcerated
			Tumor
	Stromal	Subcolumnar	In an ectopy
			In a polyp
		In the residua of re-epithelialization	

appearance of a congestive entity (Fig. 335). Due to its cellular density, if the surface epithelium is intact, acetic acid modifies it very little, causing only a slight paleness. To the contrary, if the epithelium is missing, then classical "blurring" will appear. For identical reasons focal deciduosis fixes iodine if there are no ulcerations, but is iodine-negative if epithelium is missing.

Tumor form. This type adopts a pseudopolypoid appearance and affects an area near the cervical os (Fig. 336). Its color is reddish or purplish; it fixes iodine only slightly, except where an ulceration exists, in which case it also "blurs" with acetic acid. On occasion it is necessary to differentiate the tumor form of deciduosis from a true polyp (by its site of implantation and the absence of a pedicle), a nabothian cyst modified by pregnancy (by the different vascularization and consistency, and by blurring) and an endometrioma (absence of bleeding, slight congestion). On the other hand, as we have already stated, the coexistence of deciduosis with endometriosis is possible (Bret, Coupez and Grepinet).

Ulcerated form. Usually this evolves from one of the other types. Without preparation its appearance differs very little from that of the others (Fig. 337), but after the acetic acid test, which coagulates its serofibrinous exudate, an image of "white frost" appears and is typical of this lesion. This white spot is at times difficult to distinguish from a stable atypical scar, but generally it has an unmistakeable appearance. Silver nitrate confirms the absence of epithelium at this level. As are all ulcerations, it is iodine-negative and of imprecise and irregular contours.

The *superficial* or *epithelial deciduosis* has the colposcopic appearance of a red congestive zone, which is changed to white after treatment with acetic acid. The lesion resembles polished crystal. Its edges are ill defined, and it tends to be situated in the periphery of an ectopy of pregnancy. Schiller's test is slightly positive.

It is not always easy to distinguish this type of deciduosis from a "stable atypical scar," even though the latter tends to have more precise edges and greater visual density. On the other hand, plaques of deciduosis exhibit glandular orifices, which the atypical re-epithelialization and its sequelae do not.

The *polyp* observed during pregnancy may have originated during the pregnancy or previous to conception. However it must be admitted that these formations are, outside of pregnancy, very rarely observed before the age of 40. It appears that glandular hyperplasia, edema and mechanical ectropion, have been responsible for exteriorizing a hypertrophic strip of endocervix which has changed into a polyp (Fig. 338).

From a colposcopic viewpoint, polyps are almost always mucoid. Acetic acid reveals the classical columnar papillae of an ectopy. Due to its recent exteriorization, it rarely shows metaplastic plaques. Phenomena of decidualization are frequent. Deciduosis of a polyp begins in its most external part in the form of a white spot which extends progressively along the length and width of the polyp, including its pedicle. It may adopt any of the tones of white, from nacreous to ivory (Fig. 339).

It is very important to know this image in order to avoid confusing a polyp with the expulsion of a fragment of decidua, which implies an unhappy prognosis for the incipient gestation (Fig. 341), or with the total or partial necrosis of a polyp. The differential diagnosis is obtained by identifying the pedicle of the polyp, observing that it is smooth and intact, and confirming its implantation in the cervical canal (Fig. 340) by gentle traction. This maneuver is impossible if the lesion is a fragment of decidua, which would come away at the first attempt at traction. In the case of a necrotized polyp, the tissue becomes fragmented by the forceps, the whitish color is dirty, and the surface is very irregular.

Modifications Observed in Lesions Existing Prior to Gestation

Ectopy and Pregnancy. In the course of gestation important colposcopic modifications take place at the level of preexisting ectopies. These are caused by edema of the stroma, glandular hyper-

(*Text continued on page 245*)

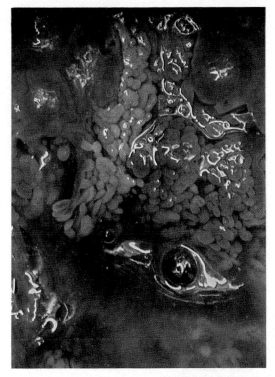

Figure 331. Ectropion of pregnancy, accompanied by an intense cystic glandular hypertrophy of the surrounding metaplastic epithelium.

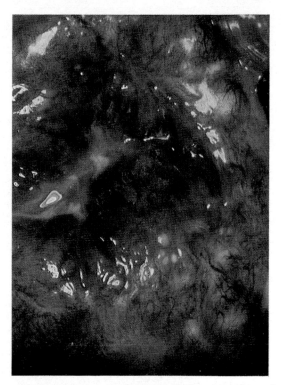

Figure 332. Cystic glandular hypertrophy and hyperplasia at the cervical os. In this case mechanical ectropion does not exist.

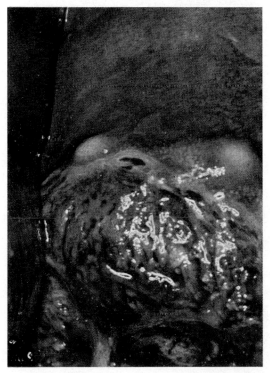

Figure 333. Flat form of deciduosis in the periphery of an ectopy, after the acetic acid test.

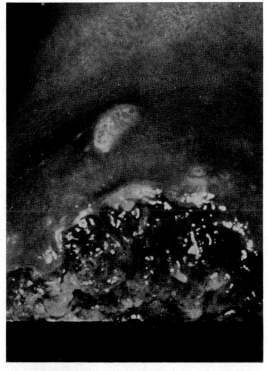

Figure 334. Focal deciduosis, of small size, but forming a marked elevation above the exocervical surface.

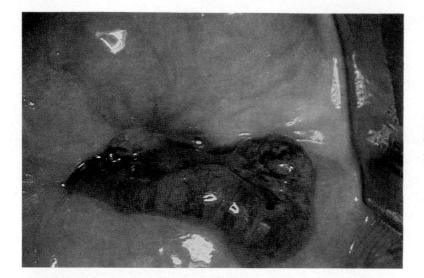

Figure 335. Colposcopy, without preparation, of a focal form of deciduosis. After the test with acetic acid, the reddish congested area turned whitish.

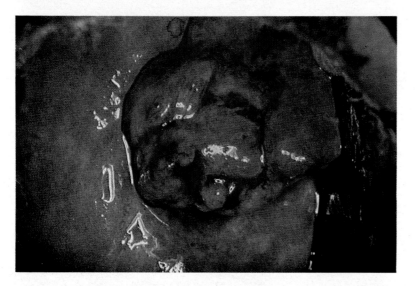

Figure 336. Pseudopolypoid tumor form of a very striking deciduosis.

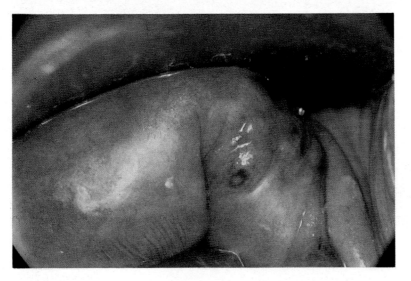

Figure 337. Colposcopy, without preparation, of an ulcerated form of deciduosis.

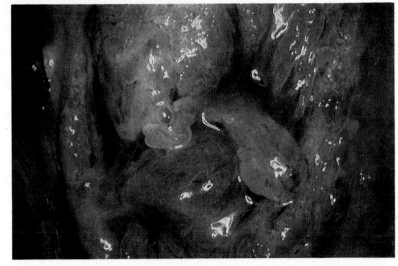

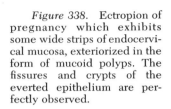

Figure 338. Ectropion of pregnancy which exhibits some wide strips of endocervical mucosa, exteriorized in the form of mucoid polyps. The fissures and crypts of the everted epithelium are perfectly observed.

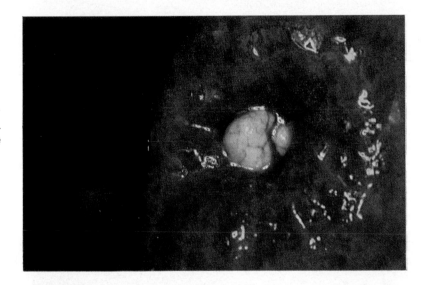

Figure 339. Decidualized polyp with a white nacreous appearance.

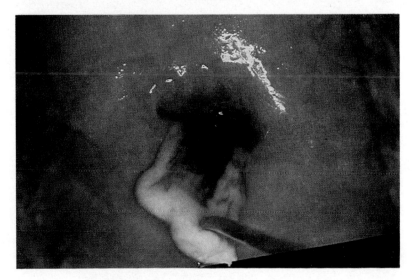

Figure 340. Traction on the polyp reveals a non-decidualized pedicle, which is the clue in its differentiation from decidua.

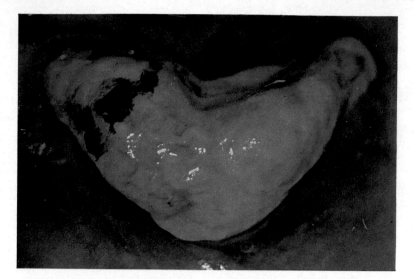

Figure 341. Decidua in the process of expulsion (green filter).

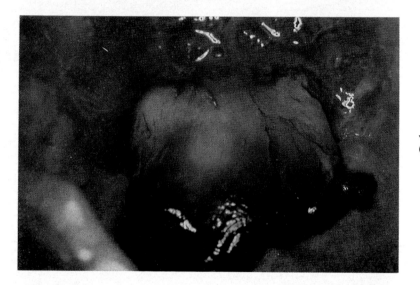

Figure 342. Decidua with necrosis of its extremity (8 months' gestation).

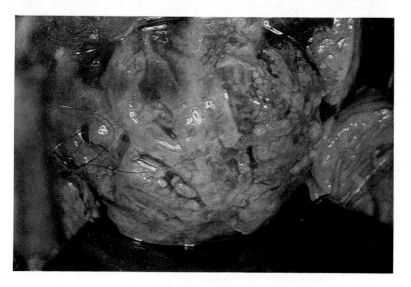

Figure 343. Ectopy existing prior to pregnancy may be so changed during gestation as to suggest a malignant process.

plasia and hypertrophy, and phenomena of decidual transformation. Pregnancy increases the volume of the columnar papillae considerably, to the point of converting them into pseudopolypoid lesions. Infection is also very frequent, and colposcopic observation, already complicated by the presence of a particularly adherent mucus, is made even more difficult by the hemorrhagic fragility of those papillar elements.

The glandular crypts are elongated and deformed, the crevices become deeper and more irregular, and the ectopy may take on a suspicious appearance to one not accustomed to doing colposcopic examinations during this period (Fig. 343). Decidual infiltration beneath columnar epithelium, which is harder to detect than that under stratified epithelium, is transformed after the treatment with acetic acid into white granular prominences of variable size that adorn the ectopy (Fig. 344).

Re-epithelialization is interrupted in ectopy undergoing repair, and generally there is an increase in the area of the ectopy because of ulceration of glandular cysts in its periphery.

The opened glands considerably increase their activity, which explains the crumbling of the zones of re-epithelialization of which they form part. The epithelium is destroyed by maceration (increased secretion of the glandular elements) and ulceration (bursting of glandular cysts). If a strong decidual reaction is added to this picture, with the appearance of whitish plaques of poorly defined contours, the ectopy may be difficult to distinguish from an atypical transformation.

Atypical Re-epithelialization and Pregnancy. Gestation may considerably change the appearance of the evolving or residual atypical re-epithelialization. Edema and congestion almost always modify the external contour of these lesions, causing the loss of sharpness in the colposcopic view. The appearance of some congestive plaques and the phenomena of basal hyperplasia made evident by whitish zones, may lead to a suspicious diagnosis (Fig. 345). Growth of an ectopy may add to the changes at the edge of an atypical re-epithelialization,

making it difficult to spot. For the same reason a stable atypical scar may come to resemble a zone of re-epithelialization, because it has become juxtaposed with a recently exteriorized plaque of columnar epithelium (Fig. 346).

For all these reasons, processes considered benign before pregnancy may take on a more serious appearance in the course of pregnancy making histologic and cytologic examination necessary (Fig. 347).

Atypical Transformation and Pregnancy. During pregnancy it is practically impossible to guess the origin and grade of the histologic lesion which constitutes the substrate of a zone of atypical transformation. It may have developed in the course of gestation or it may have existed earlier. Any observed colposcopic lesion may imply a serious histologic atypia or a benign lesion. Only prolonged and careful observation will provide the answer.

From a colposcopic viewpoint, there are no images specific to the atypical transformation of pregnancy. It is always a very complex lesion in which the white spots, mosaic and ground structure are intermingled. Its edges are not sharp, and along with leukokeratotic zones, congestive, erosive or ulcerated areas are observed.

Generally, intense keratinization is not seen; the lesion is usually a simple red zone without preparation, which shows its optical complexity only after treatment with acetic acid (Figs. 348 and 349).

The patterns of circles and drops are frequent and denote the abnormal metaplastic activity of the glandular orifices (Fig. 350). We have often seen, in the midst of many white spots, oval elements limited by a fine red punctation, which are less geometrical than the mosaic structure and notably resemble a mosaic-like vaginitis. Schiller's test, besides demonstrating that the whole lesion is iodine-negative, shows that its true boundaries greatly exceed those indicated by the acetic acid test.

Intraepithelial Carcinoma and Pregnancy. There exist different and controversial viewpoints in regard to the association of in situ carcinoma and pregnancy.

(*Text continued on page 249*)

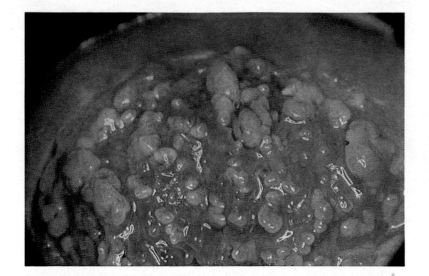

Figure 344. Decidual ectopy. In this case the decidual infiltration is localized to the stroma, situated under the ectopic columnar epithelium. Granules of ectopy have a characteristic whitish color.

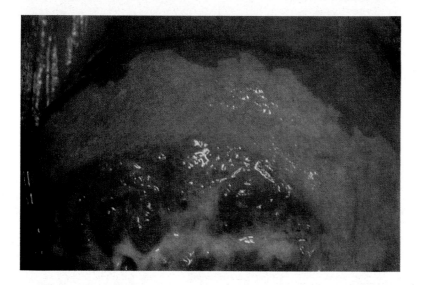

Figure 345. Zone of atypical re-epithelialization driven back toward the periphery by an expanding ectopy of pregnancy. These lesions may lose their sharp edges during gestation and be accompanied by congestive zones which make them suspicious.

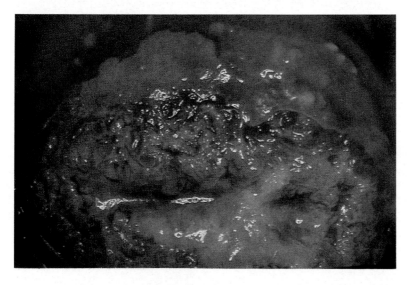

Figure 346. Zone of atypical re-epithelialization, considered as residual and stable before gestation (stable atypical scar), which when repelled by the ectropion of pregnancy takes on the appearance of an evolving atypical re-epithelialization.

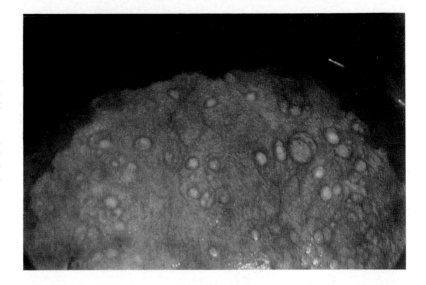

Figure 347. Stable atypical scar, transformed by pregnancy. Its edges have lost sharpness at various points, numerous patterns of circles and drops have appeared, and some congestive areas are seen. The picture leads one to think about a zone of atypical transformation.

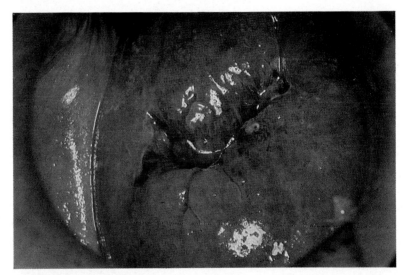

Figure 348. Zone of atypical transformation, seen without preparation. The lesion already existed before the pregnancy and changed very little during gestation. Note that before the acetic acid test it might be mistaken for a common ectopy.

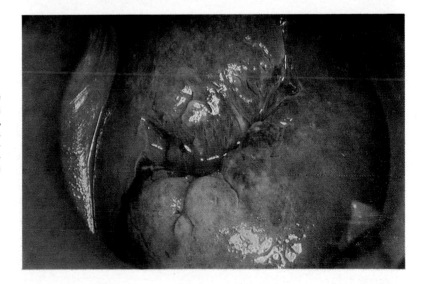

Figure 349. The same zone of atypical transformation seen in the preceding figure, after the acetic acid test. A bizarre admixture of leukokeratotic, congestive and erosive zones, with imprecise contours, is now seen.

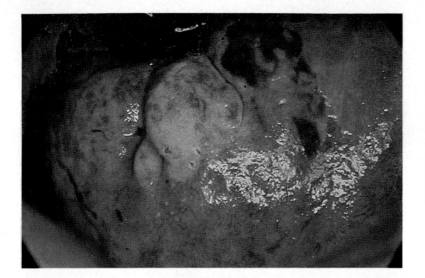

Figure 350. Colpophotograph at high magnification of the lower lip of the cervix, the same one seen in Figures 348 and 349. A great white spot is observed, containing glandular orifices. There are also superimposed images of mosaic structure, red congestive zones, and erosive zones, and imprecise or practically invisible edges.

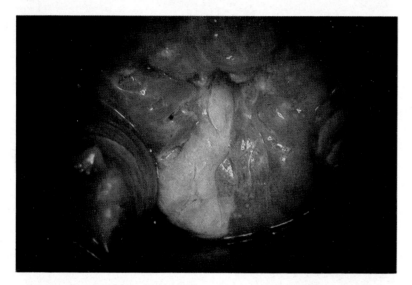

Figure 351. Colposcopic appearance of the zone of atypical transformation corresponding to the histologic lesion of Figure 353. A leukokeratotic plaque is seen with some images of circles and droplets, difficult to see at this magnification. The congestive zones are very subdued and the contours of the lesion are relatively well marked. At this time the gestational age was 35 weeks.

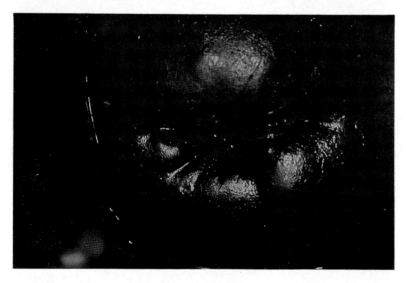

Figure 352. Colposcopic appearance of the same cervix as in the preceding figure, at two years after childbirth, and after the application of Lugol's solution. The lesion, which had been considered to be an intraepithelial carcinoma, has totally regressed. When this examination was performed, the patient was again pregnant (six weeks). Routine histologic studies excluded a "recurrence."

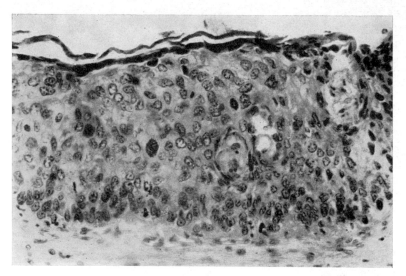

Figure 353. Histologic section of a zone of atypical transformation, discovered in the course of the third month of gestation. The diagnosis was intraepithelial carcinoma.

The impossibility of establishing common criteria arises from the following facts:

1. There is no common histologic nomenclature. Each author's concept of any given atypia incorporates some morphologic characteristics which do not correspond with those included by others.

2. Investigators do not hesitate to give a lesion another name if it evolves in some way other than had been assumed at first examination.

3. There is a tendency to eliminate by conization many of the atypical lesions discovered during gestation, and this obviously impedes follow-up.

4. Few investigators have used colposcopy to follow the course of cervical atypia, whereas this would permit serial biopsies under perfect control.

Experience accumulated over more than 17 years by one of us (Coupez) in the study of gestational cervical atypias as related to intraepithelial carcinoma by means of colposcopic, cytologic and histologic observations, suggests that there are three pathogenetic possibilities:

1. The lesion existed prior to pregnancy, and no important histologic modifications are produced as a consequence of pregnancy.

2. The lesion existed prior to pregnancy but is aggravated by pregnancy, though the histologic substrate continues substantially unmodified.

3. The lesion appears for the first time in the course of the pregnancy.

The first possibility explains the existence, during pregnancy, of zones of atypical transformation, with the same colposcopic characteristics as in nonpregnant women. These are generally extensive lesions, with a tendency toward leukoplastic keratinization. Histologically they are almost always well differentiated.

If the second situation is present, the most common colposcopic appearance is that of a "transformed dysplastic scar." Although red congestive, erosive and even ulcerated zones are observed, the contours of the lesion continue to be clear-cut. Histologically, basal cell hyperplasia which ascends unchanged to the last epithelial layers is usually diagnosed; only in the uppermost layers is maturation encountered.

Lastly, when the carcinoma has originated during pregnancy, it may adopt the appearance of an atypical re-epithelialization (with relatively sharp edges and situated in the margins of an ectopy) or of an incipient atypical transformation. This may take the form of "white drops" and extends from the ectopic glandular orifices or from homogeneous white plaques that originate around the transition zone. The histologic substrate is variable, but there is never a mature and well differentiated epithelium.

EVOLUTION OF THE LESIONS AFTER DELIVERY

The evolution of cervical lesions that are developed or aggravated by gestation is reversed in postpartum uterine involution. As is logical, it is conditioned by the abrupt change in hormone levels and the return to the histologic conditions that prevail in the nonpregnant woman. In three or four weeks the modifications of the stroma, the glandular epithelium and the stratified epithelium will have disappeared and the cervix will present only the sequelae of delivery and images of regressing changes of pregnancy.

Of all the lesions appearing for the first time during pregnancy, deciduosis is the first to disappear. Generally it does not leave any signs, but decidualized endometriosis returns to its original colposcopic appearance.

Cystic glandular hypertrophy also disappears rapidly and is usually not visible at the postpartum examination. Mechanical ectropian generally regresses in two to three months following delivery. However, if the ectropion is of considerable size and there is notable local infection, a definitive exteriorization of the squamo-columnar transitional zone may be produced.

Ectopy existing prior to and aggravated by pregnancy seldom resumes its prior appearance. Although the exuberance and size of the papillae are notably reduced, the dimensions of the lesion diminish very slowly, especially when the phenomena of normal re-epithelialization are not initiated until several months after delivery. However, any problems of identification which may have arisen during gestation disappear.

Atypical re-epithelializations, like dysplastic scars, quickly resume their previous appearance. In six to eight weeks after childbirth, the superimposed congestive zones have disappeared and the lesions once more have precise boundaries.

Due to the trauma of childbirth and the subsequent local infections, many of these lesions completely disappear within two weeks after delivery.

Evolution of Suspicious Lesions after Delivery

To be considered here are those lesions, supposedly related to intraepithelial carcinoma, in which we have recognized three evolutional possibilities (p. 249). Atypical lesions observed during gestation, but which existed prior to pregnancy, should not be expected to regress after delivery. We have had the opportunity to follow two lesions of this type which colposcopically adopted the form of an atypical transformation (white spots with superimposed images, visible only after treatment with acetic acid, accompanied by red congestive and erosive zones, without sharp edges). After childbirth, the lesions persisted practically unmodified, but they tended to ascend within the endocervical canal, which obliged us to intervene.

Lesions existing prior to pregnancy (generally atypical re-epithelializations of the residual type), but apparently aggravated by pregnancy, tend to resume their previous colposcopic characteristics after delivery. Through colposcopy we have observed three lesions considered to be in situ carcinoma. Each was a transformed dysplastic scar. Less than five months after delivery, the colposcopic appearance had lost all signs of aggressivity, the lesions had recovered their sharp outlines, and the congestive or erosive areas had disappeared. Cytologic study then revealed the Papanicolaou's Class II and biopsy showed benign regular dysplasia on histologic examination.

Lastly, one has to be equally prudent in the face of a diagnosis of assumed in situ carcinoma, developed during pregnancy, with the colposcopic appearance of a re-epithelialization or atypical transformation. Generally these are lesions that existed prior to pregnancy. The infection which accompanies gestation provides them with the characteristics of a long-standing lesion (Figs. 351 and 352). The eight cases which we have been able to observe rapidly regressed after delivery, and their disappearance was complete from colposcopic, cytologic and histologic viewpoints.

In conclusion, it is difficult to predict the evolution of a serious epithelial lesion discovered during pregnancy. In our opinion, regression is the rule in the case of formed atypias, or those aggravated by stimuli of pregnancy. Identification of this characteristic is difficult, but it is possible when certain colposcopic images are observed (modified dysplastic scar or atypical re-epithelialization of ectropion). In other cases only careful observation after delivery, using colposcopy simultaneously with cytology and histology, will permit us to reach a valid conclusion. The duration of these observations should not exceed three months for those lesions that do not improve substantially after delivery. In effect, we have proved that regressions (colposcopic, histologic and cytologic) are always produced before that time and that only transformed dysplastic scars may need a longer period to attain complete histologic normalization. Persistence of histologic and cytologic alterations beyond that time should oblige one to abandon the expectant management, even though colposcopy demonstrates a certain regression.

We have followed 18 patients with these characteristics, one of them involuntarily, for five years. On two occasions we observed an invasive carcinoma, at eight months and five years after childbirth.

MANAGEMENT

From the known evolution of lesions discovered in the course of pregnancy, the proper approach to management follows logically. Deciduous, mechanical ectropions and the majority of the polypoid formations regress after childbirth. The other lesions of a benign type (aggravated ectopy, atypical re-epithelialization and stable atypical scar) will recover their earlier characteristics, and management will be the same as under "normal" (nonpregnant) conditions (see the respective chapters).

If a suspicious lesion has been diagnosed, and if the histopathologic diagnosis of severe dysplasia or intraepithelial carcinoma has been made after delivery, three situations are possible.

1. The lesion has totally regressed. In this case we recommend combined cytologic and colposcopic examination every six months for two years, and then annually.

2. The lesion has regressed histologically (simple dysplasia), but colposcopically continues to show a stable atypical scar. We recommend destruction by electrocoagulation after six months of regularly benign cytology.

3. The lesion has not regressed, either histologically or cytologically, after three months. It is prudent to perform an amputation of the cervix, with serial histologic study, despite the fact the colposcopic report tends to improve.

REFERENCES

Bercu-Bardicef, L., Luca, V., and Pascu, F.: Deciduoza colului uterin. Obstet. si Ginec., 9:449, 1962.

Berger, J., and Gruninger, B.: L'évolution des atypies aggravées au niveau du col utérin décelées "in graviditate." Gynéc. Obstét., 58:168, 1959.

Boutselis, J. G., and Ullery, J. C.: Intraepithelial carcinoma of the cervix in pregnancy. Am. J. Obstet. Gynec., 90:593, 1964.

Bret, J.: Expulsion de caduque au cours de la grossesse: Aspect colposcopique. Rev. Franç. Gynéc. Obstét., 54:227, 1959.

Bret, J., and Coupez, F.: Cancer du col et grossesse: Corrélations cytologiques et colposcopiques. Rev. Franç. Gynéc. Obstét., 52:177, 1957.

Bret, J., and Coupez, F.: Role de la colposcopie dans le dépistage du cancer du col au cours de la grossesse. Semaine Hôpitaux Paris, 33:4241, 1957.

Bret, J., and Coupez, F.: Colposcopy on normal and abnormal cervices during pregnancy and the postpartum period. Acta Cytol., 3:61, 1959.

Bret, J., and Coupez, F.: A propos du carcinome in situ au cours de la grossesse: Régression des dysplasies cervicales suspectes (Évolution clinique. Aspects colposcopiques). Gynéc. Obstét., 59:538, 1960.

Bret, J., Coupez, F., and de Brux, J.: Déciduose du col utérin: Aspects cliniques et colposcopiques. Gynéc. Obstét., 58:199, 1959.

Campos, J., and Soihet, S.: Histologic changes in the uterine cervix during pregnancy and the diagnosis of carcinoma in situ. Surg. Gynec. Obstet., 102:427, 1956.

Carrera, J. M., and Dexeus Trias de Bes, S.: El cuello uterino durante la gestación: Estudio colposcópico, citológico e histológico. Rev. Esp. Obstet. Ginec., 29:401, 1970.

Coupez, F.: Endométriose du col utérin. Entretiens Bichat Gynéc., 287, 1966.

Coupez, F.: Col et grossesse. Entretiens Bichat Gynéc., 331, 1969.

Danforth, D. N.: The squamous epithelium and squamocolumnar junction of the cervix during pregnancy. Am. J. Obstet. Gynec., 60:985, 1950.

de Brux, J., and Dupré-Froment, J.: La régression des lésions cervicales au cours de la grossesse (Étude histologique et cytologique). Gynéc. Obstét., 59:566, 1960.

de Brux, J., Panopoulos, C., and Coupez, F.: Morphologie et évolution de 106 atypies cervicales observées au cours de 12.300 grossesses. Rev. Franç. Gynéc. Obstét., 66:671, 1971.

Epperson, J. W. W., Hellman, L. M., Galvin, G. A., and Busby, T.: The morphological changes in the cervix during pregnancy, including intraepithelial carcinoma. Am. J. Obstet. Gynec., 61:50, 1951.

Fanghänel, M.: Über das Verhalten und die Rückbildung der Portio vaginalis uteri post partum im kolposkopischen Bild. Zbl. Gynäk., 88:409, 1966.

Fioretti, P., Bonzani, A., and Andriani, A.: Associazione dell'esame colposcopico e colpocitologico nella diagnosi precoce del carcinoma del collo dell'utero in gravidanza e puerperio. Arch. Ostet. Ginec., 68:725, 1963.

Fluhmann, C. F.: The histogenesis of squamous cell metaplasia of the cervix and endometrium. Surg. Gynec. Obstet., 97:45, 1953.

Gabriel, H., Gilli, J.: Verrier, J. P.: Esai de dépistage systématique du cancer du col utérin en début de grossesse. Rev. L. An. Méd., 12:809, 1965.

Galloway, C. E.: The cervix in pregnancy. Am. J. Obstet. Gynec., 59:999, 1950.

Gil-Vernet, E., Alvarez Zamora, L., Terrades Balet, J., Fortuny Estivill, A., and Royo Tomás, J.: Modificaciones epiteliales atípicas de la portio en las embarazadas. Toko-Ginec. Práct., 22:101, 1963.

González Merlo, J., Jiñuelas, S., and Montalvo, L.: Estudio citológico de las atipias epiteliales del embarazo. Toko-Ginec. Práct., 23:371, 1964.

Greene, R. R., and Peckham, B. M.: Preinvasive cancer of the cervix and pregnancy. Am. J. Obstet. Gynec., 75:551, 1958.

Hamperl, H., Kaufmann, C., and Ober, K. G.: Histologische Untersuchungen an der Cervix schwangerer Frauen. Arch. Gynäk., 184:181, 1954.

Hayden, G. E.: Carcinoma of the cervix associated with pregnancy. Am. J. Obstet. Gynec., 71:780, 1956.

Hinde, F. C.: Cervical biopsy in pregnancy. J. Obstet. Gynaec. Brit. Comm., 71:707, 1964.

Jones, E. G., Schwinn, C. P., Bullock, W. K., Varga, A., Dunn, J. E., and Buell, P.: Carcinoma of the cervix uteri during pregnancy: A study of the combined effect of a trichomonacide, a broad-spectrum antibiotic, and a long-acting progestin on dysplasia and in situ carcinoma of the cervix. Am. J. Obstet. Gynec., 89:285, 1964.

Jones, E. G., Varga, A., Leff, J. G., Schwinn, C. P., Slate, W. G., Wargin, J. T., and Bullock, W. K.: Efficiency of multiple biopsy for cancer detection during pregnancy: A progress report. Obstet. Gynec., 26:70, 1965.

Kaplan, A. L., and Kaufman, R. H.: Diagnosis and management of dysplasia and carcinoma in situ of the cervix in pregnancy. Clin. Obstet. Gynec., 10:871, 1967.

Lepage, F., and Schramm, B.: La déciduose du col de l'utérus. Gynéc. Obstét., 54:550, 1955.

Masin, M., and Masin, F.: Desorption technic in differential diagnosis of cervical dysplasias during pregnancy and post partum. Acta Cytol., 9:213, 1965.

Molitor, K.: Uteruskarzinom und Gravidität. Zbl. Gynäk., 86:54, 1964.

Moore, J. G., Wells, R. G., and Morton, D. G.: Management of superficial cervical cancer in pregnancy. Obstet. Gynec., 27:307, 1966.

Moreno, L.: El cuello uterino durante el embarazo. Rev. Obstet. Ginec. Venez., 24:21, 1964.

Moreno Navarro, J., and Torres, A.: Aspectos colposcópicos de la portio gestante. Toko-Ginec. Práct., 22:62, 1963.

Murphy, E. J., and Herbut, P. A.: The uterine cervix during pregnancy. Am. J. Obstet. Gynec., 59:384, 1950.

Nesbitt, R. E. L., Jr.: Benign cervical changes in pregnancy. Clin. Obstet. Gynec., 6:381, 1963.

O'Leary, J. A., Munnell, E. W., and Moore, J. G.: The changing prognosis of cervical carcinoma during pregnancy. Obstet. Gynec., 28:460, 1966.

Orr, C. J. B., and Pedlow, P. R. B.: Deciduosis of the cervix manifesting as antepartum hemorrhage and simulating carcinoma. Am. J. Obstet. Gynec., 82:884, 1961.

Peckham, B., Greene, R. R., Chung, J. T., Bayly, M. A., and Benaron, H. B. W.: Epithelial abnormalities of the cervix during pregnancy. Am. J. Obstet. Gynec., 67:21, 1954.

Peterson, W. F., Stauch, J. E., Toth, B. N., and Robinson, L. M.: Routine vaginal examinations during labor: A comparative study with bacteriological analysis. Am. J. Obstet. Gynec., 92:310, 1965.

Probst, R. E., and Mier, T. M.: First trimester pregnancy and carcinoma of the cervix. Missouri Med., 61:446, 1964.

Reagan, J. W., Bell, B. A., Neuman, J. L., Scott, R. B., and Patten, S. F.: Dysplasia in the uterine cervix during pregnancy: An analytical study of the cells. Acta Cytol., 5:17, 1961.

Richart, R. M.: Cervical neoplasia in pregnancy: A series of pregnant and postpartum patients followed without biopsy or therapy. Am. J. Obstet. Gynec., 87:474, 1963.

Richart, R. M., and Barron, B. A.: A follow-up study of patients with cervical dysplasia. Am. J. Obstet. Gynec., 105:386, 1969.

Roddick, J. W., Jr., and Crossen, P. S.: Invasive carcinoma of the cervix complicated by pregnancy. South. Med. J., 59:417, 1966.

Russo, A., and Macchioni, B.: La deciduosi del collo dell'utero: Contributo colposcopico. Minerva Ginec., 14:1128, 1962.

Samuel, S.: Sulla deciduosi della portio uterina: Problema di diagnosi differenziale con il cancro. Riv. Ostet. Ginec., 18:346, 1963.

Schmitz, H. E., Isaacs, J. H., and Fetherston, W. C.: The value of routine cytologic smears in pregnancy. Am. J. Obstet. Gynec., 79:910, 1960.

Sénèze, J., Wolff, J. P., and de Ikonicoff, L. K.: Cancer du col et grossesse: A propos de 28 cas. Gynéc. Obstét., 65:13, 1966.

Stone, M. L., Weingold, A. B., and Sall, S.: Cervical carcinoma in pregnancy. Am. J. Obstet. Gynec., 93:479, 1965.

Suppi, G.: Il problema diagnostico dell'epithelioma iniziale del collo dell'utero in gravidanza. Ann. Ostet. Ginec., 88:33, 1966.

Wada, T., and Imamura, Y.: Metaplastic epithelial changes in the cervix of pregnant uterus. Clin. Gynec. Obstet. (Tokyo), 15:505, 1961.

Waldrop, G. M., and Palmer, J. P.: Carcinoma of the cervix associated with pregnancy. Am. J. Obstet. Gynec., 86:202, 1963.

Wied, G. L.: Epithelial abnormalities on the ectocervix during pregnancy (Symposium). J. Reprod. Med., 4:1, 1970.

Williams, T. J., and Brack, C. B.: Carcinoma of the cervix in pregnancy. Cancer, 17:1486, 1964.

Youssef, A. F., and Fayad, M. M.: The post-partum vaginal smear. J. Obstet. Gynaec. Brit. Comm., 70:32, 1963.

Chapter Ten

PRACTICAL
COLPOSCOPY

In the course of this last chapter we wish to summarize, in a practical and schematic manner, the different stages of the colposcopic examination applied to the most frequent cervical findings. We will not review all of the colposcopic problems already studied, nor will we list their morphologic details. Our purpose here is only to introduce the reader to a system which has given us consistently good results.

To review the fundamental steps of the colposcopic examination:

1. Successive observations first without preparation, then after the acetic acid test, and subsequently after the application of Lugol's solution.

2. Identify all the visible patterns on the exocervix, the cervical os and, when possible, the inferior portion of the endocervical canal.

3. Arrive at a diagnosis, endeavoring to incorporate the various images observed within a well defined picture (ectopy in the course of typical re-epithelialization, zone of atypical re-epithelialization, stable atypical scar, etc.).

4. For practical purposes, classify the lesion as benign (well identified), doubtful or suspicious (unidentifiable).

5. Decide upon a course of therapy: (a) None required if the lesion is recognized as benign and asymptomatic. (b) Immediate therapy if it is a benign lesion, but produces symptoms. (c) Hormonal, antibacterial or mixed treatment, with follow-up examinations, if the lesion is doubtful. (d) Immediate cytologic and histologic investigation if the colposcopic picture is suspicious or identifiable only with difficulty.

Table 66.   Examination of a Clinically Normal Cervix

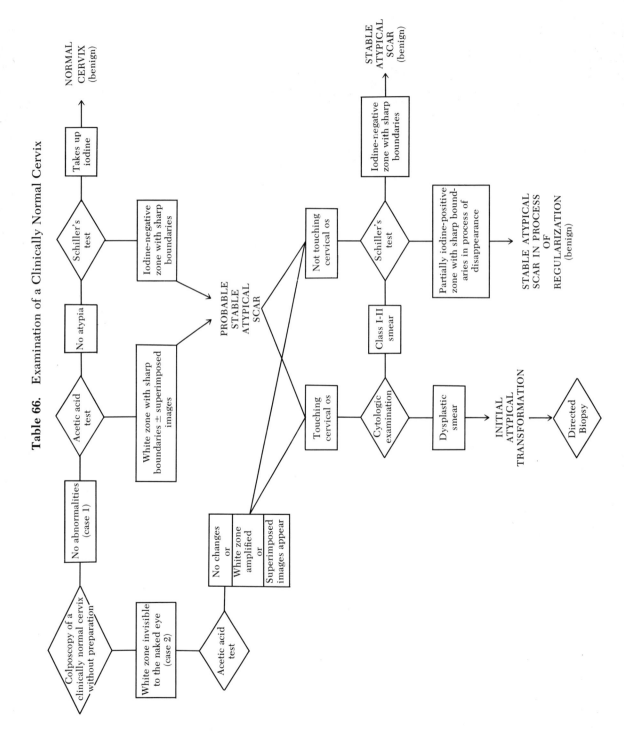

EXAMINATION OF A CLINICALLY NORMAL CERVIX

CASE 1

After colposcopic examination without preparation, the exocervix and the cervical os do not show any anomalies, and the acetic acid test is done.

A. *No atypia appears.*

In this case it is necessary to apply Lugol's solution, which may reveal (1) a totally iodine-positive cervix up to the squamo-columnar zone of transition, in other words a normal exocervix (p. 15), or (2) a cervix with a zone that does not fix iodine, or that fixes it in an irregular manner, signifying residual atypical re-epithelialization. If an area is frankly iodine-negative, with sharp edges, it is a stable atypical scar (p. 160). If, on the contrary, it takes up iodine only partially, the description is "atypical scar in the process of regularization," which invariably has a benign character (p. 161).

B. *A white zone is discovered*, with clear-cut outlines, sometimes with superimposed images of mosaic or ground structure. This is undoubtedly a stable atypical scar. The visual intensity of the lesion depends on the grade of parakeratosis of the superficial cellular layers. Schiller's test shows it to be iodine-nega-

tive. It may be considered benign if it does not touch the zone of squamo-columnar junction. If it does not encroach upon this transitional area, and especially if it involves the endocervix, it cannot be considered a stable lesion, and cytologic or histologic examination is necessary before treatment (p. 160).

CASE 2

Examination of the unprepared cervix reveals a discrete white zone, with sharp boundaries, and sometimes with superimposed images. The acetic acid test is done.

The appearance of the lesion may be the same, or its characteristics may be better evaluated, or new whitish zones, formerly invisible, are observed. Schiller's test will exactly establish the limits of the atypia. The degree of visual intensity enables a judgment of its superficial keratosis or parakeratosis. If it is not accompanied by any red zone, and is separated from the anatomical cervical os, it should be considered as a stable atypical scar. However, just as was indicated in Case 1, it should be submitted, prior to its destruction, to a cytologic or histologic examination.

Table 67.   Examination of a Cervix that Presents a Red Zone at Clinical Examination

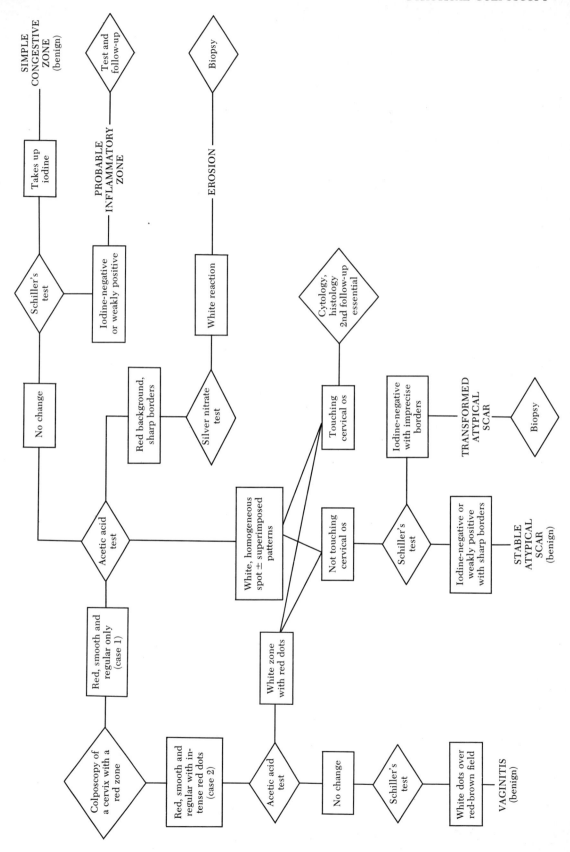

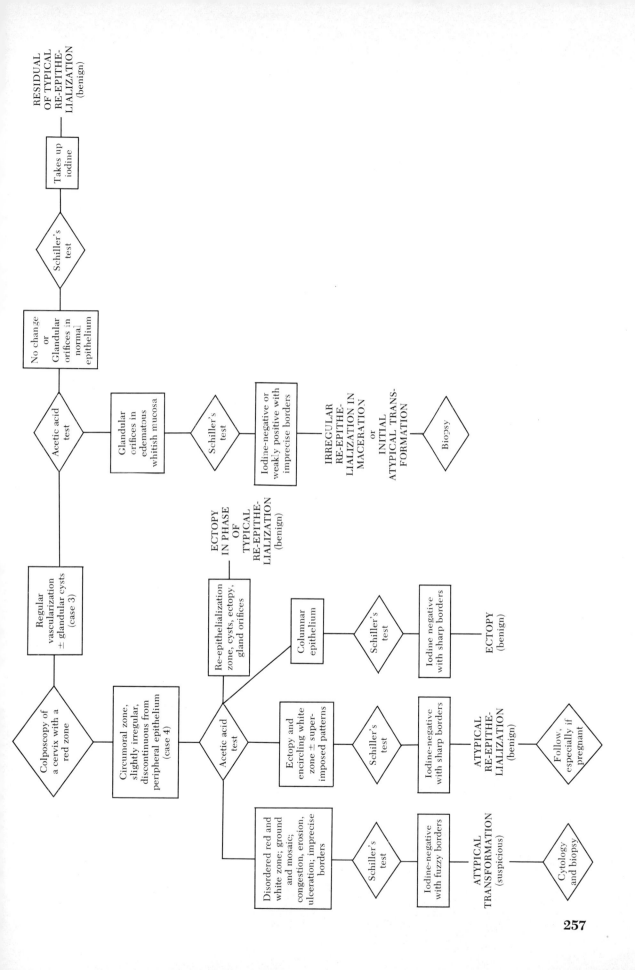

COLPOSCOPY OF A CERVIX THAT PRESENTS A RED ZONE AT CLINICAL EXAMINATION

CASE 1

The clinical examination and direct colposcopy both demonstrate a smooth and regular red zone, without distinguishing characteristics. The acetic acid test offers several possibilities.

A. *No changes are observed,* in which case Schiller's test may demonstrate (1) that the lesion takes up iodine normally and is a simple congestive zone, a well identified and benign lesion (p. 42), or (2) that it is iodine-negative, or takes up iodine very faintly. This may be an inflammatory lesion, which demands adequate treatment and later re-examination (p. 31).

B. *Clear edges of the red zone are revealed.* The silver nitrate test should be performed; if a whitish reaction appears, denudation of the stroma is confirmed. As this image is compatible with diverse colposcopic types of lesions, the tissue should be studied cytologically and histologically (p. 42). Even when these examinations are negative, repeat examinations are recommended after adequate treatment.

C. A white spot appears, either homogeneous or with superimposed images. If after Schiller's test the lesion irregularly fixes iodine and some precise limits are observed, the diagnosis of congestive atypical scar in the process of regularization may be entertained. This is a benign lesion (p. 161). On the other hand, if the lesion is frankly iodine-negative and its contours are very clear, it is a congestive atypical scar. It is a benign lesion that may be subjected to treatment without further examinations, if it does not touch the cervical os. On the contrary, it requires microscopic studies if it is in contact with the os, or lies partly within the endocervix.

CASE 2

A smooth and regular red zone has no particular characteristics at the clinical examination, but demonstrates intense red dots at the colposcopic examination without preparation.

A. *Few changes are observed upon application of acetic acid.*

In this case Lugol's solution will demonstrate that the zone totally or partially takes up iodine and that it appears littered with white dots, which stand out very well over a brown-red background. This is vaginitis (p. 31), a well identified and benign lesion.

B. *A white zone appears, splotched with red dots.*

If Schiller's test shows the whole zone to be iodine-negative with blurred outlines, the lesion is established as ground structure on a congestive, atypical scar. This lesion falls into the "doubtful" category and demands cytologic and histologic study in any case, and particularly if it is near the cervical os. On the contrary, if silver nitrate demonstrates a sharp-edged lesion, microscopic examination is necessary only if the zone is near the os.

CASE 3

A smooth and regular red zone with atypical vessels and glandular cysts is found at the colposcopic examination without preparation.

After the acetic acid test the following may be observed.

A. *No variation.* In this case, Schiller's test will demonstrate that the whole zone uniformly takes up iodine, and the lesion is the glandular and vascular sequel of an old typical re-epithelialization (p. 106). This is a benign and well identified lesion.

B. *Glandular orifices appear upon an apparently normal mucosa.* The whole zone is iodine-positive, except around the glandular orifices, where iodine-negative circles appear. This is also the sequel of a typical re-epithelialization (p. 114) and is equally benign.

C. *Glandular orifices appear in the midst of an edematous mucosa, more or less whitish, without precise limits.*

If iodine negativity or only weak positivity can be shown in the whitish zones lacking sharp outlines, an irregular re-epithelialization in maceration must be suspected (p. 122). Because the diagnosis is not certain and this lesion may be mistaken for an initial atypical transformation, cytologic and histologic study is obligatory.

CASE 4

A circumoral red zone, of slightly irregular surface, in evident discontinuity with the stratified epithelium of the rest of the exocervix.

The examination without preparation on occasion permits the observation of some papillar elements within the cervical mucus. Positive identification is not always possible. With the acetic acid test, the colposcopic observation may discover:

A. *A plaque of columnar papillae, in the form of a bunch of grapes, which may adopt one of two appearances.* The first is ectopy directly limited by a stratified epithelial edge. Schiller's test confirms the location of the interepithelial line. The lesion in this case is an ectopy in its purest form, with no reparative tendency (p. 81). This is a well defined and benign lesion.

The second form is ectopy bordered by a whitish opalescent zone, which separates it from the normal stratified epithelium. In its interior, glandular orifices, islets of ectopy and retention cysts, are seen. The diagnosis is ectopy in the course of typical re-epithelialization (p. 94). Lugol's solution confirms the finding and will demonstrate the irregular and fragile margins of the lesion.

If that white zone is narrow, such as a slender strip in the periphery of the ectopy, it is due to the fact that the process of re-epithelialization is just beginning. If, on the contrary, it is wide, with central metaplastic plaques, the re-epithelialization is in a more advanced stage. Finally, if the ectopic plaque is in juxtaposition to the anatomic cervical os, re-epithelialization is in its terminal phase (p. 112). In all cases this is a well identified and benign lesion.

B. *Appearance of two totally different images*, one plaque of ectopy encircling the os and one or more white spots in the periphery of the ectopy. The appearance of the spot is homogeneous or includes pictures of ground or mosaic structure. While its boundaries with the rest of the squamous epithelium of the exocervix are sharp and definite, the boundaries with the ectopy are less evident. Such spots may occupy one or more sectors of the outer edge of the ectopy.

Schiller's test will be negative, for both the ectopy and the white spots. The latter are externally limited by a border provided with special sharpness, which contrasts with the poorly defined limits of the zone of normal re-epithelialization. This lesion is an atypical re-epithelialization of the ectopy (p. 146). It is a well identified lesion, of generally benign characteristics, but it should be followed, especially during gestation.

If the white spots are small, and in the periphery of the ectopy, the atypical re-epithelialization is just beginning. If they appear as wide plaques, occupying a good portion of the former red zone, the process is in an advanced phase. And if the ectopy is reduced to the immediate proximity of the os, progressively drowned by the typical and atypical re-epithelialization, it is nearer to the stage of stable atypical scar (p. 154).

C. *The red zone is replaced by an irregular admixture of white spots and red zones.* The white spots are distributed without order, possess a strong visual intensity, and if they present superimposed patterns, the images are very obvious (ground structure in coarse dots; mosaic in elevations limited by a wide vascular network or a fine red punctation).

The glandular orifices are also very visible and are generally accompanied by images of circles or white drops. Their limits are poorly defined.

The red zones are congestive, sometimes erosive, and many times hemorrhagic, lacking the characteristic papillary images of bunches of grapes. They lack sharp margins or limits.

In toto, such a lesion demonstrates no similarity with a pure ectopy, or ectopy in the process of typical or atypical re-epithelialization. It originates at the cervical orifice and does not present any precise delimitation from the normal stratified epithelium.

With Schiller's test, the lesion is iodine-negative, with irregular and fragile contours. The limits now observed very often exceed those of the red zone observed without preparation. The lesion may be identified as a zone of atypical transformation, a highly suspicious lesion

Table 68. Colposcopy of a Cervix with One or Several White Spots Visible at Clinical Examination

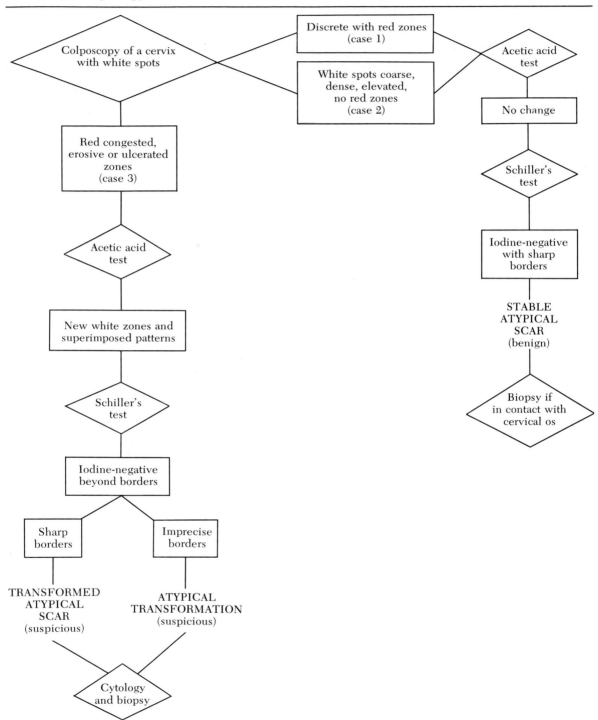

which requires immediate cytologic and histologic study (p. 164).

In some cases acetic acid or Lugol's solution reveals images similar to those described, but situated in the midst of a lesion that has clearly defined limits. This probably is a transformed atypical scar (p. 161). The cause of its transformation (neoplastic process or infection) is not always identifiable by colposcopy, and it should be subjected to microscopic study.

D. *The edges of the irregular red zone are at a different level than the rest of the exocervix.* Careful examination of the red zone cannot demonstrate typical granules of ectopy, and on the other hand, the edges of the zone are much more evident than those of a true erosion. The silver nitrate test is positive, while Lugol's solution demonstrates the iodine negativity of the lesion and its accentuated limits. This is an ulceration that leaves the stroma exposed. It is a difficult lesion to identify etiologically, and it requires biopsy (p. 42).

COLPOSCOPY OF A CLINICALLY VISIBLE WHITE SPOT OR AN AGGREGATE OF WHITE SPOTS

CASE 1

The white spots are small and are not accompanied by any congestive, erosive or ulcerated red zone.

The examination without preparation immediately identifies a glandular (nabothian) cyst or a trickle of adherent mucus. It also verifies the absence of vascular irregularities and shows that the white spots are clearly visible modifications of the stratified mucosa: loss of its smooth and usually brilliant appearance, and the adoption of a granular and dull elevation. Eventually it is also possible to observe pictures of mosaic or ground structure.

The acetic acid test does not modify the visible lesion but enhances its contours and may cause the appearance of new white spots with or without superimposed images.

Schiller's test is negative, with precise limits, for all the visible atypias and for all those which appear with the acetic acid test. On some occasions it reveals new iodine-negative or irregular plaques.

Such lesions are stable atypical scars, of benign character (p. 160) and do not require cytologic or histologic examination, unless they are in contact with the endocervix.

CASE 2

The white spots are coarse and dense and show an elevation above the normal exocervical mucosa. They have the characteristics of clinical leukoplakia. No congestive or ulcerated zone accompanies them.

The examination without preparation confirms the absence of vascular irregularities and sometimes reveals other smaller white spots, not visible to the naked eye.

The acetic acid test does not modify the visible lesion but makes its outline more precise and may produce new white spots with or without superimposed patterns.

Schiller's test is totally negative at the level of the white spots. The margins of the lesion, despite the density of the spots, are not very sharp. However, the contours established by Lugol's solution are close to those of the atypia observed without preparation or after the acetic acid test.

These are more or less keratinized stable atypical scars, benign and well identified lesions, which require microscopic examination only if they come into contact with the cervical os (p. 161).

CASE 3

The white spots are accompanied by red zones.

The colposcopic examination without preparation determines the characteristics of the clinical images: the white zones are small or frankly leukoplakic. They have some sharp or irregular boundaries. There exist at times pictures of very accentuated mosaic or ground structure, with vascular punctation. The red zones cannot be characterized in this stage of the examination, but it is the best time to study the visible vascularization. It is possible to observe a range from totally normal vessels with extensive ramifications, as seen in typical re-epithelialization, up to very atypical vessels, of irregular caliber and anomalous course. The colposcopic picture is that of a diffuse atypia, lacking in clear boundaries with the rest of the normal cervical epithelium.

The acetic acid test may not change the appearance of the lesion, or may simply provoke a pallor of the red zones and of the vascular images. On the contrary, the white spots may increase in visual density and intense superimposed patterns may appear. Glandular orifices, which tend to adopt the aspect of circles and drops, are almost always seen. Precise limits to these lesions are not observed.

When Lugol's solution is applied, the lesion is iodine-negative, with very unclear, weak contours. The boundaries indicated by Lugol's solution almost always exceed those determined by the clinical examination or after the acetic acid test.

This lesion is a zone of atypical transformation (p. 163) with epithelial keratinization. Directed cytologic and histologic study is required.

Only exceptionally is it possible to observe a lesion of this type with regular, sharp peripheral boundaries. This may be a simple keratinized and infected atypical scar, or an epithelial atypia, which will be clearly differentiated by a histologic examination. In these cases, colposcopy cannot determine the exact nature of the lesion, making histologic study necessary.

Index